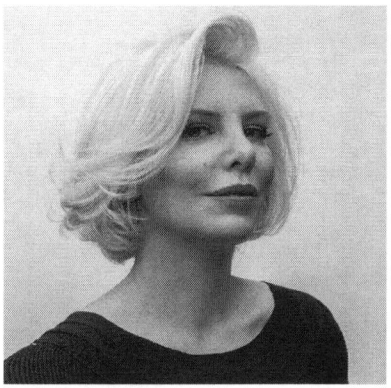
Photograph by Joel Nilsson

Kajsa Ekis Ekman is a Swedish author and journalist, born in 1980. She has written four books on women's rights, capitalism and economic crisis. Her book *Being and Being Bought: Prostitution, Surrogacy and the Split Self* was published by Spinifex Press in 2013. She lectures internationally on trafficking and surrogacy and her TEDx talk 'Everyone talks about capitalism, but what is it?' has been seen by 250,000 people. She is a critic at the Swedish major daily *Aftonbladet* and the founder of the workers' blog portal arbetarbloggen.se.

Other books by Kajsa Ekis Ekman

Om könets existens – tankar om den nya synen på kön, 2021
Bokförlaget Polaris, Stockholm
[Swedish edition of *On the Meaning of Sex: Thoughts about the New Definition of Woman*]

Sobre la existencia del sexo – Reflexiones sobre la nueva perspectiva de género, 2021
Translated by Carolina Morena
Ediciones Cátedra, Universitat de Valéncia
[Spanish edition of *On the Meaning of Sex: Thoughts about the New Definition of Woman*]

Skulden – eurokrisen sedd från Aten, 2014
Leopard Förlag. Stockholm
[The debt: The euro crisis seen from Athens]

Being and Being Bought: Prostitution, Surrogacy and the Split Self, 2013
Translated by Suzanne Martin Cheadle from *Varat och Varan*
Spinifex Press, Melbourne

On the Meaning of Sex by Kajsa Ekis Ekman is clearly written, thoroughly researched, and one of the most intelligent and impressive trawls through the madness of gender ideology to date. Anyone in two minds about whether or not trans orthodoxy causes harms won't be after reading this book.

>—Julie Bindel, journalist and author of *The Pimping of Prostitution* and *Feminism for Women*

Kajsa Ekis Ekman describes the ascent of gender essentialism, jettisoning us into a brave new world where those deemed insufficiently masculine or feminine are encouraged to take hormones and have surgery. It can only be hoped as many people as possible read this book and are made aware of the full horrors taking place in the guise of what purports to be a 'progressive ideology'. Ekman's clear analysis demonstrates how the trans movement is working to effectively dismantle feminism and guilt trip and coerce women into their own erasure. One day we will look back in wonder on a time when people were ready to recognise a person's sex on the basis of their say-so, ignoring the evidence of their own senses and disregarding cautionary instincts developed to safeguard women and children from male sexual predators.

>—Anna Kerr, Principal Solicitor, Feminist Legal Clinic

In this book, Kajsa Ekis Ekman uses her piercing intelligence to provide an excellent overview of how we have come to such a sorry pass, in which men who pretend to be women and their supporters have been able to smash feminism and overturn women's rights. She focuses on issues that have not yet been treated by other feminist critics with such forensic attention, such as why 'transmen' are ignored and treated with contempt, as women always are, while their 'brothers', the transvestites, have become the pin-up girls of culture. In a gripping chapter on the creation of the 'cis-person', Ekman examines what happens to women when they are downgraded and erased by transgender politics, to great and frightening effect. Kajsa Ekis Ekman has written a fascinating book.

>—Sheila Jeffreys, author of *Penile Imperialism: The Male Sex Right and Women's Subordination*

Kajsa Ekis Ekman has provided what so many people confused by gender identity theory need: A critical assessment that is fair and blunt, analytically precise and unafraid of challenging both liberal AND patriarchal dogma. *On the Meaning of Sex* is a brilliant examination of the intellectually incoherent and anti-feminist ideas of gender identity theory. Ekman's clear thinking and clear prose are a much-needed antidote to the muddled conversation about sex and gender in mainstream culture. Many of us encounter gender identity theory and think, "But that doesn't make any sense." Ekman's account of history and science explains why in a way that helps everyone, including people who identify as trans.

—Robert Jensen, Emeritus Professor, University of Texas at Austin; author of *The End of Patriarchy: Radical Feminism for Men*

On The Meaning of Sex chronicles this century's return of regressive stereotypes of women to western culture through a close examination of transgender ideology and the scientific hokum being churned out of academic institutions and corporate media that reverse the advances made by the Enlightenment where science has been erased by the cult of emotion and misogyny. Ekman brings a refreshing analysis to how the creation of the 'trans person' necessitates the conterminous invention of the 'cis-person' that together cannibalise the biological and political realities of women and girls in order to 'gender wash' male violence as 'female' within a movement that portrays itself as 'progressive' when it is anything but.

—Julian Vigo, anthropologist, journalist, writer, editor of *Savage Minds*

ON THE MEANING OF SEX

Thoughts about the New Definition of Woman

Kajsa Ekis Ekman

Translated by Kristina Mäki

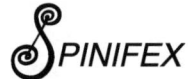

We respectfully acknowledge the wisdom of Aboriginal and Torres Strait Islander peoples and their custodianship of the lands and waterways. Spinifex offices are located on Djiru, Bunurong, Wadawurrung, Eora, and Noongar Country.

First published by Spinifex Press, 2023

Spinifex Press Pty Ltd
PO Box 5270, North Geelong, VIC 3215, Australia
PO Box 105, Mission Beach, QLD 4852, Australia
women@spinifexpress.com.au
www.spinifexpress.com.au

First published in Swedish by Bokförlaget Polaris as
Om könets existens – tankar om den nya synen på kön
Translated from Swedish by Kristina Mäki
The publication of this book has been supported by a translation grant from the Swedish Arts Council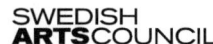

Copyright © Kajsa Ekis Ekman, 2023
Copyright © Translation Kristina Mäki, 2023

The moral right of the author and translator has been asserted.

All rights reserved. Without limiting the rights under copyright reserved above, no part of this publication may be reproduced, stored in or introduced into a retrieval system, or transmitted, in any form or by any means (electronic, mechanical, photocopying, recording or otherwise) without prior written permission of both the copyright owner and the above publisher of the book.

Copying for educational purposes
Information in this book may be reproduced in whole or part for study or training purposes, subject to acknowledgement of the source and providing no commercial usage or sale of material occurs. Where copies of part or whole of the book are made under part VB of the Copyright Act, the law requires that prescribed procedures be followed. For information contact the Copyright Agency Limited.

Edited by Renate Klein, Pauline Hopkins and Susan Hawthorne
Index by Aviva Xue
Cover design by Deb Snibson
Typesetting by Helen Christie, Blue Wren Books
Typeset in Albertina
Printed by McPherson's Printing Group

 A catalogue record for this book is available from the National Library of Australia

ISBN: 9781925950663 (paperback)
ISBN: 9781925950670 (ebook)

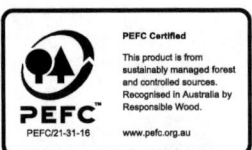

Acknowledgements

First and foremost, I would like to thank Renate Klein, Susan Hawthorne and Pauline Hopkins at Spinifex Press – without you this book would not have been made available to English-speaking readers. Thank you for allowing feminist thought to travel across borders! Working with you is always a pleasure and it is reassuring to know that you will not be satisfied until the end result is immaculate. For the English translation, I would like to thank Kristina Mäki, who worked tirelessly on the translation and with a determination to always find the exact word in the ever-changing landscape of the gender debate. I would also like to thank the Swedish Arts Council for contributing to the translation costs, making sure Swedish authors are heard in the international debate.

Contents

Introduction	1

Part 1: Seventy-One Genders – A Revolution in the Making

1. "We're Expanding the Concept of What It Means to Be Human"	9
2. "Transwomen Are Women – But What Is a Woman?"	12
3. Boys Climb Trees, Girls Make Bead Necklaces: The Return of Stereotypes	18
4. Chasing the Gendered Brain	25
5. Gender Is in the Eye of the Beholder	42
6. 2007: The Order of Modernity	50
7. 2017: The Gender-Congruent Person	55
8. Help – My Son Loves Pink!	62
9. An Invisible Theory	71
10. The History of Sex : One-Sex and Two-Sex Theories	76
11. Return of the One-Sex Theory	83
12. What Happens to Biological Determinism When There Is No Body?	85
13. How Feminism Started Loving Gender	89
14. How Patriarchy Incorporated Its Dissidents	100

Part 2: One Pill Makes You a Girl, One Pill Makes You a Boy – The 71 Genders Become Two

15. When States Reassign Their Citizens' Sex	119
16. "Doctors are Salivating at the Prospect of Applying Puberty Blockers"	125
17. They Will Probably Become Infertile, But That's the Price You Pay – The New Era of Sterilisations	135

18. When States Convert Homosexuals	144
19. What Is a Man without a Penis?	149
20. Younger, Faster, Happier?	153
21. Hormone Evangelists in the Pharmaceutical Industry	160
22. Tumblr, Trans and Trauma – Testimonies from Teens	171
23. Mastectomy or Death: Harnessing the Threat of Suicide	182
24. The Industry Under Pressure	202

Part 3: The One Sex Theory

25. A Tale of Trans People?	207
26. Woman: A Dangerous Word	209
27. Vagina: A Dangerous Word	218
28. The Creation of the Cis-Person – or How We Fell in Love with Gender Roles	222
29. Gender Self-Identification	235
30. A Room of One's Own	238
31. Unspeakable Violence	247
32. Every Man's Right	250
33. Invisible Trans Men	253
34. Open Female Spaces, Closed Male Spaces	257
35. "The End of Women's Sport as We Know It"	262
36. "It Started with the Realisation that Women Do Not Exist" – A Fatal Blow to Equality Policies	275
37. "She Deserves a Kick in the Ovaries"	280
38. Sex, Race, Class, or … An Exception to Intersectionality	292
39. Nature/Nurture – A Dialectical View	304
40. Notes on the Word 'Woman'	309
References	313
Index	329

Introduction

If one looks up the word sex in the *Encyclopaedia Britannica*, one finds the following explanation: "… the sum of features by which members of species can be divided into groups – male and female – that complement each other reproductively."[1] Sex is here a reproductive category and nothing else. This definition does not say anything about what men and women should look like, how they should behave, or what they should feel – the most important point appears to be that there are two sexes and that they are capable of reproduction together.

Consulting the Swedish public health service website in 2019 however, one gets a completely different answer. Under the heading "What is sex?" it says, "Your sex is not determined by your body or what's written in your passport. What's important is what sex you feel like."[2] Similarly, we find the following on a website that provides information about menstruation:

> In order to menstruate you need to have a uterus, but being born with a uterus doesn't necessarily make you a woman. Only you can determine which sex to identify as.[3]

An increasing number of institutions are adopting the view that sex has nothing to do with the body, and this view is becoming official policy in several western countries. Sex – or gender – has become an identity with

---

1 <https://www.britannica.com/science/sex>.
2 <https://www.1177.se/liv--halsa/konsidentitet-och-sexuell-laggning/konsidentitet-och-konsuttryck/>.
3 <https://pablodigtallvar.se/en/menstruation-and-trans>.

a life of its own and referring to a person as a woman or man based on their genitals is now clearly a faux pas – we are not to assume anything without asking, because sex cannot be seen on the outside. The US magazine *Teen Vogue* reminds us that not even the presence of a massive, hairy beard can be taken as evidence of someone being a man.[4] Several councils, organisations and pre-schools recommend that the day start with everyone stating their preferred pronouns.[5] Despite the fact that the body suddenly has become unimportant, whether one considers oneself a woman or a man is still of utmost importance and potentially offending someone by using the wrong pronoun is to be avoided at all costs because this is seen as harmful to a person's sense of self.

The first country in the world to implement a law on self-determination of gender was Argentina. Canada, Norway and Denmark followed suit (as did the state of Victoria in Australia), and in these countries the legal procedure for supposedly changing one's sex is now straightforward, akin to registering a change of address. A similar change is being suggested in Sweden. "Changing your legal sex should be a quick and simple process that should not necessarily require contact with healthcare services,"[6] wrote the Social Affairs and Culture and Democracy Ministers in 2018. They went on to say that

> [T]he new law should first and foremost take into account how the individual identifies themselves. It is only the individual who can know how s/he identifies.

The proposal is being presented as a modernisation of the laws on gender identity. In fact, the two ministers state that they are finally tabling a modern law on gender identity and apologise for it having taken so long. Lotta Vahlne Westerhäll, the sole investigator in the inquiry entitled 'The Legal Definition of Sex and Medical Sex Reassignment', along with the inquiry's secretary wrote in the Swedish daily *SvD*:

---

[4] Trésor Prijs. (1 June 2018). 'How my beard affects my gender identity as a trans femme'. *Teen Vogue*.
[5] <http://www.diva-portal.org/smash/get/diva2:1063959/FULLTEXT01.pdf>.
[6] Alice Bah Kuhnke and Annika Strandhäll. (18 May 2018). 'Att byta juridiskt kön ska bli snabbt och enkelt'. *SvD Debatt*.

Any person who wishes to change their registered sex should be able to do so freely. Nor should any requirements or prerequisites regarding medical intervention or care be imposed.[7]

The Australian Government reasons in the same way and put forward a similar proposal in 2018. The sex change process ought to be

... merely administrative in nature, straightforward, timely, and not incur undue financial and legal burden.

The Australian proposal includes the suggestion that sex be removed from birth certificates. Sex has thus become an irrelevant detail, while gender is considered of utmost importance. The reason given for making this change in the law is that the appearance of sex at birth on birth certificates is said to cause pain and suffering and that "... the experiences of trans, gender diverse and intersex people are at the heart of this review."[8]

Several sporting organisations like the IOC (International Olympic Committee), WSER (Western States Endurance Run) and the NCAA (National College Athletics Association) have followed suit and changed their rules so that it is now the way a person *identifies* and not their *actual biological* sex that determines which category they compete in. Sometimes not even hormone treatment is required. The athletes in the junior category of the Swedish Championships in gymnastics can choose whether they want to compete in the women's or men's category, regardless of their legal sex, following a decision taken by the Swedish Gymnastics Association in November 2020.[9]

An increasing number of institutions and businesses have adopted the idea that it is now no longer biology that determines sex but self-identification. Since 2013, the Associated Press has recommended that journalists use preferred pronouns.[10] The US National Speech and Debate Association explains in its code of conduct that one should be careful not to use the wrong pronoun. It's not about biological sex or physical

---

7   Therese Bäckman and Lotta Vahlne Westerhäll. (9 April 2019). 'Ändra juridiskt kön bör bli enklare', *SvD Debatt*.
8   Project 108 Discussion Paper: Review of Western Australian legislation in relation to the recognition of a person's sex, change of sex or intersex status, Law Reform Commission of Western Australia 2018.
9   Lisa Edwinsson. (29 November 2020). 'Gymnaster får välja tävlingsklass oavsett kön – upp till och med JSM-nivå'. *DN*.
10 <https://www.languagewire.com/sv/lw/tema/en-viktig-forandring-i-ap-stylebook>.

appearance and it's always best to ask to avoid being a threat to someone's safety:

> An individual's biological sex assigned at birth does not determine their gender. [...] In practice, don't assume that a person's gender presentation corresponds with their pronoun usage. At first, listen carefully for referential details in which a person may self-disclose their pronouns. If you would like to establish a connection to someone, you might say, 'I use them/their pronouns. May I ask what pronouns you use for yourself?'[11]

This encouragement to use preferred pronouns might be dismissed as a matter of politeness, but the policy changes also mean that a man who has committed violent crimes and later begins to identify as a woman is described as a 'woman' by the media. The changes also mean that men are being moved into women's prisons if they identify as women.

The new definition of sex is also beginning to be used in healthcare, where written material has removed references to women in its literature about giving birth and breastfeeding, since "… women are no longer the only people who can give birth."[12] Many women's organisations have also begun to adopt the new definition. For example, the organisation Kvinnor och funktionshinder (Women and Disability in Sweden) decided in 2016 that

> [O]ur association is and will remain a women's association. However, we won't be excluding people based on which sex organs they have, or which sex they are assigned at birth. If someone introduces themselves as a woman, then she is a woman. No one apart from a person themselves has the right to assign a sex to anyone else.[13]

But even if the body does not determine gender under the new definition, it has not therefore become irrelevant for the proponents of this new theory. On the contrary, it has become even more important. According to gender identity theory, a person can be split in two: brain and body, two parts which have completely different understandings of what sex the person is. It is argued that the brain has gotten the grip, while the body doesn't get it, is 'the wrong body' and should therefore submit to the brain's will and

---

11 'Best practices for pronoun use', National Speech and Debate Association.
12 <https://www.dailymail.co.uk/news/article-5112377/Midwives-ordered-call-women-labour-PERSONS.html>.
13 <http://www.kvinnor-funktionshinder.se>.

be changed. This change used to be called sex change, was later referred to as sex reassignment surgery, and is now known as gender reassignment surgery, or in Sweden: gender confirming surgery.

The implication inherent in these linguistic changes is that the brain is the correct sex and the body has to be changed in order to confirm the brain's sex. Over the last ten years, there has been an explosion in the number of young people diagnosed with gender dysphoria – the number in Sweden has increased by 2913 per cent.[14] For the best results, doctors recommend that treatment begins before puberty and the Swedish National Board of Health and Welfare, as have many state health boards across the west, has been recommending puberty blockers to children who are unsure which gender they belong to. Thousands of clinics have sprung up around the world in which children can get medical treatment to resemble the opposite sex and the age limits for gender reassignment have been lowered in several countries.

Gender identity theory has been recognised and accepted in Sweden by parties across the political spectrum and in the UK, it has been supported by the Conservatives, the Greens and Labour, although this seems to be shifting. In the Argentinian Senate, the proposal to make sex a question of self-identification was voted through by 55 votes in favour, none against and two abstentions. By way of comparison, when the proposal for legalising abortion was voted on five years later, 38 votes were against it and 31 were in favour.[15]

We are dealing with a new theory on sex that has become hegemonic and commonplace in a short period of time. In just ten years, countries, sporting organisations, the media and international organisations in the west have accepted and adopted this view. At the same time, scarcely any in-depth discussion about it has taken place. What does gender identity theory actually entail? What ideology is expressed by it? And what consequences will it have? And for whom?

---

14 Socialstyrelsens statistikdatabas (Swedish National Board of Health and Welfare Statistical Databases). (Accessed 25 November 2020). Diagnoser, Endast specialiserad öppenvård, Antal patienter, F64 Könsidentitetsstörningar, Riket, Ålder 10–19, 2007–2019 (Database search for number of patients with gender dysphoria in Sweden 2007–2019).

15 <https://www.perfil.com/noticias/politica/despenalizacion-del-aborto-asi-vota-cada-senador.phtml>.

PART 1

SEVENTY-ONE GENDERS – A REVOLUTION IN THE MAKING

CHAPTER 1

"We're Expanding the Concept of What It Means to Be Human"

When we first encounter gender identity theory, it looks very pleasant indeed. It is presented to us as a narrative about opening our minds and thinking beyond restrictive norms. We're told that, for a long time, we've misunderstood what gender actually is. This erroneous thinking has caused much suffering but we're now beginning to open our eyes and understand that whether we are men or women has nothing to do with our sex organs and is in fact about how we feel.

Sex is now said to be fluid and not as fixed as we previously thought. And we're told that there are actually 23 genders, or 71 according to Facebook. *National Geographic, Scientific American* and Swedish Social Services all state unanimously that gender exists on a 'spectrum'.[16] You can be somewhere in between a man and a woman, completely outside either of these categories, or be a combination of any or all of these at the same time. Every individual knows best how he or she (or they!) feel(s) and no one has the right to assign a sex or gender to anyone else.

On the face of it, this looks like a feminist utopia and a reactionary nightmare: the dissolution of gender has finally arrived! What woman hasn't wished that men could walk a mile in her shoes? Or, as the Swedish

---

16 <https://natgeo.se/vetenskap/manniskor/national-geographic-skriver-historia-med-ett-starkt-nummer-om-kon-och-konsidentitet> and Amanda Montañez. (1 September 2017). 'Beyond XX and XY: The Extraordinary Complexity of Sex Determination'. *Scientific American*.

Left Party put it in a bill in 2015, "we're moving away from the current binary model and expanding the concept of what it means to be human."[17]

Jay Stewart, founder of the UK-based Gendered Intelligence and the Entrepreneur of the Year in 2016, explains that we're on the cusp of a gender revolution.[18] This is a revolution that requires us all to open our eyes and undertake a "mind-set reset," understanding that we don't need different rights and laws for different people because "sex isn't what we are but what we do."

A group of Finnish artists explain it thus at their exhibition in Helsinki:

… the binary constructs of sex are challenged, we're starting to see new terminology and voices that are claiming their right to define how things are discussed … Above all else, it's about exposing different forms of oppression and inclusion and exclusion.[19]

The language used here appears to be copied straight from women's movement materials: 'challenge', 'claim the right', 'new terminology', 'expose oppression'. *National Geographic*'s report entitled 'The Gender Revolution' notes: "… freed from the binary of boy and girl, gender identity is a shifting landscape." The report is accompanied by a picture of a person on their way into an operating theatre alongside the quote: "no one can stop me from being who I am." The cover shows a nine-year-old child with pink hair, pink clothes and the caption: "The best thing about being a girl is that now I don't have to pretend to be a boy."[20]

The story we're told is both all-encompassing and singularly specific: everyone needs to reset their brain, while at the same time the issue is described as one that only concerns 'trans people'. As the new narrative coincides with the increasing visibility of trans people in the media, the two things are often conflated so that individual people's journeys and gender identity theory appear to be one and the same thing.

Newspapers and magazines report on people who can finally 'become who they are'. The choice of wording is important – you *are* therefore not who you are but must *become* who you are. The real self is your gender and

---

17 Motion till riksdagen (Bill tabled in Parliament) 2015/16:49 by Jonas Sjöstedt et al. (V): 'Förstärkta rättigheter för transpersoner'.
18 Vanessa Baird. (1 October 2015).'The trans revolution', *The New Internationalist*.
19 Eva Lamppu. (16 May 2017). 'Kulturdebatt: Är genusrevolutionen verklighet eller bubbla?', *Svenska Yle*
20 *National Geographic*, January 2017.

gender is no longer a social construct that patriarchy imposes on people but an individual's identity that is set in stone.

A Swedish influencer asserts that the day she had her gender reassignment surgery was the happiest day of her life.[21] A Swede who transitioned to being a man states, "I'm more true to what I want to do and I've never written better music," while another Swede who transitioned to become a woman says that it is easier to display emotions as a woman – "I feel so much better now than I did five, ten, fifteen years ago."[22]

These articles often end with statements about how gender is not related to the body but is located in the *brain*, and that in order to achieve happiness, the body must be adjusted to fit the brain. The message is clear: if the reader sympathises with the personal journey they read about, they must also accept the new gender identity theory.

The story we are being told uses words like tolerance and acceptance of diversity. We hear of proud parents who love their children 'just the way they are'. Much of this narrative and terminology is familiar to us and reminds us of the struggle for gay rights. In other words, it appears to be a no-brainer, because who could be against allowing people to be themselves? It must surely be a good thing that laws are updated so that everyone has access to appropriate health care, to be able to express themselves fully and that people update their vocabulary so as to not hurt others? This is no doubt, as Annika Strandhäll (Sweden's Minister for Social Affairs 2017–2019) claimed, a matter of modernisation? Of being on the right side of history – and aren't we by definition, as long as we're against the narrow-minded? If these positive arguments aren't enough to convince you, here's a word of warning from *The Guardian* columnist Owen Jones in his piece entitled 'Anti-trans zealots, know this: history will judge you':

> History is a savage judge of those who resisted the onward march of gay rights. I doubt it will be less damning of those who bitterly fight trans rights.[23]

---

21   <https://omni.se/influeraren-mathilda-berattar-foddes-i-fel-kropp/a/4qKAM9>.
22   Erik Galli. (8 February 2018). 'Vi frågade svenska transpersoner om det bästa med att vara trans', *Vice*.
23   Owen Jones. (15 December 2017). 'Anti-trans zealots, know this: history will judge you', *The Guardian*.

CHAPTER 2

"Transwomen Are Women – But What Is a Woman?"

If sex is no longer biology, what is it then? The new theory's knee-jerk response to this is that sex or gender can be anything you want it to be and shouldn't be defined. One thing, though, is clear and is repeated over and over again: gender is *not* the body and the fact that so many people continue to equate having XX chromosomes with being a woman is extremely problematic. Rachel Cohen, campaign manager at the UK LGBTQ charity Stonewall writes, "Being trans is not about 'sex changes' and clothes – it's about an innate sense of self."[24] A US handbook for parents of trans teens explains:

> We do not choose our gender identity; rather, our gender identity emerges from within. It is believed to be an inherent aspect of a person's makeup and cannot be regulated or determined by others.[25]

Gender is portrayed like some sort of mystical essential oil that wells up from our insides and is tied neither to culture nor to the physical body. The only thing that matters is how the individual feels. Everyone is hereafter encouraged to discover their true gender.

---

24 Rachel Cohen. (July 2018). Quoted in David Pilgrim, 'Reclaiming reality and redefining realism: The challenging case of transgenderism'. *Journal of Critical Realism*, Vol. 17, No. 3, pp. 308–324.

25 Stephanie Brill and Lisa Kenney. (2016). *The Transgender Teen: A Handbook for Parents and Professionals Supporting Transgender and Non-Binary Teens*, p. 40. Jersey City: Cleis Press.

According to this view, sex is not observed at birth. Instead, the phrase 'sex *assigned* at birth' is used, making it seem like midwives carry out some kind of arbitrary act, handing out sexes to people randomly. The term 'sex assigned at birth' also makes a phenomenon such as sex-selective abortion completely incomprehensible, if sex is assigned at birth, what would pre-birth selection be based on? The term 'assigned sex' has, however, replaced 'sex' or 'biological sex' in most US, and many European, official documents.

Assuming that nothing 'is', how can we then 'be' anything? And how does one know what one is? Several books on the matter initially stick to something resembling a deliberate lack of principles: gender can be anything at all. David Pilgrim, a British professor of clinical health, calls this idea that I *am* because I *want to be* "ontological vandalism."[26] A desire becomes synonymous with a fact. In an answer to Pilgrim in the *Journal of Critical Realism*, author and queer activist Jason Summersell writes:

> Yes, chromosome count is important for one's classification if one's objective is to identify whether someone has a Y chromosome because one is trying to decide whether they suffer from Turner's syndrome in which the Y chromosome is absent. However, it is not important if one wants to decide how to address wedding invitations. For the latter classification, we need to know whether invitees see themselves – really ontologically see themselves – as male, female, or non-specific.[27]

Thus Summersell distinguishes between chromosomes and identity, with identity being something completely individual that can only be determined by one's own feelings. Sex is here reduced to wedding invitations and preferred pronouns (considerations of the same calibre as whether we should address someone formally or informally), and we're told that it is of the utmost importance that we use correct pronouns for people. Anything else will be offensive. But what is it about sex that has the capacity to offend? Why is it such a sensitive subject? And when we

---

26 David Pilgrim. (July 2018). 'Reclaiming reality and redefining realism: The challenging case of transgenderism'. *Journal of Critical Realism*, Vol. 17, No. 3, pp. 308–324.
27 Jason Summersell. (August 2018). 'Trans women are real women: a critical realist intersectional response to Pilgrim'. *Journal of Critical Realism*, Vol. 17, No. 3, pp. 329–336.

'ontologically see ourselves as something' – what is that something, and what does it consist of?

Summersell's essay is entitled 'Trans Women are Real Women', which has turned into somewhat of a contemporary battle cry. Not many people seem interested in whether trans men are real men and Summersell doesn't touch upon that matter. The important thing, it seems, is to decide who is a woman. There is no difference between trans women and real women, writes Summersell, and therefore all quotas put in place for women should also include those born male:

> Rather than side-lining trans women as 'not representative', their concerns should be explicitly considered, in exactly the same way, and for exactly the same reasons, that the concerns of black women, mature women and disabled women should be explicitly considered.[28]

He seems to be saying that everyone is a woman and that there's nothing special about this group. Trans women and women are exactly the same.[29] This would mean that trans women and trans people don't exist – but in the next breath, Summersell seems to be saying that there *is* a difference between women and trans women after all:

> … there is no contradiction in the claim that one is an ontologically real person with a prostate (some would say a man) for the purposes of one context (e.g. a prostate examination), an ontologically real woman for the purposes of another context (e.g. one's daily life), and an ontologically real trans woman in yet a third context (e.g. a trans women support group).[30]

If trans women are women, why do we need support groups specifically for trans women? To explain this, Summersell argues that there is a difference after all – but this difference can only be claimed by trans women. We all recall from our math classes that what's on one side of the equal sign must be exactly the same as that on the other and that this fact remains

---

28 Ibid.
29 This is a very strange comparison to make – is there anyone who thinks that black, elderly and disabled women are not women? It looks as though Summersell is mixing up definitions and hierarchies because even if black, elderly and disabled women are discriminated against, this is not the same thing as saying that they aren't women and therefore mistaking them for men. In this case they wouldn't have been discriminated against as women in the first place.
30 Jason Summersell. (August 2018). 'Trans women are real women: A critical realist intersectional response to Pilgrim'. *Journal of Critical Realism*, Vol. 17, No. 3, pp. 329–336.

even if we swap what's on the left with what's on the right. But when Summersell says that trans women are women, he does not mean that women, therefore, are trans women. Thus, a separate group called women does not exist, but a group called trans women does. This leads to the conclusion that whenever we talk about women, we also mean those born as men, but whenever we talk about those women born as men, we are not referring to those born as women. This is a somewhat asymmetrical equation and any woman who tries to disagree, finds herself trapped in a labyrinth. If she wants to fight for her rights, Summersell can only reply that she is discriminating against other women, women who are, moreover, even more oppressed than she is. She cannot therefore stand up for her own sex without being accused of fighting against members of this very sex.

According to Summersell, there is no contradiction in a person being a woman, a man and a trans person in different circumstances. Having a prostate is something pretty concrete, but matters become a lot less clear when he asserts that anyone can be an ontologically real woman in their "daily life."

Ontology is the branch of philosophy that deals with the nature of existence. Ontological inquiry strives to find the essence of things, for example what it is that makes a stone a stone. So what makes a woman a woman? Summersell argues that there is nothing essentially female or male in our bodies, but implies instead that there is some kind of inner feminine essence in the way women live their lives.

I am very interested in how Jason Summersell thinks women live our daily lives. Is there something special one must do in order to live an essentially female life? He has already said that it isn't about the body, so we can assume that everything related to menstruation, pregnancy and buying one's first bra is out of the equation, so what then are we left with? When I wrote to him to ask what an ontologically real woman does in her daily life, in his answer he quipped that, "one can do whatever one wants as long as it isn't illegal LOL."[31] So the last clue leads us to an empty box – no definition can be found there either. You can, thus, according to Summersell, identify as something, and therefore *be* that something, but this something does not exist and cannot be defined.

---

31 Email correspondence Kajsa Ekis Ekman with Jason Summersell, Autumn 2018.

In an editorial in the Swedish daily *Dagens Nyheter*, Lisa Magnusson writes that the idea of "gender fluidity" has made a lot of feminists so "scared, angry and resentful" that they've sought refuge in feminism's old enemy: biological determinism. Magnusson is in favour of a wider definition of woman that includes everyone:

> One is not born a woman, Simone de Beauvoir wrote, one becomes a woman. This has been a central tenet of modern feminism. [...] Some become women later than others in the eyes of society, while others never do. The category 'women' is diverse and not easily defined. [...] Feminism as a movement is not about biology but about an ideological purpose: equality. Everyone should be welcome.[32]

Simone de Beauvoir's quote is routinely thrown into the debate, even by reputable academics like Catharine MacKinnon, to the extent that one wonders whether it is the only thing that people have managed to remember from *The Second Sex*. The fact that one is not born a woman but becomes one is being used here to say that anyone can become a woman, both men and women. Nevertheless, as feminist professor of literature, Toril Moi, writes:

> This is simply not the case. For Beauvoir, a woman is someone with a female body from beginning to end, from the moment she is born until the moment she dies, but her body is her situation, not her destiny.[33]

Simone de Beauvoir never meant that 'woman' was just a construct that could be created out of thin air, but that woman was a person whose oppression by patriarchy was defined by her being a woman. Since we are people with a self – and the self is important in de Beauvoir's thinking – it is not possible to see woman as just a 'role' one assumes, as people react and act based on their situation. The famous quote is as follows in its entirety:

> One is not born, but rather becomes, woman. No biological, psychic, or economic destiny defines the figure that the human female takes on in society; it is civilization as a whole that elaborates this intermediary product between the male and the eunuch that is called feminine. Only the mediation of another can constitute an individual as an *Other*.[34]

---

32 Lisa Magnusson. (18 February 2018). 'Feminism är ideologi, inte biologi', *Dagens Nyheter*.
33 Toril Moi. (1999). *What Is a Woman?* p. 76. Oxford: Oxford University Press.
34 Simone de Beauvoir. (2009). *The Second Sex*, p. 330. Translated by Constance Borde and Sheila Malovany-Chevallier. New York: Vintage.

For de Beauvoir, there was nothing difficult about defining woman: a woman is a person born with a female body. Regardless of how a woman dresses, lives or thinks, she is a woman. Saying that one is not born a woman is shorthand for *the subordination which society sees as being the lot of women is determined by society, not biology.*

Biological determinism is thus not a belief that biology exists, but making the connection between woman – a physical fact – and so-called femininity – a social characteristic. It is defined as follows by the Swedish Psychological Guide: "… explaining psychological phenomena through physiology and principles of evolutionary biology." It is therefore the connection between body and behaviour that is biologism. The idea that a person born with a woman's body is suited to certain types of work or displays certain behaviour is biologism. *The idea that there is such a thing as 'female' behaviour in the first place, that those born as women ought to behave in the way that society determines as female and that those who behave in this way are women* is biological determinism.

In *The Second Sex*, de Beauvoir argued against this idea by showing that the behaviours we consider female and male are cultural constructs.

According to Magnusson, however, biologism is saying that a woman is a woman. To be defined as a woman you now no longer need to be a woman and the definition can extend to anyone at all. Following this logic would require abolishing all classifications, since they are all biologist: why can only sheep be called sheep? Why shouldn't a cow be allowed to be a sheep? Why should a car not be called an airplane? Shouldn't everything be welcome in the category 'car'? Shouldn't CEOs be welcome to be part of unions in the name of equality?

The point is that the word woman is nothing other than the word we use for the group of people born with XX-chromosomes and egg cells, just like sheep is the word for a certain type of animal. If the word woman does not refer to a person born with XX-chromosomes and egg cells, it must refer to something else. When Magnusson claims that some people 'become' women later in life, what exactly do they do to become women? Something is being left unsaid here, but having emptied the term woman of meaning, Magnusson falls short of filling it with a new one.

CHAPTER 3

Boys Climb Trees, Girls Make Bead Necklaces: The Return of Stereotypes

Nothing can float around freely forever, not even theories. Sooner or later, they'll have to land – the question is where. If we remove the material base that previously provided the grounding for the definition of sex, we are left with little other than stereotypes and cultural norms. These are now to replace sex chromosomes as the basis for the definition of sex.

One such definition is found in the British Association for Counselling and Psychotherapy (BACP) handbook on *Gender, Sexual and Relationship Diversity*:

> It is important not to assume, for example, that being a woman necessarily involves being able to bear children, or having XX sex chromosomes, or breasts. Being a woman in a British cultural context often means adhering to social norms of femininity, such as being nurturing, caring, social, emotional, vulnerable, and concerned with appearance. However, of course, not all women adhere to all these things. For example some neurodiverse women (on the autistic/aspergic/ADHD spectrums) may struggle to express emotions, or with social situations.[35]

---

[35] British Association for Counselling and Psychotherapy. (2017). 'Good practice across the counselling professions 001'. *Gender, Sexual, and Relationship Diversity* (GSRD).

Sex should thus, from now on, be defined as behaviour and not as biology. Being a woman is, henceforth, a way of being. You are a woman if you adhere to certain characteristics, not because you were born with a female body. Sex has gone from being an objective fact to being a personality trait. The BACP doesn't say who, or what, determines these characteristics or why being "vulnerable" is female, just vaguely references "social norms." One is gripped by a sudden urge to object that it is not women, after all, who can be knocked out by a single blow below the belt. However, the point is not to argue with these characteristics, but to note the return of essentialism, minus the biology.

'Women' are thus, according to this definition, all those who are vain, weak and caring, unless of course they are on the spectrum and fail at being women. The question which the BACP doesn't answer is: if they have removed biology as a basis for the definition of woman, what definition are they relying on when they claim that women with Asperger's syndrome are *women*?

When the Swedish author Fredrik Ekelund came out as transgender in his sixties, he revealed in an interview that his female self is called Marisol and described the difference between his male and female selves:

> As Fredrik, I constantly want to perform and achieve things. Marisol is calmer, more harmonious, letting the world come to her. To use a football metaphor, I don't play offense as much as Marisol. If I'm passed the ball as Fredrik, I've only got one thing on my mind: scoring. But had I been Marisol on the field, I would probably have been happy with a few neat dribbling moves.[36]

The author divides himself into two selves. One self has a Swedish man's name, the other a Spanish woman's, and these two selves have clear roles – the man is active, the woman passive, the man acts, the woman waits, the man scores, the woman just plays to look good and is satisfied with "a few neat dribbling moves" – alas, not too many!

Yet he is not actually speaking about two different people, but one and the same: himself. Ekelund is simply saying that he's a complex, multi-faceted person. He has a desire to be passive, good-looking and vain. In his writing, he explains how this desire became so strong that he couldn't

---

36 Kristin Nord and Emma Larsson. (23 September 2018). 'Fredrik Ekelund: Jag vill alltid gråta när jag sminkar av mig'. *Sydsvenskan*.

live without expressing it. The key thing is that *he doesn't want to express these characteristics as a man*, locating them instead in an imaginary woman, thus expelling them from his male self.

Ekelund goes on to describe some "affected gestures that I use. My woman says that it's really fussy and silly and that no woman does this. To which I answer, maybe not but all women would like to."

What does he mean by saying that all women would like to behave in an affected way? Who decided this? Who is it that actually has a drive to behave like this? In this case, it's a man, yet he ascribes this desire a female gender and goes so far as to speak on behalf of *all* women. Naturally, he knows better than 'his' woman.

The Swedish children's book *Jag är Linus, en pojke med snippa* (*I am Linus, a Boy with a Minnie*) by Camilla Gisslow starts with a little girl standing naked in front of a mirror. Strewn around her on the floor are toy airplanes, cars, fishing rods and a doll on the bed. There's a poster on the wall that reads "I'm going to be a police officer when I grow up." The girl looks at her naked body discontentedly and says, "Everyone thinks I'm a girl because I have a minnie!" On the next page, she's wearing a blue police officer's uniform, a tanktop and shorts and a cap emblazoned with 'Police'. She says smilingly: "You can be a boy even if you have a minnie!" Further on, she tells us: "I got angry with my mum when she bought dresses for me. I didn't like my hair … I wanted short hair!" At the end of the story, she's transformed into Linus and has short hair, a Batman jumper and scratched and bleeding knees. Her preschool celebrates the transformation with cake and by changing the name on her chair, coat hook and toothbrush to Linus. On the last page, she – now he – is climbing a tree, smiling and saying, "Now I feel I am myself."[37]

The following year, Gisslow published an almost identical book called *Jag är Bella – en flicka med snopp* (*I am Bella, a Girl with a Willy*). This time, it's Wasim who's standing naked in front of a mirror surrounded by birds in cages, dolls and building blocks, and who wants to have purple skirts and long hair, not wear shirts and ties. He also gets a big cake at preschool when he becomes a girl. His mum, depicted in a hijab, and the imam at the mosque, both welcome his new identity as Bella.[38]

---

[37] Camilla Gisslow. (2017). *Jag är Linus-en pojke med snippa*. Järfälla: Tallbergs Publishing.
[38] Camilla Gisslow. (2018). *Jag är Bella-en flicka med snopp*. Järfälla:Tallbergs Publishing.

The books are identical: the story is the same, even the sentences are the same, with the keywords swapping places. The message is that sex is not about genitals, but about *style*. There are two styles available: if you like one, you're a girl, if you like the other, you're a boy. Both books are about finding the right role, not about questioning these roles. Meanwhile, the world around the child stays the same: in this world, mothers wear a hijab or short skirts and heels, and men are religious leaders.

So far, so similar. But we soon discover that there's a big difference between the role of the girl and that of the boy. When the girl becomes a boy, she suddenly has a future. Linus not only gets to dress differently, he also has a future career (police officer), he climbs trees, builds tree houses and dangles his legs sitting up in the tree. He plays games and lives dangerously, evidenced by the trickles of blood on his knees. In the last picture, he reaches up toward a higher branch, where we see a pair of shorts-clad legs. The boy is literally on his way to the top.

The child who becomes a girl has no future career, however. Bella having a job is not even mentioned in the book. She's shown making bead necklaces with the other girls, wearing an apron and helping her mum with the cooking, braiding her hair, wearing a tiara and going along to the mosque. Her relationship to agency is characterised by the absence of doing; when her dad arrives with a tool box and wants to play, Bella stands there in silence, upset and turning her back. The underlying message? Girls do not play with tool boxes. She isn't even active when she's buying ice cream but a man orders for her while she smiles serenely in the background. Only one picture shows her moving: she's riding a bike, her gigantic skirt billowing.

Camilla Gisslow received the Diversity Index Award and has been nominated for the Svenska hjältar (Swedish Heroes) list published by the paper *Aftonbladet*. She's the mother of a trans boy and has founded a successful consulting business that provides training to authorities on LGBTQ matters. Her motto is "every person is unique" and the nomination states that she shows how you "can be a person beyond your sex."

But isn't the message in her books exactly the opposite? What it is really saying is that a girl's task is to dedicate herself to her appearance, be quiet and help in the kitchen, while a boy has a future, a career and an active life. Not since the 1870s have children's books as reactionary as these been seen in print. In 1945, when Pippi Longstocking declared herself to be the world's strongest girl and could chase away thieves and police officers, lift a horse and live without parents, she showed a utopian future compared to Gisslow's vision.

The US teaching tool 'The Genderbread Person', which is used in American schools, explains sex through an image of a human body. Anatomical sex is what's between your legs while gender identity is located in your brain/mind. Sexuality or attraction, as the poster calls it, is in your heart, and gender expression is your actions, clothing and demeanour.[39] The writer, activist and Ted Talk phenomenon Sam Killermann brags that his poster has been downloaded hundreds of thousands of times and that this has made him somewhat of an authority on gender. Killermann states that gender identity is "how you internally interpret the chemistry that composes you." He does not explain how one can interpret one's chemistry, but does state that this interpreting is complete by the age of three. "It is generally accepted that our gender identity is formed by the age of three and that it's very difficult to change it after that." However, Killermann explains that gender identity should be seen as something distinct from gender expression:

> You wake up wearing baggy gray sweatpants and a T-shirt. As you walk into your kitchen to prepare breakfast, you're expressing an androgynous-to-slightly masculine gender. However, if you see your partner in the kitchen and decide to prowl in like Halle Berry from Catwoman, then you are expressing much more femininely [sic]. You pour a bowl of cereal, wrap your fist around a spoon like a Viking, and start shoveling Fruit Loops into your face, and all-of-a-sudden you're bumping up your levels of masculinity. After breakfast, you skip back into your bedroom and playfully place varying outfits in front of you, pleading with your partner to help you decide what to wear. You're feminine again.[40]

So being manly, according to Killermann, involves wearing T-shirts and baggy trousers, shovelling cereal into your face and holding your spoon "like a Viking." Being feminine is prowling around like a cat, being in the bedroom thinking about clothes and being so indecisive that you have to ask your partner for help performing such a mundane task as getting

---

39 <https://www.genderbread.org/resource/genderbread-person-minimal-3-3>.
40 Sam Killermann. (2017). 'Breaking through the binary: gender explained using continuums'. <https://www.genderbread.org/wp-content/uploads/2017/02/Breaking-through-the-Binary-by-Sam-Killermann.pdf>.

dressed. Personally, I don't know any person of any sex who does any of this (who places their clothes in front of them "playfully"?), but Killermann obviously thinks having loads of free time and wandering around aimlessly are feminine characteristics. And for those of you who thought breakfast was something you ate to get nutrition – you're terribly mistaken. Meeting your basic needs is actually something manly, as Killermann clarifies.

Killermann's little lecture is supposed to signal to us that he's open-minded and flexible. He points out several times that it's wrong and old-fashioned to assume that there are only two sexes and he wants to highlight how diverse and multifaceted individuals are. But in his understanding, this diversity isn't created by freeing oneself from categories of gender. On the contrary, he locks all human action into the categories masculine and feminine. You can't even get out of bed without being gendered. The human beings of the future should therefore be interpreting and gendering themselves constantly, find their gender identity and then continuously gender their every expression. The individual is expected to jump between expressions – yet the expressions themselves are not open for discussion.

But hold on a minute. Wasn't gender meant to be dissolved? Wasn't this new ideology supposed to be about questioning old patterns and "daring to be yourself?" Lo and behold, when we scratch the surface, the story has suddenly changed tack. Gender is on the contrary very fixed and determined, just not by the body, but by our behaviour. Here we immediately come face to face with a biological determinism minus the biology, where feminine and masculine are ascribed certain behaviours and characteristics. These appear to be disconnected from the body and exist in their own, ethereal world. Prohibited, from now on, is the connection Vagina = woman; authorised, from now on, is the connection vain, vulnerable, affected = woman. We were intially presented with a story about 'openness' and 'acceptance' regardless of gender, something that resembled the narratives of the gay rights movement and feminism so closely that we didn't pay much attention. When we now turn around to take a closer look, something completely different has happened.

Gender roles are back without us having noticed! It's just that sex and gender have swapped places. Gender is now *real* and sex is the *construct*. Sex is said to be 'assigned' at birth, that is, a social construct that society applies by force to the child. Gender identity, on the other hand, is said to be innate. This is nothing but gender essentialism: gender as an essence regardless of the body.

Gender is not dissolved at all, contrary to what we first thought. It is in fact exactly the opposite. Gender reigns supreme, having defeated sex, and the pillar it is standing on is nothing but the same old stereotypes. What we're seeing is a kind of ideological reshuffle. Gender identity theory borrows fundamental terms from feminism, but attributes *opposite meanings to these terms*. The term social construct is retained, pledging allegiance to feminist theory, as well as the term biological sex, which used to denote what is fixed and immutable – but these two terms have swapped places with one another. Now, gender roles constitute the real sex. Womanhood is no longer about having a uterus, but pink ribbons and dolls. Masculinity is no longer synonymous with having a penis but with war and machines. And, these gender roles, it is said, are innate.

CHAPTER 4

Chasing the Gendered Brain

Can one, however, really be 'born in the wrong body'? Does the brain have a gender identity, in the first place, and is that identity unrelated to the sex of the person? Researchers have fired the starting gun in the race to find the gendered brain and the scientist who manages to locate it can expect to be showered in world-wide acclaim and funding. People are being taken into labs to have their teeth measured and their genitals stimulated and the brains of deceased trans people are being carefully studied.

A similar search to unravel the mystery of sex unfolded in the 1980s and 90s – though at the time it was the difference between men's and women's brains that was meant to be proven. No consensus was reached on the matter and the hype eventually died down, only to return as a key component of gender identity theory. We're being told yet again that female and male brains exist, just that they are not always located in female and male bodies.

Writing in the Swedish daily *Aftonbladet* in 2018, molecular biologist and science writer Henrik Brändén claims that gender identity is determined by the levels of foetal testosterone. If testosterone levels are high, a male gender identity will develop, while if lower, a female gender identity will develop:

> The amount of testosterone in a few small nerve bundles in the brain's oldest parts determine how strong two reflexes become. One of these sets

off a quintessentially female sexual movement (arching) and the other a quintessentially male sexual movement (humping.)[41]

Brändén goes on to say that often, though not always, male foetuses are exposed to a stronger testosterone bath. However, this can also happen to many female foetuses. This exposure will then determine the extent to which the foetus develops "archetypal female or male characteristics" such as "verbal ability, the ability to mentally rotate geometrical shapes, and interest in people versus interest in things," as well as whether one is turned on by men or women. It is thus "natural to be born in the wrong body," Brändén asserts.

The question is: if it's natural, what part about it is *wrong*? Let's assume for a minute that Brändén's hypothesis is correct: the foetus that's 'bathed' in testosterone will develop into a person who humps and can mentally rotate geometrical shapes. (I'm not really clear on which gender Brändén thinks likes "things" and which he assumes to have "verbal ability"). Let's assume that a certain amount of girls are born and develop in this way. This seems reasonable – after all, 'cowgirl', the position in which a woman climbs on top of a passive man and humps up and down, is described in the *Kamasutra* and is reported by *The Independent* to be men's favourite position. Perhaps all women who enjoy this position have been exposed to a lot of testosterone in the womb? As well as all women who are interested in maths and science? Even so, what Brändén fails to prove is whether it's actually these women who become transgender – or if this even applies to people at all. In the article, Brändén speaks of human foetuses, but in his book, *Själens biologi och vår fria vilja* (The Biology of the Soul and Our Free Will) it transpires that he's actually only referring to studies on rats. It is a well-known fact among endocrinologists that parallels cannot be drawn between humans and rats on this particular issue because male rats have an oestrogen effect in their central nervous systems due to higher levels of testosterone, which is not the case in humans.[42]

Brändén nevertheless claims that nature determines a person's gender identity. But if gender identity isn't connected to biological sex at all, why

---

41 Henrik Brändén. (1 February 2018). 'Naturligt vara född i "fel kön"', *Aftonbladet Kultur*.
42 Charles E. Rosselli and Scott A. Klosterman. (1 July 1998). 'Sexual differentiation of aromatase activity in the rat brain: effects of perinatal steroid exposure'. *Endocrinology*, Vol. 139, No. 7, pp. 3193–3201.

call it *gender* identity, and divide it into male and female? Isn't it actually a completely different kind of identity; couldn't he simply call it a humping identity? Not so, according to our molecular biologist, because humping and mounting are *male* movements, and those women who mount their partners therefore have "male reflexes" in the "oldest parts of their brains." He reaches this conclusion by referring to "archetypes." So we're back to a thesis that relies on the existence of *cultural archetypes* to be proven. In his book, Brändén claims that

> [T]he fact that [a person's] gender identity does not need to match [their] genitals can also be seen when we look back in history. There are several stories dating back to Sweden's time as a superpower in the 1600s of women adopting male roles and earning a living as soldiers. One of them, Ulrika Eleonora Stenhammar, said as a child that she was uninterested in learning female tasks and instead preferred to ride horses and go hunting.[43]

What Brändén shows with his observation is, in fact, that *sex* has no automatic connection to *gender*. Just because you're born with a vagina doesn't mean that you can't ride horses, go hunting and fight. In fact, in modern-day Sweden, nine out of ten horseback riders are female and the majority of these are teenage girls.[44] Brändén has simply confirmed the basic thesis of feminism: your genitals shouldn't determine your fate. The difference is that, instead of using examples like these to show how arbitrary gender roles are, Brändén implies that Stenhammar was not a real woman, going so far as to conclude that she didn't *perceive herself as one*.

As further evidence for his theory, we are treated to the following examples: the Portuguese coming across "frightening characters" (Brändén's term) in the Amazon who, despite their female genitalia, had short hair and waged war with bows and arrows. Also, he says that "it is generally agreed" that the 17th century Swedish queen Kristina had "typically 'male' interests during her upbringing."[45] The question remains: what is it that's *male* about these interests – history, languages and science – if there are many women around the world who share them? Why is it so important that these women be viewed as deviant?

---

43 Henrik Brändén. (2020). *Själens biologi och vår fria vilja*, p. 276. Lund: Celanders Publishing.
44 <https://www.ridsport.se/Omoss/Statistik>.
45 Brändén. (2020). p. 276.

Let's, for the time being, accept Brändén's hypothesis about men's and women's brains being different, and let's say that many women are born with brains that resemble male brains and many men are born with brains that look more like women's brains. This entails a spectrum of behaviour: some women are by nature more aggressive, more prone to humping etc. *Would this then not be a natural part of femininity?* The discovery that there are women and men of many different kinds could be used to broaden the ideas held about their respective characteristics. We could conclude that a certain number of women are born to hunt and be rocket scientists, as this is determined by the exposure to testosterone in the womb and no one can change this! We could establish that this is a completely natural characteristic for women, and thus abolish the idea of gender once and for all. If new biological research shows that 'gender' is *not* connected to sex, why even speak of them as synonyms? Instead, the opposite happens. Brändén uses the same findings to narrow the definition of woman, not to open it up. He argues that women who do not fit a preconceived model of 'woman' are born in the wrong body. They are not actually women, and should be moved from this category and fully be described as and indeed *become* men.

This recurring discrepancy turns out to be one of the foundations of gender identity theory: Sex is said to be unrelated to gender – which is exactly what feminists have always said; that gender is an arbitrary cultural construct – yet we are told they somehow need to be aligned, and that society needs to intervene and make sure they do.

So, where is gender identity located, if not in biological sex? The advocates of gender identity theory don't seem to have reached an agreement on this matter. For Brändén, it's determined by hormone exposure; for biopsychologist Thomas E. Bevan, it's about finger length. Bevan owns a company that conducts research into the biopsychology of trans people for the US military. In his book, he states:

> There are various biomarkers that support the idea that being transgender is due to biologial genetics. For both males and females, a prominent biomarker is the ratio of lengths between the second and fourth finger. Transgender people have been shown to have different ratios from non-transgender people.[46]

---

46   Thomas E. Bevan. (2017). *Being Transgender: What You Should Know*, p. 54. Westport, Connecticut: Praeger.

Bevan is referring to research on 50 trans men and 68 trans women with a control group of 37 people in New York. The trans men (women) had finger lengths similar to those of 'cis' men, and in the trans women (men), no difference was observed when compared to 'cis' men. The researchers muse about whether the proportions between the length of the index and ring finger could be an indicator of masculinity in women but guard against stating this outright by writing that "… data on 2D:4D ratios in transgender individuals are scarce and contradictory."[47] A group of German researchers, however, claim to have found the opposite: trans women's finger length proportions are closer to those of women, while those of trans men are not similar at all to the proportions seen in men.[48] These conclusions were drawn based on a study of 226 people.

Both teams of researchers think they've found *something* despite their conflicting results. The question is: what exactly? Even if they noticed a difference in the length of the index and ring finger, they would still need to prove that this was what *caused* transsexuality or was caused by it, which would mean that the difference would be present in all transsexuals.

One of the pioneers in the field of gender identity of the brain is the Dutch neurobiologist Dick Swaab. He claims that there are indications that gender identity can be traced to a tiny spot in the hypothalamus: subnucleus INAH3. This spot is often slightly bigger in men than women and having studied 42 deceased people's brains, of whom 13 were trans people, Swaab noticed that INAH3 in trans women was closer in size to that of women while the area in trans men was similar in size to that in the men.[49] In men, this area is slightly larger than in women, but women who

---

47 M. Leinung and C. Wu. (June 2017). 'The biologic basis of transgender identity: 2D: 4D finger length ratios implicate a role for prenatal androgen activity'. *Endocr. Pract.* Vol. 23, Issue 6, pp. 669–671. Doi: 10.4158/EP161528.OR. Epub 2017 23 March. PubMed PMID: 28332875.
48 Harald J. Schneider Johanna Pickel and Gunter K. Stalla. (2006). 'Typical female 2nd–4th finger length (2D:4D) ratios in male-to-female transsexuals – Possible implications for pre-natal androgen exposure.' *Psychoneuroendocrinology*, No. 31, pp. 265–269.
49 Dick Swaab and Alicia Garcia-Falgueras. (November 2008). 'A sex difference in the hypothalamic uncinate nucleus: relationship to Gender Identity'. *Brain*, 131 (Pt 12), pp. 3132–3146.

identified as men had a larger INAH3 and men who identified as women had an area that was smaller.[50]

The very same area of the brain, subnucleus INAH3, was also the subject of great research interest in the 1990s, when researchers were trying to find a genetic cause for homosexuality. At the time, it was pinpointed as a genetic marker for male homosexuality. Neuroscientist Simon LeVay found that male homosexuals had a smaller INAH3 subnucleus when compared to heterosexual men and his research received significant attention all over the world. Homosexual men all over the US sent the study to their parents to show that their sexuality was innate. The Swedish daily *Dagens Nyheter* commented that the findings could cure homophobia because those who accepted homosexuality as genetically determined tended to be more tolerant.[51]

LeVay's findings were heavily criticised by those who argued the analysis was binary and did not leave room for bisexuality, and by feminists, especially lesbians, who said that they *chose* to be lesbians. Research on what causes homosexuality has now fallen out of fashion. Other studies contradicted LeVay's findings and he has since stated that he had been misunderstood.[52] The searching around in dead people's brains for the root of homosexuality seems to have stopped. Nor was it ever an easy task: the area in question makes up at most 0.000009 per cent of the brain's mass and is a little dot not even big enough to fill up the 'o' in macho.[53] However, in 2008, Swaab claimed that this dot was what would help solve the mystery of – not sexuality, but gender identity! The dot develops in the same way in boys and girls up to the age of four, when the amount of cells seems to stop increasing in girls, but not in boys.

Swaab's study got plenty of attention – the roots of gender identity had finally been found, headlines proclaimed. Swaab quickly gathered

---

50   Shawna Williams. (1 March 2018). 'Are the brains of transgender people different from those of cisgender people?' *The Scientist*.
51   <https://www.dn.se/arkiv/debatt/dn-debatt-okad-tolerans-mot-homosexuella-ny-undersokning-mest-positiva-ar-de-som-menar-att/>.
52   William Byne et al. (September 2001). 'The interstitial nuclei of the human anterior hypothalamus: an investigation of variation with sex, sexual orientation, and HIV status'. *Hormones and Behaviour*, Vol. 40, No. 2, pp. 86–92. See also <https://www.scientificamerican.com/article/massive-study-finds-no-single-genetic-cause-of-same-sex-sexual-behavior/>.
53   David Nimmons. (1 March 1994). 'Sex and the brain'. *Discover Magazine*.

his insights in a popular science book entitled *We Are Our Brains*, which sold 100,000 copies and contains thoughts on basically anything and everything. Women are not turned on by naked men, medical students always have dominant mothers and a moribund soldier always cries for his Mother – Swaab seems to be able to explain the whole enchilada. Soon enough, though, criticism of his study on trans people started to appear. Firstly, it turned out that he had to increase the number of participants in order to achieve the desired result. The first study detected no difference between trans women and men, whereupon Swaab added more people and the difference could now be seen. The only issue was that all of his 13 trans people had undergone hormone treatment. Three Spanish researchers scrutinised Swaab's report and concluded that hormone treatment accounted for the difference:

> In a first report, MtFs [males to females] had a brain weight that did not differ from that of the studied male and female control specimens. When more subjects were included in the study, it was found that brain weight was almost significantly lower than those of control males, but did not differ from those of control females. As was seen above, this 'in between' position for the MtF brain weight seems to be a consequence of the cross-sex hormone treatment and not a phenotypic characteristic of the MtFs; rather, it would be the dramatic effect of estradiol and antiandrogen treatment on their gray matter.[54]

When scientists at the Karolinska Institute re-did the study on living people who had not undergone hormone therapy, they got the opposite result. Ivanka Savic and Stefan Arver studied 48 heterosexual men and 24 trans women who were attracted to women. They found no differences at all in their brains – all areas of the brain were identical for men and trans women. They state:

> Like HeM ['cis' men], MtF-TR [trans women] displayed larger GM volumes than HeW ['cis' women] in the cerebellum and lingual gyrus and smaller GM and WM volumes in the precentral gyrus. Both male groups had smaller hippocampal volumes than HeW. As in HeM, but not HeW, the right cerebral hemisphere and thalamus volume was in MtF-TR lager than the left. None of these measures differed between HeM and

---

54 A. Guillamon, C. Junque and E. Gómez-Gil. (2016). 'A review of the status of brain structure research in transsexualism'. *Archives of Sexual Behavior*, Vol. 45, No. 7, pp. 1615–1648. Doi:10.1007/s10508-016-0768-5.

MtF-TR. MtF-TR displayed also singular features and differed from both control groups by having reduced thalamus and putamen volumes and elevated GM volumes in the right insular and inferior frontal cortex and an area covering the right angular gyrus. The present data do not support the notion that brains of MtF-TR are feminized.[55]

Despite the fact that Swaab proved that hormones may have affected a miniscule spot in the brain of only 13 trans people in terms of being closer in size to that of women, his study has been cited tens of times more than Savic and Arver's. For the stressed-out journalist who's assigned an article on the trans question and needs a quote from an expert to close with, Swaab willingly provides. He's not afraid of opening his mouth and supplies quotes such as, "Thanks to neuroscience we know that gender identity is established in the brain before birth for the rest of your life. But there are people who doubt this, just as there are those who think the Earth is flat."[56]

Another branch of research in this field studies stress levels in trans people. They're taken into labs, asked to undress, touched on various parts of their genitals and their reactions are then measured using magnetoencephalography. The University of California carried out a study in which eight trans men and eight 'cis' women had their breasts and hands touched with a plastic finger. Two of the trans men reported they identified more as 'genderqueer' than as men but none of them liked having breasts. All the 'cis' women reported wanting to have breasts. The researchers, Laura Case and colleagues, discovered that the trans men's sensory responses to having their breasts touched were lower than the women's.[57] According to their research, MRI scans even revealed that some trans men experienced feelings of stress and unease/discomfort at having their breasts touched. The study does not say whether the subjects had worn binders (clothing that compresses and reduces breast sensation). Nevertheless, the researchers conclude that the make-up of the brain

---

55 Ivanka Savic and Stefan Arver. (November 2011). 'Sex dimorphism of the brain in male-to-female transsexuals'. *Cerebral Cortex*, Vol. 21, pp. 2525–2533, <doi:10.1093/cercor/bhr032>.

56 Kevin Van Vliet and Dick Swaab. (September 2019). 'Ik wou dat die Nashville-verklaring er niet geweest was'. *HP De Tijd*, 1.

57 Laura K. Case et al. (July 2017). 'Altered white matter and sensory response to bodily sensation in female-to-male transgender individuals'. *Archives of Sexual Behavior*, Vol. 46, No. 5, pp. 1223–1237.

itself is different in trans men, and not that the psychological discomfort activates certain parts of brain:

> These findings suggest that dysphoria related to gender-incongruent body parts in FtM individuals may be tied to differences in neural representation of the body and altered white matter connectivity.

With this sentence, Case et al. have made the mind-blowing discovery that eight individuals who do not like having breasts do not like having their breasts poked and prodded in a lab. Their study certainly does not prove gender identity to be innate, yet it is indiscriminately cited by activists and researchers wanting to prove that gender is located in the brain. Neurologist Stephen V. Gliske at the University of Michigan goes so far as to base his new theory on the origins of gender on it:

> I denote this new theory as the multisense theory of gender dysphoria. This new theory focuses on function, including sense of gender and its inputs, rather than male/female dichotomy in anatomic size and shape (the focus of the opposite brain sex theory) […] The underlying neurobiology would influence how much an individual feels chronic distress, how much they desire to act in a manner consistent with their gender role, and how much they feel the gendered aspects of their body belongs to them.[58]

According to Gliske, the University of California study proves gender identity to be innate. Only it isn't a question of the size or shape of the brain, as Swaab maintains, but sensory perception. In one anthology, this same study is even wielded as a weapon against the far-right![59] Consequently, we are even further removed from the eight people in the lab at the University of California, two of whom were not even sure they wanted to be men and identified as 'genderqueer'. We could also not be further from the issue of trans rights: it could most definitely be possible to acknowledge the existence of gender dysphoria without having to prove that gender is innate.

---

58 Stephen V. Gliske. (2 December 2019). 'A new theory of gender dysphoria incorporatingthe distress, social behavioral, and body-ownership networks'. *eNeuro*, Vol. 6, No. 6. Doi: 10.1523/Eneuro.0183-19.2019.
59 Tristan Fehr. (2020). 'Essentially a Lie: Challenging Biological Essentialist Interpretations of Transgender Neurology'. In Louie Dean Valencia-García, *Far-Right Revisionism and the End of History: Alt/Histories*. London: Routledge.

Yet another theory is thrown into the works by a group of Chinese researchers who contradict Gliske and Swaab, claiming that the RYR3 gene could be the missing piece of the puzzle. The RYR3 gene is "clearly identifiable in the brain and regulates the release of calcium from intracellular storage." In their study of nine trans women and four trans men, the team found a genetic variation in the RYR3 gene.[60] Based on this finding, they argue that trans people do not in fact resemble the opposite sex, but display their *own* genetic variation, which cannot be found in the population at large. These researchers are therefore proponents of the idea that being trans is an identity in and of itself. (However, they have not studied the extent to which the genetic variation presents in the subjects' family members and/or relatives.)

A similar thought process is followed by seven Spanish researchers who think they have spotted a pattern among trans people: they often have more older brothers than 'cis' people, though this only seems to be the case when the trans person is homosexual in relation to the sex they were born as. The researchers are however unable to say what the reason for this might be.[61]

In contrast to the Chinese group's findings, 13 US and Dutch researchers claim that gender identity itself is hereditary.[62] In a research overview published in *Behavioural Genetics*, they evaluated studies of pre- and primary school children, which were classified in a list.[63] The list is called PSAI, or Pre-School Activities Inventory, and has been used globally by researchers, pre-schools and psychologists since 1993 to study gender role behaviour in young children. Children's play is observed by parents or staff, who are encouraged to look for the following characteristics and activities:

---

60   Fu Yang, Xiao-hai Zhu, Qing Zhang, Ning-xia Sun, Yi-xuan Ji, Jin-zhao Ma, Bang Xiao, Hai-xia Ding, Shu-han Sun and Wen Li. (2017). 'Genomic characteristics of gender dysphoria patients and identification of rare mutations in RYR3 gene'. *Scientific Report*, Vol. 7, pp. 8339.
61   E. Gómez-Gil, I. Esteva, R. Carrasco et al. (2011). 'Birth order and ratio of brothers to sisters in Spanish transsexuals'. *Archives of Sexual Behavior*, Vol. 40, pp. 505–510. <https://doi.org/10.1007/s10508-010-9614-3>.
62   Tinca J. C. Polderman, P. C. Baudewijntje Kreukels, Michael S. Irwig et al. (January 2018). 'The biological contributions to gender identity and gender diversity. Bringing data to the table'. *Behavior Genetics*.
63   <https://www.psychometrics.cam.ac.uk/services/psychometric-tests/psai>.

Masculine:
- Playing with a tool set
- Engaging in fighting
- Playing at having a male occupation (e.g. a soldier)
- Shows interest in snakes, spiders or insects
- Showing interest in real cars, trains or airplanes
- Likes to explore new surroundings
- Climbing (e.g. fences, trees, gym, equipment)
- Engaging in sports and ball games

Feminine:
- Avoids getting dirty
- Avoids taking risks
- Playing with girls
- Pretending to be a family character (e.g. parent)
- Playing house (e.g. cleaning, cooking)
- Likes pretty things
- Dressing up in girlish clothes
- Plays with tea sets

The researchers claim to have found a pattern: monozygotic twin brothers display similar behaviour more often than dizygotic twins. If one identical twin likes trains, so does the other, and if they like playing with tea sets, so does their twin. This finding leads the researchers to claim that gender identity is hereditary. Whether the twins in the study are trans people remains to be seen. The researchers did not find any physical differences in the twins. Despite only having found differences in personality, their conclusions are about gender identity: "Masculinity is defined in terms of 'aggressivity/aggression, dominance and independence' and femininity in terms of being 'warm, emotional and caring'." Independent girls and warm and caring boys thus have 'atypical gender identities' even before they themselves are aware of it. We can only conclude that the discovery of other cultures would be news to these researchers.

In the 1980s and 90s, researchers chasing the gendered brain were stumped by a similar problem, namely that they found so many exceptions – cases in which people behaved in entirely unexpected ways. Today's researchers setting out to prove that gender identity is innate have done away with this inconvenient problem: they can simply state that all girls who do not behave in a typically girly way actually have a male gender identity and vice versa.

However, they come up against a different problem, thoughtfully described by Gliske: one cannot write off the role of culture. Does our culture decide what constitutes girly clothes or is this somehow determined in the brain? Predictably, the question of causality is the biggest cause of conflict in this field of research.

In addition, as a group of researchers from Georgia State University argue, it is difficult to draw conclusions about innate characteristics based on adult brains. These scientists studied animals that were divided into female and male groups and subjected to different treatment. Among the animals receiving the same treatment, one could clearly see the brains becoming similar. Since the brain is the most adaptable organ in the body, it displays 'epigenetic markers' caused by life experience.[64]

Gina Rippon, Professor of Cognitive Neuroscience at the University of Birmingham dismisses most of the research on gender identity as simple "neurotrash." She maintains this is practically a question of 'garbage in, garbage out': poor research with vague results that the media converts into banal soundbites like "women love chocolate" and "we only use 10 per cent of our brain." In her book *The Gendered Brain – The New Neuroscience that Shatters the Myth of the Female Brain*, Rippon shows that modern research has not found anything that could be termed "the female brain."[65]

In 2015, Daphna Joel and others at Tel Aviv University carried out brain scans of 1400 people. The researchers explain that, if the brain were dimorphic like sex organs, differences would overlap only in very few cases and these differences would be mutually exclusive. However, this is not the case in either white or grey brain matter and every individual actually has their very own mosaic: "... regardless of the cause of observed sex/gender differences in brain and behavior (nature or nurture), human brains cannot be categorized into two distinct classes: male brain/female

---

64 Laura R. Cortes, Carla D. Cisternas and Nancy G. Forger. (2019). 'Does Gender Leave an Epigenetic Imprint on the Brain?'. *Frontiers in Neuroscience*, Vol. 13. Doi: 10.3389/fnins.2019.00173.

65 Gina Rippon. (2019). *The Gendered Brain: The New Neuroscience that Shatters the Myth of the Female Brain*, p. 92. London: Penguin Vintage.

brain." In 92–100 per cent of cases, it is not even possible to determine whether the brain belongs to a man or a woman.[66]

Nor are matters so straightforward when it comes to the (in)famous "gender spectrum." Cordelia Fine from the University of Melbourne, whose book *Testosterone Rex* was awarded the Royal Society Science Book Prize 2017, explains that high levels of testosterone do not automatically result in lower levels of oestrogen. A person can have a lot of both hormones or little of both – testosterone also has the paradoxical characteristic of converting into oestrogen, resulting in boys often developing breasts during puberty.[67]

If gender identity could be found in the brain, identifying a person's true gender would be an easy task. There would be no need to look between the legs of newborn babies and consultations before gender reassignment surgery would be equally unnecessary. Were gender identity fixed, innate and biological, it could be determined by means of a simple test: newborns' brains could be scanned to find out whether they were girls or boys. Yet no such brain scan or DNA test exists. What does exist are hypotheses and tendencies, contradicted by other hypotheses and tendencies.

So far, all scientific studies on gender identity conclude that the results are inconclusive and that nothing can be stated with certainty. In other words, science does not know whether something called gender identity even exists!

On the other hand, one thing is clear: something called *sex* definitely does exist. Thirty per cent of our 21,000 genes are differentially expressed depending on whether they are found in a man (XY) or in a woman (XX).[68] They are the same genes, but they are expressed differently depending on sex. They regulate processes such as skeleton growth, sperm production, kidney function, thickness of the heart muscle, height and fat production.

---

66 Daphna Joel et al. (15 December 2015). 'Sex beyond the genitalia. The human brain mosaic'. Proceedings of the National Academy of Sciences. <http://www.pnas.org/content/112/50/15468.abstract>.

67 Cordelia Fine. (2018). *Testosterone Rex: Myten om våra könade hjärnor*, p. 122. Translated by Linus Kollberg, Göteborg: Daidalos. *Testosterone Rex: Myths of Sex, Science and Society*. London: Icon Books.

68 Moran Gershoni and Shmuel Pietrokovski. (2017). 'The landscape of sex-differential transcriptome and its consequent selection in human adults'. *BMC Biology*, Vol. 15, No. 7.

For instance, XX-chromosomes determine whether genes will send a signal to the skeleton to create broader hips, while XY-chromosomes determine whether the Adam's apple grows. Finally, while one cannot see whether a brain is female or male, it is often an easy task to see whether a person has female or male sex organs. Sex is, moreover, mutually exclusive. A person cannot both have the ability to give birth and to impregnate. It is an either-or system known as sexual dimorphism, a characteristic of all mammals for the past 178 million years. What we call 'sex' began 600 million years ago, when the reproductive process evolved from cells splitting themselves into two (with only one progenitor) to the combination of two cells, first the isogamic way with two equal cells uniting, and later the anosigamic way, with large gametes[69] uniting with small gametes. Ever since, we divide mammals into two sexes: the one with large gametes is called female and the one with small gametes is called male.

There is nonetheless a small group of people in whom sex development does not take place in the same way. These people are born with DSD, or Disorders of Sexual Development, a group of conditions involving variations in hormones, reproductive glands or chromosomes that affect sexual development. This might involve a lack of testosterone production or lack of an enzyme leading to an excess of male sex hormones. It can also cause difficulties in determining a newborn child's sex, something that happens to approximately 0.02% of all newborns. Nevertheless, these people still belong to one of the two biological sexes. What used to be called 'true hermaphroditism' – when a person is born with both testicular and ovarian tissue – does not mean that the person has both XY and XX chromosomes.

Furthermore, the term 'intersex' is misleading, as it means 'between the sexes' and thereby might imply the existence of people who lack a biological sex, which is not true. The most common DSD occurs to biologically female children with 46 XX chromosomes whose external genitals have masculine characteristics. This is called CAH (congenital adrenal hyperplasia) and does indeed release a flood of testosterone in utero. However, the individuals whose sex development actually does differ from that of females in society at large, seldom have gender dysphoria. Not a single study on the topic has found a link between this

---

[69] José Errasti and Marino Pérez Álvarez. (2022). *Nadie nace en un cuerpo equivocado*, p. 33. Deusto Publicaciones.

flood of testosterone and the desire to be a man.[70] In fact, 95 per cent of girls with CAH do not have gender dysphoria, with the percentage who do being just a little higher than in the general population. It is important to realise that we do not know whether this is because they were mistaken for boys as newborns, which happens to many girls with CAH in countries with poor access to health care.

Henrik Bråndén also wants to wade into the debate about CAH and directs us to a study by the well-known German psychologist Heino Meyer-Bahlburg, who shows that women with CAH are attracted to women more often than other women.[71] From this, Bråndén draws the conclusion that the foetal exposure to testosterone has implications for "subjective gender identity."[72] Apparently, it tells us something about *sexual orientation*, namely that most women with CAH become heterosexual, but that a slightly higher number become homosexual and bisexual when compared to the control group. However, the conclusion that lesbians have a male gender identity is entirely of Bråndén's own concoction. Bråndén seems to be mixing up sexual orientation and gender identity here – as so many do, unfortunately.

As a matter of fact, no causal link exists between high levels of testosterone and a desire to be a man. Some studies indicate that exposure to higher levels of testosterone during foetal development may affect physical features and abilities, but nowhere is it proven that this in itself would result in a feeling of *being* a man. *The point is, if the hypothesis about biological gender identity were correct, it would first and foremost be intersex individuals who became trans.*

Women with high levels of testosterone and men with low levels should be those who exhibit a tendency to allegedly 'change' sex. However, an intersex body does not seem to mean an intersex brain. On the contrary,

---

70 A.B. Dessens, F.M. Slijper and S.L. Drop. (August 2005). 'Gender dysphoria and gender change in chromosomal females with congenital adrenal hyperplasia', *Archives of Sexual Behavior*, Vol. 34, No. 4, pp. 389–397. Review. PubMed PMID: 16010462.

71 H.F. Meyer-Bahlburg, C. Dolezal, S.W. Baker and M.I. New. (February 2008). 'Sexual orientation in women with classical or non-classical congenital adrenal hyperplasia as a function of degree of prenatal androgen excess'. *Archives of Sexual Behavior*, Vol. 37, No. 1, pp. 85–99. Doi: 10.1007/s10508-007-9265-1. PMID: 18157628.

72 Bråndén. (2020). p. 270.

research shows that it is mainly people with no sex development disorder who become trans. Here, researchers frantically scrape around for any physical signs that could possibly be cited as a reason: a dot in the brain's grey matter, a different type of play in the sand pit, a physical revulsion for breasts, a longer ring finger. The fact remains that such links are not found in the group of people who actually present differences in sex development.

The 30 per cent of genes that are expressed differently in men and women do so solely because of our XX and XY chromosomes. Sexual characteristics are, in other words, directly related to sex. The popular idea that the body is somehow divided into an 'outside' and an 'inside', and that there would be an inner biological gender with a life all of its own, is therefore not true. It is a biological impossibility since the body is genetically programmed. If men could biologically be women, they would *be* women.

Despite this, popular science treats the matter as though it were a foregone conclusion. Books about gender identity assert that gender is located in the brain. Diane Ehrensaft, the author of *The Gender Creative Child*, resolutely addresses parents stating it is wrong to say that a baby born with a vagina is a girl, because "gender doesn't belong between their legs but between their ears."[73]

In the handbook *The Transgender Child* (also written for parents), the entire brain is described as "a gendered organ."[74] Gender identity is "formed in the brain," claim the authors and gender specialists Stephanie Brill and Rachel Pepper, and "most agree that it is most likely determined before we are born."[75] What is meant by "most"? Which research they are relying on and which part of the brain they are talking about is not elaborated. Instead, they state that the gender of one's brain is "determined by the individual alone."[76] Indeed, all one needs to do is observe "hairstyles, body language, ways of walking and moving through space, clothing preferences, and styles of play."[77]

---

73 German Lopez. (2016). 'How to know if your child is transgender, according to an expert'. *Vox* 26/6.
74 Diane Ehrensaft. (2016). *The Gender Creative Child*. New York: Workman Publishing.
75 Stephanie Brill and Rachel Pepper. (2008). *The Transgender Child: A Handbook for Families and Professionals*, p. 14. Jersey City, New Jersey: Cleis Press.
76 Ibid. p. 4.
77 Ibid. p. 23.

The good old gender roles are back as proof of gender identity – no sooner was the brain's role introduced than it disappeared into thin air. The constant references to the brain serve a particular purpose: they lend a scientific air to theories on gender identity. The handbooks cited above give the impression that science and research has reached a consensus. But do not hold your breath for anything like a scientific method to test these hypotheses. Yet Brill and Pepper authoritatively conclude that "there is nothing anyone can do to change a child's gender identity" as it is "a core part of self."[78]

All manner of popular science articles even go so far as to claim that gender identity can be seen in animals. These claims are based on animals displaying gender-typical behaviour, though they concede that many behaviours in animals "do not fit neatly into those categories."[79]

The idea that the brain has a gender is thus yet again starting to gain ground. Endocrinologist Joshua Safer, who prescribes hormones to children and young people at Boston's Center for Transgender Medicine, claims that "the acceptance of gender identity as biological has entailed a dramatic paradigm shift. It will take time for the medical community to adapt."[80] In the Swedish newspaper *Svenska Dagbladet*, Hanna Söderström (who describes herself as a "rightwing transsexual blogger") writes, "I am a woman because the brain I was given by nature is female and because the environment I live in perceives me as a woman."[81]

---

78 Ibid. p. 4.
79 Amanda Leigh Mascarelli. (31 July 2015). 'Gender. When the body and brain disagree'. *Science News for Students*.
80 Erik Augustin Palm. (28 March, 2017). 'Transdokumentär för cis-publik', *Ottar*.
81 Hanna Söderström. (16 January 2012). 'Juridiskt kön inte samma som biologiskt', *SvD Debatt*.

CHAPTER 5

Gender Is in the Eye of the Beholder

Not all proponents of gender identity theory are biological determinists – some opt for a social constructivist approach and claim that anyone who is regarded as a woman, is a woman. When wanting to garner points with feminists, proponents of gender identity theory often provide the following explanation: anyone can be a woman because gender is a social construct. In the book *Ett transfeministiskt manifest* (A Transfeminist Manifesto), trans activist and film critic Maria Ramnehill argues that a woman is "anyone who is treated like a woman":

> All other definitions are irrelevant and unnecessary for feminism as feminism's aim is the emancipation of all those who are treated like women. There is no 'is' in feminism, only 'is interpreted as'.[82]

Ramnehill goes on to say that there are "a few old school feminist dykes from the 70s" who don't agree and who need to "grow up" since "the only thing they've learned from feminism is how to limit other women's lives."[83] To this, one could counter that if there 'is' no such thing as a woman, then it should not be possible for there to 'be' any old school feminist dykes from the 70s either. Whether there 'are' men or not, Ramnehill does not go into.

This author is representative of a third tendency in gender identity theory. According to this view, it is not the individual who determines her own identity (as argued by Cohen) nor are genes, hormones and humping gender markers. Here, the social environment is key. If others see a person

---

82   Maria Ramnehill. (2016). *Ett transfeministiskt manifest*, p. 85. Stockholm: Atlas.
83   Ibid. p. 86.

as a woman and treat her accordingly, then she 'is' a woman. This definition allows Ramnehill to use the feminist idea of gender as a social construct and thereby avoid both the embarrassing biological determinist trap present in the gendered brain argument as well as the neo-liberal notion that everyone is automatically what they want to be, while still retaining the idea that gender is an identity. The idea goes as follows: if others see me as a woman, they'll treat me the way they treat you – we therefore have the same experiences.

This reasoning does carry some weight, especially when forming alliances based on experiences. History and contemporary times certainly provide examples of such alliances. For instance, some trans women in the prostitution industry have fought alongside the women's movement to abolish the sex industry. The experience of having been treated both like a man and a woman doubtlessly provides valuable insights about patriarchy. This is evidenced by French survivor Anne D'arbes' account of how prostitution played out completely differently depending on whether she was seen as a man or woman: as a male prostitute, D'arbes states, one is treated like an equal; as a female, one is abused and hurt.

In certain women-only spaces like women's shelters and changing rooms, Ramnehill's principle has long been standard practice – people are generally not required to show ID when they enter the women's or men's changing room or when they access support at a women's shelter. A man who passes as a woman doesn't create any feelings of discomfort. The reverse is also true: a woman walking home alone at night being followed by a bearded individual isn't going to have time to find out whether the man was born a woman and is actually a trans man. These experiences affect and shape us: the feeling *someone is afraid of me* is one that many men live with and this feeling is shared by trans men. Equally, *someone's following me, maybe he's going to try to rape me?* is an experience shared by women and trans women. After many years, a person who has gone through gender reassignment surgery will have gathered a set of experiences similar to people born in that sex, and will have much in common with them. If experiences arise as a result of the treatment we receive in society, and this treatment depends on the body we have, then presumably those who inhabit a woman-like body have women's experiences. Ramnehill's argument is interesting when read through the lens of de Beauvoir's thinking on the body as a *situation* as well as Butler's theories on *interpellation* – we become a subject through being named (as one).

Still, as a definition, it does not hold water. The legal definition of sex impacts equality and anti-discrimination laws, statistics, sport and several other areas of life. Replacing the concrete, biological definition of sex with one based on a subjective interpretation as Ramnehill suggests, is lacking and problematic in several ways.

Firstly, its logic is circular. If *x* is that which is treated as *x*, we still haven't answered the question: what is *x*? Were we to apply the same reasoning to other categories – a chair is that which is treated as a chair, a dog that which is treated as a dog, a terrorist the person who is viewed by others as a terrorist and a Swede a person seen as a Swede – we can immediately see the weakness of the argument. We would have to determine how a woman, a dog, a chair and a terrorist are treated before we could say that a person or thing is one of these. A circular thesis ends up being meaningless without external reference points.

To say that 'a chair is something that is treated like a chair', we first need to establish how a chair ought to be treated. Presumably, we'd come up with the following: a chair is something you sit on. Following this definition, do I become a chair if someone sits on me? Does a chair stop being a chair if it sits on a person instead of the other way around? Does someone actually become a terrorist if the media says so? If a majority of people believe that a person born in Sweden to foreign parents is not Swedish, is this thus the case? How should a woman be treated? Is there a certain way to treat a person which allows us to say: you have been treated in the way women are treated and therefore you must be a woman? Do authorities therefore need to carry out surveys to find out who has been treated like a woman and what would the criteria for such a survey be?

Secondly, we'd need to establish who would have the final say in determining which people are part of which category. After all, people can be 'seen' in many different ways depending on who is doing the 'seeing'. It is not always the case that people state loud and clear 'I see you as …', but these judgments are also interpreted in their turn by the individual subject to them. If a trans woman is groped, it isn't always easy to determine whether the perpetrator was after a trans woman or a woman, and thus whether the groping was motivated by transphobia or sexism. Some trans women seem to take male attention as proof that they are seen as women, but many men have a particular interest in trans women. In the end, this is an unwieldy definition which would require a constant and incessant collation and interpretation of society's reactions for the individual to answer the question *who am I?*

In addition, the definition hands all the power to the gaze of others, making the self completely powerless. If society thinks that a person in the position of a colonised subject is a dog, is this the definition that the state should adopt? Is there no place for resistance to the view of others? Does a stranger have the right to invalidate our own understanding of our identity?

However, the biggest problem with Ramnehill's definition is that it doesn't stand on its own two feet, but relies on the unquestioned notion that a general idea of what a woman looks like exists. According to this view, a man is seen as a woman if he can 'pass' as one, that is, the extent to which he physically resembles a woman. In practice, this is about how much surgery he's had, how he dresses, his height, hands and how well he's managed to adjust his voice. If he can't manage this, then he isn't seen as a woman and, according to Ramnehill's definition, is not a woman. This definition is completely dependent on a prototype of 'woman', and this prototype cannot be anything other than a biological, natal woman's body. A man who wants society to see him as a woman will presumably not be that successful in his endeavours if he has five breast implants added or enlarges his Adam's apple. Ramnehill's thesis relies entirely on the existence of a point of reference. This point of reference is the female body.

Here is yet another theory that cannot float around in thin air but has landed right on mummy's bosom. Even Ramnehill appears not to subscribe to this theory wholeheartedly. This is evidenced by the recurring indignation at people who 'misgender'.[84] However, if the key is the opinion of others, 'misgendering' would be impossible. As per Ramnehill's assertion above, "there is no *is*, only *is interpreted as*," it follows that those who are treated as men, are men.

Other parts of Ramnehill's writing also reveal an essentialist understanding of gender. For example, the book says about Chelsea Manning that "a transwoman was never actually a man." Ramnehill claims that Manning was always a woman, even during the time that the world knew

---

84 <https://www.ottar.se/artiklar/rasande-uppg-relse-med-transfobi>.

him as Bradley.[85] This statement brings us back to gender as something that 'is', regardless of the body, society or clothing.

Ramnehill's texts oscillate between labelling gender as something completely irrelevant – "what is female gender identity other than an invention" and "biological sex is a social construct" – only to say in the next breath that trans women are "the lumpenproletariat of patriarchy" because they cannot give birth and therefore cannot "carry out the main form of female employment in patriarchy."[86] On the one hand, Ramnehill is denying the specific oppression that women experience while, on the other, highlighting the specific experience of trans women. In Ramnehill's thinking, there is a difference between women and trans women after all, but the difference only applies so as to evidence trans women's suffering. Ramnehill claims:

> While some feminists only analyse gender from the point of view of the socially constructed body of medical science, we transfeminists liberate the body from gender and let each individual create their gender on their own terms. We're building utopia, day by day, body by body, oestrogen patch by oestrogen patch.[87]

This statement appears to contradict the original thesis. On the one hand, those who pass as women are women, on the other hand everyone creates their gender on their own terms. Both of these assertions cannot be true at the same time, though. It's impossible to both *freely* create your body *and* pass as a woman. This short extract contains other oddities, too. Ramnehill refers to biology as *socially* constructed by *medical science*, while the hormone-treated body is said to be free of gender, existing somewhere beyond it. Surely, however, if there's something that's created by medical science it's the oestrogen patch?

Ramnehill's texts are often rhetorically constructed around an 'us' and a 'them'. On the one side, there's utopia, liberation, one's own terms, emancipation and a doing away with norms, on the other there's the old school 70s dykes (of whom there are only 'a few', anyway), medicine, social constructs and biologism. These words appear to have been chosen more

---

85 Ramnehill, 2016, p. 40.
86 Ramnehill, 2016, p. 87.
87 Ramnehill, Maria. (2014). 'För nyanslöst för en progressiv kvinnorörelse'. *Feministiskt perspektiv*, Vol. 20, No. 6.

for their capacity to ignite positive or negative associations than for their usefulness as analytical tools.

One could argue that it's pointless, even cruel, to pick apart these clumsy attempts at creating a theory since it might primarily be a tool for explaining a personal choice. If an individual wants to tinker with their body and find arguments in favour of doing so, perhaps these arguments won't always be the most logical ones and why should we care? Similar contradictions are found in other emblematic contemporary statements, for example when a woman has her lips done because she 'doesn't care what others think of me' or when athletes compete in the olympics 'just to compete against myself'. The difference is that these contradictions are at the heart of gender identity theory, which is about to be converted into the basis of legislation in many countries. If a man wears women's clothing, looks at himself in the mirror and thinks, 'Wow. This is how I want to look, now I'm just missing a pair of breasts' or if someone poses naked on the internet to 'show body positivism', there isn't much anyone can say about it. Ramnehill's book, though, is not called 'My Journey' but 'A Transfeminist Manifesto' and what is being proposed here is nothing other than a new definition of sex.

Catharine MacKinnon, US law professor and veteran campaigner against sex discrimination, has a similar argument to Ramnehill's. She positions herself against those who want to define women as those who are born women.

> Anybody who identifies as a woman, wants to be a woman, is going around being a woman, as far as I'm concerned, is a woman […] How one becomes a woman is not, I think, our job to police.[88]

This statement begs to be lauded for its generosity – everyone is welcome to be a woman if they want! However, it doesn't answer the question of what this something that we can want to be, go around being and identifying as, actually *is*. How can we identify as something that cannot be defined? Is there no core, or rather, what is the core? According to MacKinnon, simply defining what a woman is would be policing. In the next breath, though, she proceeds to do exactly this. MacKinnon observes that "what we live as 'woman' is a social construction of male supremacy":

---

88 Cristan Williams. (27 November 2015). 'Sex, gender, and sexuality. An interview with Catharine A. MacKinnon'. *The Conversations Project*.

My particular question was OF WHAT is sex socially constructed? The answer I gave, and still believe, is sexuality. Sexuality is itself not biological, but social, so the constructing is also the constructed, which makes sense since there is no place outside society.

So, being a woman is being a bottom in bed. The essence of gender is sexual oppression and anyone who assumes the position of the oppressed can be a woman. Our essence is oppression. In her claim that *nothing* exists outside society, MacKinnon is applying an extreme form of social constructivism. Materiality is therefore nothing, language everything, thus biological sex means nothing and gender everything.

If the only difference between men and women is their status in the sexual hierarchy, and if this hierarchy is entirely 'constructed', why is it that those with a certain role in reproduction, namely giving birth, always end up at the bottom of the hierarchy? If it has – as MacKinnon argues – nothing to do with biology, it is an utterly incredible coincidence! Further along in the interview, we discover that MacKinnon hasn't done away with the term biological sex after all. Her view is that sex discrimination exists and that it is not the same as gender discrimination:

> To be discriminated against based on being a trans woman or trans man is sex-based discrimination. It's either based on sex per se or it's based on what is perceived as the lack of fit between gender and sex, and both of those are discrimination.[89]

What is 'sex per se' and what's the difference between this and what MacKinnon calls 'gender'? If everything is a social construct, there wouldn't be any sex 'per se'. If women and trans women are exactly the same, there shouldn't be any discrimination of trans people that's different from discrimination of women. In such a situation, no one would be able to tell who was a woman and who was a trans woman. Yet MacKinnon is now claiming that discrimination of both women and trans women is based on biological sex – something that didn't exist only moments ago.

We are apparently dealing with a theory that purports to abolish key concepts only to then rely on them being retained because without them, the whole theory would collapse. Perhaps MacKinnon can see this herself as she quickly abandons theory – unusual for MacKinnon – and starts

---

89 Catharine A. MacKinnon and Durba Mitra. (2018). 'Ask a Feminist. Sexual harassment in the age of #MeToo'. *Signs Journal*, Vol. 4, No. 6.

throwing out personal anecdotes masquerading as evidence. She says she's met many trans women who "really inspire" her, whilst there are biological women who aren't feminists at all. In this case, the former are more "her team," she concludes. Apparently, biological women do exist after all – still, the definition of a woman now seems to be 'being liked by Catharine MacKinnon'.[90]

The spokespeople of gender identity theory all agree that gender has nothing to do with sex organs, but there is no consensus on how it should be defined. Those who maintain that gender identity is located in the brain fail to establish any scientific way of finding it, while those who support self-identification can't finish a sentence without falling back on stereotypes. Those who say that gender is in the eye of the beholder, do not let the beholder decide in the end. Finally, those who say that gender is a social construct cannot join up their reasoning without relying on biology.

---

90 Cristan Williams. (27 November 2015). 'Sex, gender, and sexuality. An interview with Catharine A. MacKinnon'. *The Conversations Project*.

CHAPTER 6

2007: The Order of Modernity

Despite the fact that research has failed to pin down exactly what gender identity is, gender identity theory has become enormously popular. In just a short space of time, governments and institutions throughout the western world have begun to view sex as an identity and not as material reality. In Sweden, this change has only taken ten years. It suffices to compare two government inquiries on the trans issue to see the giant leap that was taken between 2007 and 2017. In 2007, there was a government inquiry on sex reassignment conducted by special investigator and Appeal Court lawyer Lars Göran Abelson with expert assistance from senior doctors, lawyers and professors. They produced a 268-page report, 'Sex Reassignment – Proposals for a New Law', which included the view that:

> [O]bjectively speaking, it can be said that a man is an individual with external sex organs with a particular appearance, has a certain combination of chromosomes and a particular set of endocrine glands. A woman can be defined in a similar way. Another definition is the ability to become a father as opposed to a mother of a child.[91]

The report's authors went on to say that sex is something that children learn to identify early on and that they know "sex is unchanging over time and is not dependent on what activity one engages in (a boy does not

---

[91] Betänkande av könstillhörighetsutredningen. (2007). 'Ändrad könstillhörighet – förslag till ny lag', SOU (Official State Enquiries). Enquiry No. 16, p. 15.

become a girl if he plays with Barbie dolls)."[92] This is a material definition of sex as chromosomes, not gender roles. The inquiry clearly separated sex from gender, the latter "being/the basis of the socially constructed view of feminine and masculine."[93] In other words, sex is the body, while gender is the Barbie doll. The two are not the same thing and are not necessarily linked.

However, the inquiry authors did acknowledge that great suffering can result if an individual's sex and gender do not coincide. Regardless of why this happens, they concluded that individuals should be helped to align the two, which was actually the impetus for conducting the inquiry in the first place.

The objective of the inquiry was clearly narrow, focusing only on the number of people who wanted to change their sex, which "has increased considerably over the past years" yet by 2007, there were only around 60 individuals in the country per year who applied for sex change.[94] The inquiry was thus focused on these 60 transsexual individuals and their well-being – it did not set out to change the general definition of sex.

Transsexuality was defined as a psychiatric condition in which one feels born in the wrong sex. It was said to affect between 1 in 10,000 and 1 in 15,000 people. The report's authors did not make any claims about the causes of transsexuality but did say that it may be caused by hormones during foetal development.[95] They also identified a cure: surgery. After surgical intervention, they said, the patient "no longer suffers from the condition" and is now known as a former transsexual. According to this 2007 report, being transsexual is an identity that one only inhabits prior to the operation. The aim of reassignment surgery is to improve the mental health of individuals suffering from long-term psychological afflictions.

The inquiry authors claimed that the majority of people who undergo surgery feel better afterwards. They placed great emphasis on the difference between primary and secondary transsexualism – the former is said to entail always having felt like one is born in the wrong body (sex), and is mainly said to affect lesbians, while the latter has a sudden onset and affects mainly older heterosexual men who often display traits of

---

92 Ibid. p. 39.
93 Ibid. p. 39.
94 Ibid. p. 11.
95 Ibid. pp. 45–48.

fetishism.[96] Notably, heterosexual women and homosexual men were not discussed in the inquiry.

The report's authors recommended that careful attention be paid when diagnosing, because many of those presenting with the condition of transsexualism can have other, underlying diagnoses and issues. When it comes to young people, they advised waiting until they turn 18 before undertaking any surgical interventions: "It is never advisable to begin sex reassignment treatment on young people living in dysfunctional families. Such situations need to be managed and resolved before treatment begins."[97] Hormones should be assigned "with caution" to young patients and their prescription should only occur if five criteria are met. These criteria included the child "having demonstrated a pattern of gender non-conforming throughout their entire childhood," no underlying mental health diagnoses being present and the agreement and consent of the family.[98] The inquiry's recommendations made clear that a full assessment of the family was necessary in all cases involving children "as other emotional and behavioural issues and unresolved problems are common obstacles in the child's environment."

The authors further recommended that:

i) an individual who has transitioned be allowed to change their first name;
ii) an individual does not need to have felt transsexual since youth in order to change sex but that feeling this way "for a considerable length of time" should be enough; and
iii) an individual should no longer have to be unmarried to change sex.[99]

However, they also stated that anyone undergoing this change should be 18 and that endocrine glands should be removed from all individuals wanting to change sex because "this is in accordance with the wish that virtually all transsexuals have" and to "eliminate the possibility of a person registered as a man giving birth."[100] The inquiry authors said that even though this would be unlikely to happen in reality, it was important to avoid such situations. They advised that even if a transsexual person does

---

96 Ibid. p. 58.
97 Ibid. p. 151.
98 Ibid. p. 153.
99 Ibid. pp. 15–17.
100 Ibid. p. 15.

not opt for sterilisation, it must be performed anyway as "practically everyone" was said to want it.

Regarding the surgery itself, it is interesting to note the investigators' concerns regarding reproduction – a woman who has transitioned to become a man must under no circumstances give birth. Even though they were certain that no one would want to do this, they were categorical about their statement that no exceptions could be made to the requirement for the removal of endocrine glands. This was in line with the inquiry's definition of a woman as someone who can be a mother, and a man as someone who can be a father. Therefore, changing sex also meant renunciation of one's role within reproduction. (This criterion was removed in 2013 and those who were sterilised were later awarded compensation.)

The inquiry also covered complications that could arise in society, such as the fact that certain activities, categories of crime, tasks and places are sex-specific. These include sport, infanticide (which only women can be charged with in Sweden since the crime refers to a mother's killing of a newborn child and implies a lower punishment than if a person other than the mother had done it), strip searches, prisons and communal showers. However, the authors didn't comment on the types of situations that could arise, saying only that the former transsexual should henceforth be considered for all intents and purposes as a member of their new sex. The only exception could be sport, which the report authors left in the hands of sports associations and organisations.

All Swedish public inquiries must include an impact assessment outlining possible repercussions of the report's recommendations on gender equality, crime prevention and a host of other categories. Still, the final chapter of the report just included a brief statement that the recommendations "won't have any consequences in the areas in question, according to our assessment."[101]

In other words, in the 2007 inquiry, sex was seen as something connected to the physical body, while gender was a social construct. Granted, there was a paradox here: on the one hand, it was said that sex is biological – i.e. playing with a Barbie doll doesn't make you a girl – on the other, performing gender correctly *was* a prerequisite for changing sex. But since this was only meant to apply to an extremely small number

---

101 Ibid. p. 243.

of people, to appease their malaise, it is as if the inquiry was making an exception to the general definition of sex versus gender. Transsexuality was viewed as a condition with a diagnosis which had a cure and which then disappeared, once the patient was cured. This has a clear modernist ring to it: all problems have a practical solution, end of story. This view doesn't change the general definition of sex, which stays firmly anchored in the material world.

This was soon to change.

CHAPTER 7

2017: The Gender-Congruent Person

Fast-forward ten years and material reality has all but disappeared. "The notion of two 'biological sexes' is a medical construct," claims a 2017 government inquiry:[102]

> In the majority of cases, sex is assigned on the basis of the characteristics of a newborn child's external sex organs and is thus based on the idea of physical characteristics as the determining factor.[103]

The inquiry then explains that assigning sex this way is not correct – physical characteristics do not determine sex, as "psychological and social gender" are equally important. What the inquiry terms 'social gender' is defined as "attributes that are commonly viewed as 'male' or 'female', for example "clothes, body language and hair."[104] This used to be called a social construct, but is no longer so in the new narrative: it is now *biological sex* which is said to be socially constructed. Gender and sex have thus switched places, gender now being the real sex, while the body has ended up between quotation marks.

The 2017 inquiry is titled 'Transgender People in Sweden' and its lead investigator is Ulrika Westerlund, former executive director of RFSL (the Swedish Federation for Lesbian, Gay, Bisexual, Transgender, Queer and

---

102 Betänkande av utredningen om stärkt ställning och bättre levnadsvillkor för transpersoner, 'Transpersoner i Sverige – förslag för stärkt ställning och bättre levnadsvillkor'. (2017). SOU (Official State Enquiries). Enquiry No. 92, p. 62.
103 Ibid. p. 61.
104 Ibid. pp. 63–65.

Intersex Rights). The document is nearly 900 pages long, its aim much wider than the 2007 one. Its objective is two-fold: "to investigate how transgender people are affected by society's cis- and heteronormativity and to identify the obstacles they face from society in living in congruence with their gender identity."[105] The focus has thus shifted from the priority stated in the 2007 inquiry of improving mental health outcomes for transsexuals, into changing social norms.

A key part of these changes involves doing away with biological sex as a category. All individuals should now be able to freely decide their gender. Gender neutral social security numbers should be implemented[106] as non-binary people can feel excluded or experience problems due to their social security number: "a change in how sex is registered in Sweden is a prerequisite for including non-binary individuals." Surveys should record gender identity, rather than biological sex, with questions formulated in the following way: "What sex are you? By sex, we mean gender identity, i.e. the gender you identify with."

Equality politics must be altered, especially references to "women and men" as these imply "a binary understanding of gender"[107] and the word "inhabitants" should be used instead.[108] Any talk of men's violence against women is binary and instead of focusing on "physical men and women," we ought to "focus on norms, gender and power."[109] Terms such as "women's healthcare" and "maternal care" are exclusive,[110] while the words mother and father also ought to be replaced with parent.[111] Furthermore, all public single-sex toilets must be made unisex.[112] The world of sport does not escape scrutiny either, and it is a problem according to the inquiry that it is sex segregated since this is based on "ideas about men and women having such different characteristics that they need to engage in sporting activities separately." The inquiry's view is that this separation by sex "upholds a

---

105 Ibid. p. 551.
106 Ibid. p. 489.
107 Ibid. p. 487.
108 Ibid. p. 146.
109 Ibid. p. 314.
110 Ibid. p. 511.
111 Ibid. p. 498.
112 Ibid. p. 158.

hetero- and cisgender norm that serves no purpose" and this should be questioned, at least when it comes to children.[113]

These recommendations do not only concern the group outlined in the inquiry's title, but society as a whole. They entail a complete overhaul of the legal definition of sex. Sex should no longer be defined as biology, but as identity. The inquiry demands that this new definition be made into law and become compulsory in education. Furthermore, public funding should be conditional so that any organisation which does not adopt this new definition will not receive public funds.[114] All public institutions ought to redefine sex as a *feeling that has nothing to do with the body*. Those who do not agree are singled out as a major problem.

This is utterly astonishing – an inquiry tasked with making life easier for a vulnerable minority group ends up stating that society should radically change the definition of sex. What do the two things have to do with each other in the first place?

The changes recommended have massive implications for equality between men and women – being able to refer to sex is a prerequisite for recognising discrimination. But instead of supplying supporting arguments for its ideological volte face, the inquiry keeps referring back to transgender people: they are said to be the *raison d'être* of the change, it is for their sake that we need to uproot and redefine any mention of men and women wherever it might be found. And how large is this group? That is not stated, but after 700 pages, it says in passing that between 1960 and 2010, 767 people applied to have their legal sex changed.[115] Since then, the group has seen a yearly 100 per cent increase,[116] however, despite this dramatic increase we are still dealing with a group that is smaller than, for example, the Roma population in Sweden. It is hard to imagine that an inquiry on the situation of the Roma people would demand a complete change in the areas of sport, locker rooms, statistics and social security numbers. Why *all* social security numbers should be changed to make 0.5% of the population feel better, is not even brought up for discussion.

Coming back to the group which the inquiry purports to be concerned with, we see that very little seems to have changed since 2007. Transgender

---

113 Ibid. p. 526.
114 Ibid. p. 524.
115 Ibid. p. 682.
116 Ibid. p. 578.

people are still seen as deviant individuals who require "correction" by society. They are defined as individuals whose "legal sex assigned at birth does not agree with their gender identity and/or gender expression" but we are not told who has assigned the different "expressions" to the genders, nor why these should "agree with" the body. But make no mistake: congruence is still the ultimate goal. The only difference is that sex-change surgery is now referred to euphemistically as "gender affirming care and treatment." Thus, surgery does not change anything, but merely *affirms* the inner, true gender by "adjusting the body so that normality is restored."[117] The treatment is seen as successful as 91.9 per cent of patients achieve "gender congruence" following surgery.[118] Although no definition of man or woman or feminine or masculine is given in black and white, the above claims make plain the inquiry's view that the human being ought to be gender congruent. That in itself is astonishing: an aim so vague it cannot even be described in words.

Yet, the measures are very concrete: in order to create the new gender, individuals should be offered free hair removal, chest binders, breast prosthetics, penis prosthetics and wigs while awaiting surgery. The fact that not all local authorities offer this at present is described as unreasonable and discriminatory.[119] Yet only individuals born male are to be offered breast prosthetics and only those born women penis prosthetics and chest binders – flat-chested women or men with a micropenis need not bother! Biological sex, which only a minute ago was dismissed as a construct, is now of the utmost relevance in deciding who requires these material prosthetics and wigs. Help is not being offered to become anyone you would like to be, you can only become the other. Those who do not conform to the norms of their own gender but would still like to remain part of it are not viewed as the state's problem and can fend for themselves.

Nowhere in this lengthy tract is there even the slightest mention that a person is fine as s/he is and ought to be accepted even when s/he doesn't fit in with society's ideas of how a girl or a boy should look and behave. Nowhere is inequality between the sexes questioned. Patriarchal violence, discrimination and the fact that men and women have such different

---

117 Ibid. p. 554.
118 Ibid. p. 593.
119 Ibid. p. 566.

positions in society and are expected to dress and behave in different ways, seems to be a given and nothing that can be changed.

Nor does the inquiry raise the questions of why an increasing number of people suffer from gender dysphoria. The major difference over the ten year period is that the focus has shifted from an alleged concern about the well-being of transgender people to viewing them as some kind of avant garde showing the way towards a new world order. This avant garde has now taken on a *political* identity, rather than it being a diagnosis, and terms such as 'former transsexual' have been done away with. One is and remains a transgender person, an eternal identity that one cannot escape.

This is, however, an avant garde that is also given the role of guinea pig. When it comes to treatment, the caution of ten years prior is gone. The number of young people with gender dysphoria has increased significantly and the reason given here is "society becoming more tolerant."[120] Citing doctors Frisén, Söder and Rydelius, the inquiry claims that early treatment of children with gender dysphoria is crucial.[121] The importance of faster access to treatment is repeated over and over. Referrals – something needed for almost all healthcare, including no-nonsense things like podiatrists, psychologists and mammograms – ought to be abolished. *Real-life experience* (RLE), which involves living full-time in one's adopted gender role prior to surgery, is now seen as unnecessary and could be distressing – it is better to just have a mastectomy right away.[122]

The risks and consequences of treatment are hardly discussed. It is noted that 41 per cent of applicants have other diagnoses, e.g. autism, anorexia, mental health needs and substance abuse issues. According to a Swedish study, 38 per cent of children with gender dysphoria have an eating disorder.[123] But where the 2007 inquiry urges caution, the 2017 one concludes that other diagnoses are no obstacle to gender affirming treatment as there isn't necessarily a causal link. The explanation now offered is that mental health issues in these cases could result from "gender minority stress" and society's "negative views of trans people."[124]

---

120 Ibid. p. 224.
121 Ibid. p.226
122 Ibid. pp. 555–556.
123 Ibid. p. 283.
124 Ibid. p. 284.

Time and again, the inquiry states that transgender individuals' mental health is worse than that of the population at large and that many have considered suicide. The inquiry does concede that individuals who have transitioned are at higher risk of committing suicide, but in the next breath, hypothesises that the high rate of psychological ill-health after surgery may be "unrelated to gender dysphoria."[125] The conclusion is thus that mental ill health *before* surgery is always a result of being transgender, while mental ill health *following* surgery is not linked to being transgender. The reason given for this is that

> proven experience demonstrates that gender affirming treatment increases gender congruence (the harmony between different aspects of gender such as gender identity, gender expression, legal gender and even the body).[126]

Gender congruence in and of itself is thus seen as a guarantee for happiness, which is an interesting philosophical claim – yet unsubstantiated.

Finally, the inquiry's view of intersex and transgender people is noteworthy. They are often talked about in the same breath and as though they were the same group, except in one regard: medical intervention. Surgery on children with intersex variations is described as a human rights violation. Citing a UN report that equates these interventions to torture, the inquiry recommends laws be implemented to stop the possibility of conducting "irreversible, normalising genital surgery and involuntary sterilisation, which leads to suffering and stigmatisation."[127] However, when the inquiry refers to similar interventions on children it has named transgender, these are called a human right. The term is now 'treatment' and is "aimed at adjusting the body so that normal conditions are achieved." This sounds oddly similar to the "normalising surgery" on intersex children condemned by the UN. The fact that surgery in this case is also irreversible and often leads to infertility no longer seems to be a concern. On the contrary, long waiting times for surgery are now cited as the main problem.[128]

The frightening thing about this 900-page inquiry report is that the core group is mainly used as a lever for the ideological argument of altering

---

125 Ibid. p. 594.
126 Ibid. p. 593.
127 Ibid. p. 547.
128 Ibid. p. 545.

society's definition of sex. When it comes to the risks and proven side effects of treatment, the inquiry displays a rather shocking indifference to the risks for trans people. It is as though their bodies, their selves and their futures are something that do not need to be taken seriously. If they become infertile, if the hormones are proven harmful, if their mental health severely deteriorates following treatment: none of this seems a major concern. So who are all these changes for, really?

In place of the legal requirement to conduct an equality impact assessment, the inquiry lets itself of the hook by briefly stating:

> The equality perspective adopted by the enquiry goes beyond mere equality between women and men. The binary view of gender that continues to be the basis for equality policy and legislation is a clear problem. [...] Therefore, the enquiry describes the impacts of its recommendations from a non-binary equality standpoint.[129]

Thus, instead of adhering to the law and analysing the impact on women and men of its recommendations, the inquiry nonchalantly dismisses the basic tenets of equality politics and its report culminates in an onslaught on equality.

---

129 Ibid. p. 839.

CHAPTER 8

Help – My Son Loves Pink!

Up until about 2 years old, she is what we would call typically boy. Rough and tumble, loved to climb, short crew cut blond hair. At about 2½, we started noticing her doing some interesting things. She loved to put pajama pants on her head, where the elastic part was here, and it would be her hair. And she'd walk around saying, 'how do you like my hair?' like every night.[130]

Sabrina says that, looking back, she should have raised him 'as a girl' from the start but it was not until she took him to the newly opened Children's Gender and Sex Development Program at the Lurie Children's Hospital in Chicago that she was given the news: her son was, in fact, a girl. That child is now a teenager and takes the puberty blocking medication Lupron, like all the other young patients attending the program. Division head Robert Garofalo enthusiastically reports that the number of individuals seeking their help has increased dramatically, to the tune of two to three families a week. Now, 0.57 per cent of all young people in the state of Illinois identify as transgender and Garofalo explains that gender is who we are: it is innate and cannot be changed.[131]

The idea that gender identity is *innate* has gained widespread traction in the US and the UK. An oft-used graphic is the colourful 'gender identity scale', used in the UK for training the police, teachers and healthcare

---

130 <https://news.wttw.com/2013/08/29/childrens-gender-clinic>.
131 <http://www.dph.illinois.gov/sites/default/files/publications/2-15-17-OHP-HIV-factsheet-Transgender.pdf>.

workers. It consists of a line with the numbers one to 12. Number one is pink and bears the image of a Barbie doll. The colours range from pastel tones to darker ones all the way up to 12, which is brown and features a picture of G.I. Joe. In the accompanying text, we learn that "Gender identity is also on a spectrum. We all have our own unique identity. Where on a spectrum might your gender identity be?"[132]

Mermaids, the organisation behind the diagram, encourages teachers to locate themselves and their students on the scale as part of their training programmes. The message is a glaring paradox: everyone has their own, unique identity but must simultaneously fit into a one-dimensional spectrum whose reference points are a Barbie doll and a soldier. It seems like we would henceforth have to forget the words Nora uttered in 1879 in Ibsen's *A Doll's House*: "I believe that I am first and foremost a human being." Now, there are no longer any human beings: girls are literally Barbie dolls.

In the colourful children's book *Understanding Transgender*, available in US school libraries, a fact box informs us:

> There is a gender in your brain and a gender in your body. For 99 per cent of people, those things are in alignment. For transgender people, they are mismatched. That's all it is.[133]

What exactly does this 'gender in the brain' consist of? The example given is a young girl who "feels odd behaving in a way that a girl is supposed to behave … she doesn't feel like a girl inside and rejects girly things, such as sparkly pink stuff, long hair and dolls."[134] According to the book, this means she is not a girl but a transgender boy. The implication is that if you think pink glitter looks nice, you are a girl regardless of your genitals. One might also be tempted to ask what is meant by the statement that in 99 per cent of cases, gender in the brain and gender in the body are *congruent*? In what way are ovaries *congruent* with pink glitter?

No time is wasted on answering this, because it is now imperative to act fast. For the girl who behaves in the above way, the book recommends puberty blockers be assigned at the first sign of puberty. This is important, as breasts and hips can cause "depression, isolation, guilt and, for some,

---

132 <https://www.spectator.co.uk/article/don-t-tell-the-parents>.
133 Honor Head. (2017). *Understanding Transgender*, p. 15. London: Watts Publishing Group.
134 Ibid. p. 6.

extreme behaviour like self-harm and even suicidal thoughts."¹³⁵ Genitals can be surgically removed later but on this topic, the book only tells children that it "can take a long time."¹³⁶

Recent years have seen a proliferation of handbooks published – I count upwards of 35 – advising parents whose children are gender non-conforming. One such handbook is *The Gender Creative Child*, in which Diane Ehrensaft advises parents to be observant of their child's behaviour and keep an eye out for anything deviant in terms of gender. "Unfortunately, we don't have a blood test" to determine gender identity, she writes, but a trained eye can observe it in children even during their first year. One example would be a little girl never wanting to wear a dress. Her parents should take her to a psychologist and if the psychologist says it is a 'phase' they are mistaken, according to Ehrensaft. Of course, you could wait and see but "don't give it too much time, because then you have a miserable child."¹³⁷

The book's title, design and cover signal diversity. The words "creative" and "child," accompanied by a photo of a child with a bob haircut in a colourful dress call to mind freedom and play. Yet the message is that girls ought to like dresses and something is wrong if they do not.

Similar advice is repeated in the handbook *The Transgender Child*: "For example, a boy with long hair who prefers to wear bright-pink shirts and soft cotton flower-print paints" is a typical example of "significantly gender-variant or gender-nonconforming."¹³⁸ The authors give the example of a boy called Alejandro: "He would toddle into his older sister's closet to put on her dresses. He would wrap his hair in scarves and towels. He was always in his mum's makeup and shoes."¹³⁹ Letting children freely explore clothing and appearance is not an alternative in these books – instead, they need to be taken to a doctor to be diagnosed.

The picture book *I am Jazz*, which in libraries is found in the under-fives section, begins with the following sentence: "For as long as I can

---

135 Ibid. p. 20.
136 Ibid. p. 23.
137 German Lopez. (26 June 2016). 'How to know if your child is transgender, according to an expert'. *Vox*.
138 Brill and Pepper. (2008). p. 24.
139 Ibid. p. XIII.

remember, my favourite color has been pink."[140] Cute pictures accompany the text about Jazz:

> Most of all, I love mermaids. Sometimes I even wear a mermaid tail in the pool. My best friends are Samantha and Casey. We always have fun together. We like high heels and princess gowns, or cartwheels and trampolines. But I am not exactly like Samantha and Casey. I have a girl brain but a boy body. I was born this way![141]

We read that Jazz has never liked cars and has always preferred princess dresses, which his parents did not allow. They forced him to wear boys' clothes and were very confused when he didn't want to. At the age of three, they went to see a doctor and "the doctor spoke to my parents and I heard the word 'transgender' for the very first time." Following the appointment, the parents changed the boy's name to Jazz and explain that he is now a she. As a she, Jazz is now allowed to wear girl's clothes and grow his hair out. The book ends in the way story books in the under-fives section usually do: "And inside, I'm happy. I am having fun. I am proud!" February 4th has been designated 'Jazz and friends national day of school and community reading', meaning that primary schools all over the US read the book.

At six, Jazz Jennings became a global celebrity as the face of transgender children. At this young age, he started a public battle to play football on a girls' team. He was even so mature as to successfully set up a charity at the age of seven and was among *Time* magazine's 25 most influential teens at 14. Jazz was soon doing makeup commercials and had his own reality TV show, which included footage of the 18-year-old's 'farewell party' to the penis. Media around the world broadcast the story of this 'inspiring' journey, albeit slightly clouded over by the fact that Jazz reports not having any "libido" and "does not know what an orgasm is."[142] The parents proudly state that they are just "supporting" their child, although their disclosure that "they suspected she was a girl long before she herself did" appears to belie their previous claim.

---

140 Jessica Herthel and Jazz Jennings. (2014). *Dial Books for Young Readers*, New York: Penguin Group.
141 Ibid.
142 <https://people.com/tv/jazz-jennings-talks-sexual-stuff-orgasm-libido-doctor-before-gender-confirmation-surgery/>.

In Chile, the world's first school solely for trans children has been established.[143] The Fundación Selenna was created by Selenna's mother, who claims that she discovered her son was transgender when he was three and told her, "When I grow up, I'm going to be a woman." She promptly took him to a child psychologist, who explained that her child was most likely transgender. Selenna is now seven and Chile's best-known advocate for trans children's rights, with a school named after him.[144] The school's website carries pictures of students with placards stating: "The state doesn't recognise my rights. I am a boy. I want a self-ID law in Chile."[145]

Over and over again the same story is told: girls who refuse to wear dresses and are therefore left at home when the family attends a wedding; boys who want dolls and flouncy skirts but aren't allowed to wear them in public because their parents are worried they'll be bullied – all up to the day when the child is declared to have been born in the wrong body. Suddenly, boys are allowed to wear dresses and the parents are relieved: they finally have an answer as to why their child was behaving so strangely. Next, the long journey through hormone treatment begins. The body must now be sculpted to match its 'true' gender.

The idea of letting the boy be a boy and still wear the dress is so unfathomable it is not even mentioned in any of the books. Just being yourself is not an option. These books also never include examples of children who like *both* trousers and dresses, or whose sartorial tastes change over time. The fact that children go through a masquerade phase between three and five, when they often play at being a range of characters from animals to Disney characters, is not mentioned. Everything is black or white, either/or. Nor do the books explain why garments with one opening for both legs are to be associated with girls, while garments with one opening for each leg are associated with boys. In the worldview of these books, this is just the way it is. The fact that the former are worn by men across Asia and the Middle East is not mentioned. And why this obsession with the colour pink as the ultimate gender marker?

---

143 Eva Vergara. (23 January 2019). 'Chilean transgender school protects children from bullying'. *AP News*.
144 Victor Hugo Robles. (26 November 2016). 'Selenna, la niña trans chilena que se convirtió en un símbolo de orgullo', *Agencia Presentes*.
145 <https://twitter.com/FSelenna/status/1131523601151266817>; <https://twitter.com/FSelenna/status/1160735225871241216>.

In her interesting book *Rosa–den farliga färgen* (Pink – The Dangerous Colour), Fanny Ambjörnsson points out that pink was in fact associated with masculinity up until the 1950s. *Ladies' Home Journal* observed in 1918 that

> the generally accepted rule is pink for the boys, and blue for the girls. The reason is that pink, being a more decided and stronger color is more suitable for the boy, while blue, which is more delicate and dainty, is prettier for the girl.[146]

Thus, a culturally and historically specific gender marker is being peddled as a fixed inner essence, originating in our DNA. The interpretation that a boy who likes wearing makeup isn't really a boy is just that: one possible interpretation among many. Another could be that he is homosexual, or that embellishing oneself is an impulse that has no gender. Yet another would be that it is a natural male impulse which has been suppressed by patriarchal culture. After all, as Darwin noted in *The Descent of Man*, the male is more attractive than the female in practically all species. Feathers, horns, song, dance and colours are the male's way of attracting females, who are often grey and inconspicuous. What if the human male also has this natural drive – expressed in the little boy's desire for colourful dresses? What if the animals are right and us humans are wrong and it's the male that's supposed to be beautiful?

Trans guidebooks, however, offer only one explanation for the beauty-loving boy: he is really a girl. Gone is the initial talk of gender being a spectrum, the dissolution of the binary system and the 71 genders. Trans guidebooks do not offer 71 alternatives for gender reassignment, only two – and the two are mutually exclusive: if you are *not* a girl, you are *automatically* a boy and vice versa.

Almost all the handbooks on the topic set out to reassure parents who think their sons are gay. They should bear in mind that homosexuality is most likely a phase: "… some transgender teens first come out as gay before recognizing that they are actually transgender."

Parents are also encouraged to "help your teen understand that they do not have to be gay to be transgender."[147] In another handbook for parents of younger children, the authors explain that a boy who likes pink dresses

---

146 Fanny Ambjörnsson. (2011). *Rosa –den farliga färgen*, p. 10. Ordfront.
147 Brill and Kenney. (2016). p. 75 and p. 171.

would have been mistakenly seen as gay in the past but now we know better – he is a girl: "… the inner mismatch is not about sexual orientation but rather about gender."[148] *Understanding Transgender*, aimed at a younger readership, provides this explanation on page 8: "Trans is not the same thing as LGB!"

> Some young transgender people may go through a time when they believe they are LGB. This is because they are attracted to a person of the same sex. But as they come to understand their situation more, they realise they are attracted to that person as their preferred gender, not as their birth gender.[149]

Homosexuality is described in these books as a previously incurable problem to which a cure has now been found: gender reassignment. Thus, being gay can again be described as a phase and a camp boy can be transformed, as *The Trans Generation* unabashedly describes, from a "gender-nonconforming boy to a gender-conforming girl."[150] Even though these books all assure their readers that there is nothing wrong with being gay, non-binary, cis or anything else for that matter, and are at pains to point out that everyone must be respected, there is nevertheless an undertone saying homosexuality is too inappropriate for the traditional family and a bit too boring for the modern one. And while homosexuality does not require any interventions, gender reassignment is a project expected to involve the entire family. All family members are encouraged to begin therapy and "explore their gender history." Parents ought to start groups and ensure schools, family and surrounding society show support and do not use the wrong name or pronouns. Above all, nothing should be questioned. Your child should take the lead, as advised in *The Transgender Teen*.[151]

Several books give examples of what parents should say to their child and stern warnings about things that must not be said under any circumstances. Using the wrong pronoun, questioning or staying silent can lead to the child self-harming or ending up in prostitution.[152]

---

148 Brill and Pepper. (2008). p. 20.
149 Head. (2017). p. 8.
150 Ann Travers. (2018). *The Trans Generation – How Trans Kids (and their Parents) are Creating a Gender Revolution*, p. 64. New York University Press.
151 Brill and Kenney. (2016). p. 26.
152 Ibid. p. 237.

In addition, asking a teen to wait before beginning puberty blockers or surgery can be extremely harmful – even when the time scale is only six months.[153] Trans guidebooks reassure the parents that the sooner a child begins hormone treatment, the easier it will be for them to pass as their new gender in adulthood. *The Transgender Child* warns parents that not starting hormone treatment early enough can result in their child needing more surgical interventions later in life. It does acknowledge that puberty blockers will lead to their child's growth being halted but concludes this is a price worth paying.[154] An American mum reports about her ten-year-old daughter, who has felt like a boy for a year:

> I am not ready to talk about medicines and surgeries; I just can't go there yet. But our doctor, and the parents in my support group tell me I should think about it.[155]

The same book mentions that a boy undergoing hormone treatment for six months runs the risk of never being able to produce fertile sperm and that, in all likelihood, infertility will follow in future, but then breezily concludes: "remember that there are many, many ways to create a family!"[156] However, most books do not even mention the consequences of the interventions.

Thus, the moral that runs through these books is that children who are not old enough to have sex, vote, drink alcohol or get a tattoo, ought to undergo significant medical interventions which risk making them infertile for life – and parents must not even ask them to wait. Those who question the ethics of interventions on minors are lectured by Ann Travers, a Canadian anthropologist:

> Western societies lean heavily on constructions of this imaginary innocence and on romanticized discourses of childhood [...] This innocence, queer scholar Sarah Chinn notes, is an impossible fantasy yet this imagined 'child' invites normative understandings of sex, gender, race, social class and citizenship.[157]

Travers puts quotation marks around the word *child*, so that the reader understands that it is a "socially constructed demographic category [...]

---

153 Ibid. p. 238.
154 Brill and Pepper. (2008). p. 217.
155 Ibid. p. 19.
156 Ibid. p. 216.
157 Travers. (2018). p. 43.

that acts as a lens through which we can see more clearly how power operates."[158] Seeing these children as innocent is, according to Travers, denying them agency and promoting an image of white, privileged, heterosexual children. If, in all this, you find yourself worrying about a concrete flesh and blood child, you are advised to think again: the child is a social construct and anyone who thinks otherwise is a hair's breadth away from being a Trump voter! Interestingly enough, quotation marks are not used on the inside flap of the book's dust jacket where Travers is cheerfully described as living in Vancouver with her partner, three children and a dog.

Trans guidebooks for parents carry the message that a boy who likes lipstick needs to be diagnosed and a girl who likes playing with cars ought to be taken to a doctor. They should change their names and sex and their bodies must be altered through medical intervention. The general public might still believe that the trans issue is about being tolerant of adults who have felt their entire lives that they want to be the opposite sex and have gone through hell to get there – but what we are witnessing here is something else entirely: children are being diagnosed as deviant for using the wrong toys.

This is not about concern for trans people. This is not openness and tolerance. It is the exact opposite. This is the return of an extremely rigid understanding of gender that pathologises and medicalises children who do not behave according to narrow gender roles. We have to go back seventy years in time to find an equally invasive theory of gender. The idea being presented by gender identity theory is that each sex should be cleansed of all individuals who don't fit in, and who thus should be deported to the other sex. The fact that this can be hailed as progressive, and supported by humanists and feminists alike, is completely incomprehensible.

---

158 Ibid. p. 42.

CHAPTER 9

An Invisible Theory

"All trans people deserve respect" is the title of a manifesto signed by 300 Swedish intellectuals. Published in the culture section of the major daily *Dagens Nyheter* in October 2020, it provides an almost perfect summary of gender identity theory. Its first characteristic is that it does not, in fact, present itself as a theory.

At a quick glance, this manifesto resembles a love letter to trans people in general: "You are important and loved. We stand with you." Words like 'loved' and 'love' are used in a generalising, almost evangelistic manner. All trans people, the letter goes on to say, "deserve equal treatment and respect." In the midst of this declaration of love, all of a sudden this *opinion* appears:

> We all believe in the power of words and want to say the following with ours: Trans women are women. Trans men are men. Non-binary people are non-binary. Transgender rights are human rights.[159]

We are not enlightened as to why this is so, what definition of woman and man is being adopted, nor why love should require the opinions expressed. We are told only that this is how things are. Those who love trans people, we are to understand, must adopt gender identity theory, i.e. that sex means nothing, gender everything, that gender is a subjective feeling, that one is the gender one feels oneself to be and that it is even possible to place oneself outside the category entirely. Failure to do so implies not

---

159 300 litteraturprofiler. (26 October 2020). 'Transpersoners rättigheter är mänskliga rättigheter'. *DN Kultur.*

acknowledging trans people's human rights. This begs the question, which rights are being referred to here? Only one is mentioned in the letter: "All trans people must have the right to healthcare based on their needs."

The letter is signed by several thinkers and writers including feminists, who otherwise view questions about sex and gender, culture and society as complex matters deserving of lengthy intellectual discussion. What a woman is and how one becomes a woman are questions that have been pondered in many a substantial volume, but now the issue is said to be simple. It is actually about the power of the word: saying that an individual is a woman is sufficient to make them one. Here we have the ideological core of gender identity theory, gift-wrapped in love.

However, this stated love bears marks of fetishising. Trans people are portrayed as valuable objects on a pedestal, to be loved for the simple reason that they are part of a particular group. Nevertheless, the only concrete thing they are said to have a right to is healthcare. We can only assume that by healthcare, the signatories mean gender reassignment surgery and hormones. No mention is made of the right to safe, evidence-based healthcare, the right to not be subjected to untested treatments, or the right to fertility. Nor is it ever stated that individuals could also simply be accepted as they are. Trans people are portrayed in the manifesto as needing to be altered by medical intervention, which implies that there is something wrong with them. Arguing that one's only right is the right to be surgically reassigned, as one has an unfitting body – is surely quite the opposite of love?

To achieve hegemony, any new theory must combine and integrate major contemporary social and political currents in a previously unseen way. Gender identity theory does precisely that: it simultaneously juggles the concepts of diversity and normality. Its narrative is multi-layered and what appears to be one thing at a cursory glance, turns out to be another on a deeper level.

In the narrative's first layer, we are told about revolution and the ongoing dissolution of gender: we are told there are 71 genders and that even these are fluid. Everyone is unique and we can be whatever we want; there is no right or wrong. It is all about love, tolerance and respect and being different is a good thing.

In the next layer, we are suddenly told that gender is to be defined according to stereotypes: girls are passive and vain while boys are determined and want to be police officers. One's sex is now one's gender, and gender is back to being a psychological category with fixed delimitations. One has to fit in, be normal and *not* break the gender mould. The boy in the dress disrupts this mould – the girl in the dress does not. While in the past, they took away the dress from the child with a penis, now they take away the penis from the child with a dress. Freedom is the keyword – freedom to be like others. We are told that liberation from social norms can be attained by wanting to be normal, about the right to be different but also that not fitting into gender norms leads to lifelong suffering. We are told about being yourself by becoming someone else, that the binary model of gender must go – and then that blue is for boys and pink for girls! Genitals have nothing to do with gender, yet they must be altered to match gender identity. Sex is no longer to be defined by biology, but gender identity is described as innate. Through combining these very contemporary ideological elements, gender identity theory succeeds in appealing to homophobic traditionalists and ultraliberal progressive postmodernists alike. The former seek normality, the latter diversity: both find it in gender identity.

This story continuously claims to be abolishing certain concepts, only to then require a prior understanding of exactly the same concepts to be comprehensible. The words woman, man and sex are obsolete, yet the story is literally drenched in the very same words. We are told that sex is assigned at birth, thereby understanding sex as non-existent prior to the midwife's act of bestowing it upon the child. However, if sex did not exist, there would be nothing for the doctor to reassign – it would just be a matter of discourse. This narrative therefore relies on the fact that we *do* actually know that biological sex exists – otherwise the word 'trans' would be incomprehensible, since its referent is biological sex. Juggling opposing concepts, gender identity theory expects us to forget about biological sex and remember it at the same time.

You would be forgiven for being confused. Indeed, most people approach the subject with their hands up: "Don't ask me, I don't know enough, this is too complex!" This attitude is apparent not just with laypersons, but also with politicians, healthcare professionals, authorities and ordinarily undaunted intellectuals. The difficulty of navigating the concepts has meant that the issue has been left to 'experts' administering training to public officials and giving out certificates. Well-nigh all the books on the topic are fronted by a glossary of terms like 'cis-normativity' and 'gender incongruence', through the studying of which we are expected to adopt a new ideology. These glossaries have the appearance of a helpful paedagogical tool but they are also authoritarian – one does not argue with a glossary.

Yet another contradiction concerns the nature of the narrative itself. Despite the fact that it makes universal claims about sex, it purports to be a narrative for and about less than one per cent of the population. Vociferous statements about men and women are bandied about, yet any attempt to unravel them is quickly met with admonishment not to meddle, as this is a matter concerning trans people. It is as though the topic of sex has become a 'read-only' document. Those who wish to discuss the consequences for women of gender self-ID laws are told they ought to 'listen to trans people', even when the topic was the consequences for women in particular..

What we are dealing with is a theory of gender/sex that does not recognise itself as theory, and has a wholly unique capacity to dissolve and become invisible the moment it is criticised. Attempts to grab hold of it and examine it are met with an insistence that the inquirer must be *against trans people's very existence* – as though trans people were synonymous with a complete set of ideas of sex/gender. This conflation is bewildering since the majority of its ideological implications concern society at large, and most of the commentators, political parties and institutions promoting the theory are not themselves transgender. Nevertheless, transgender people are used as shields to protect the theory's ideological contents from scrutiny. Each time hypotheses regarding gender as an identity are presented, trans people are referenced, as though their well-being depended on everyone adopting this theory.

Those questioning gender identity theory are met with a barrage of accusations ranging from wanting to exterminate people, being transphobic and hating diversity to bearing responsibility for teen suicide and having blood on their hands – in short, enough to have even the most thick-skinned make a swift retreat. Whenever an unsuspecting person approaches the topic, it does not take long for them to step back apologising and promising never to say anything similar again (just ask Chimamanda Ngozi Adichie, Mario López or Martina Navratilova). Just like so many others, they were taught the same lesson: the topic of sex is not up for debate. Western societies are thus in the process of adopting a new *theory* of sex, yet we are not allowed to analyse it *theoretically*. When we try, it escapes our grasp and vanishes into thin air – all we are left with is a lonely man in a skirt telling us there is no theory here, just little old me! And everyone points fingers: how dare you be against this poor, vulnerable creature?

CHAPTER 10

The History of Sex : One-Sex and Two-Sex Theories

A central tenet of gender identity theory is that the 'gender binary' must be abolished. The idea that gender is 'binary' – and that this in itself would constitute oppression – has even made its way into various government policies which make reference to binary and non-binary individuals.[160]

The word binary is adopted from digital electronics, where it refers to a system containing only the values 0 and 1, and implies a similarly symmetrical arrangement when applied to gender. Using the term binary to describe gender became popular at the beginning of the millenium. Its use in the media was scarce up until 2010, when it surged. That the conventional view of gender was 'binary' and that the binary model was bad became accepted as truth. To counter this supposedly binary model of gender, theories about the gender spectrum are now flourishing, as are ones claiming it is a fiction that human beings are a two-sex species and that subversion is possible by simply placing oneself outside the binary model of gender by calling oneself 'non-binary'. The problem is no longer the hierarchy of power between the sexes but the binary arrangement of gender.

However, as history professor Thomas Lacqueur has shown in his impressive exposé *Making Sex: Body and Gender from the Greeks to Freud* (1992), the patriarchal view of gender has, in fact, never been binary but *hierarchical*.

---

160 Arbetsmarknadsdepartementet. (1 August 2019). 'Fler satsningar för att främja hbtq-personers lika rättigheter och möjligheter'.

Male thinkers from antiquity onwards reflecting on sex departed from a *one-sex theory*. For a long time, it was not even acknowledged that woman existed in her own right: instead she was a non-man, her defining feature being the *non*.

Until the end of the 18th century, sex was not primarily described in biological terms by prominent male western and Arab thinkers. Rather, it was explained in moral and religious terms. Women and men were not viewed as opposite sexes, but as one and the same: woman was simply a lesser man. Lacqueur observes there was "only one canonical body and that body was male."[161] From Aristotle and the ancient Greek physician Galen, to the 16th century Swiss anatomist Caspar Bauhin and the Royal Physician of King Henry VIII, there runs a common ideology: woman is a mere incomplete version of man. Swedish professor of history, Yvonne Hirdman, characterises this formula: A – not A, as the 'basic formula' of gender roles.

In antiquity, bodies were thought to be composed of natural elements, in particular earth, fire, air and water. According to this view, body fluids were the determining factor in human personality, and as analogies with nature were often used to describe gender, one can indeed say that gender was viewed as a spectrum – one could be more of a man or less of a man, depending on which natural elements were strongest. As Hirdman notes:

> While man was equated with solidity, structure and heat, his body being compared to the firmness of linen fabric, woman was seen as shapeless, cold, humid and lacking in form. Her body was compared to wool, absorbing fluids and losing its shape.[162]

According to Catholic priest and anatomist Gabriel Fallopius, who discovered and lent his name to the fallopian tubes in the mid-16th century, all male body parts were also present in the female body, in an inverted form. A common opinion among physicians and thinkers was that both women and men ejaculated and produced sperm and that both sexes had to orgasm for fertilisation of an ovum to take place. Galen thought that women produced weaker sperm than men and that woman's sperm therefore left less of an imprint on the child. Hippocrates, father of medicine, claimed that 'strong' and 'weak' sperm would produce boys and

---

161 Thomas Lacqueur. (1992). *Making Sex: Body and Gender from the Greeks to Freud*, p. 63. Cambridge: Harvard University Press.
162 Ibid. p. 29.

girls respectively.[163] Other thinkers believed women capable of creating babies on their own, hypothesising that those babies would lack a soul, since it was man who contributed the 'idea' and woman the raw material.[164] Ancient Greek obstetrician and gynaecologist Soranus asserted in the second century AD that a woman's genitals were the inverted version of a man's – a commonly held opinion.

Sex was thus an ideological tale about hierarchy, with the body making an appearance merely as an illustrative example. Consequently, descriptions of the body swayed wildly between various odd explanations: women's bodies had either too much or too little fluid. At one time it was sperm and another time the soul that determined sex. The common denominator is the suffix -er: colder, hotter, weaker. Man's body is described as normal, strong and dominant, while woman is described as an inferior version. The following are Aristotle's words from *On The Generation of Animals* (350 BC):

> We have thus stated for what reason the one becomes female and the other male. Observed facts confirm what we have said. Far more females are produced by the young and by those verging on old age than by those in the prime of life; in the former the vital heat is not yet perfect, in the latter it is failing. And those of a moister and more feminine state of body are more wont to beget females, and a liquid semen causes this more than a thicker; now all these characteristics come of deficiency in natural heat.[165]

This tale continues in a similar fashion for thousands of years. The one-sex theory also meant that sex was seen as fluid, not fixed. Isidore, Archbishop of Seville in the 600s, claimed that women who devoted themselves to dancing and singing used up their fluid and could no longer menstruate, thereby running the risk of becoming men. In the 16th century, it was widely believed that those whose behaviour did not conform to their gender role ran the risk of physical transformation and 'changing over' to the other sex. Both Renaissance philosopher, Montaigne, and surgeon, Ambroise Paré, repeat the cautionary tale of Marie, the girl who jumped

---

163 Ibid. p. 55.
164 Laqueur. (1992). p. 42.
165 'On the Generation on Animals', in Jonathan Barnes (ed.), *Complete Works of Aristotle*, Volume 1: The Revised Oxford Translation, Book IV, Ch. 2. Translation by Arthur Platt. Princeton University Press (1984).

over a ditch while chasing some escaped pigs. Suddenly, a fully developed penis and scrotum popped out of her vagina. She had to change her name to Germain and live out the rest of her life as a man. Doctors actually warned girls not to spread their legs too wide apart, or they might become men just like Marie.[166]

What we have here is the epitome of idealism, and what is patriarchy if not the triumph of idealism over materialism? Idealism holds that ideas trump reality, while for materialism, reality creates ideas. The fact that a power structure can be based on something that cannot be seen or proven to exist – namely fatherhood – instead of that which is of the utmost material flesh and blood – namely motherhood – is certainly an example of ideas trumping reality, of thoughts triumphing over what the eye can see.

However, for this to happen successfully, a constant re-asserting is also required – hence two thousand years of texts devoted to explaining how woman is merely an inferior version of man. If this really were a fact, all these texts would hardly have been necessary. For example, there is no two thousand year production of texts trying to convince us that plants cannot walk. Of course, this did not mean that all people were under the impression that woman actually was an inferior type of man or that bodies could transform themselves. Materialist philosophy tends to have a firmer foothold among the working classes than in the academy, especially so in farming communities where humans witness the power of life, death and reproduction with their own eyes.

Towards the end of the 18th century, a different discourse began to develop in medical science. The Enlightenment brought about a break with religion and the medical model gained precedence, leading to the gradual growth of models based on medical science in the scientific literature on sex. In 1889, Scottish scientists, Patrick Geddes and J. Arthur Thomson, published *The Evolution of Sex*, which argued that man and woman were each other's opposites. Man is "catabolic" while woman is "anabolic": man wastes energy while woman preserves it; man is energetic while woman is lazy; man ought to work while woman should be kept outside the labour market.[167] Here, woman is no longer a lesser version of man – they are two different entities, separate sexes, which supposedly

---

166 Ibid. p. 149.
167 Quoted in Moi. (1999). pp. 17–19.

complement each other. In 1913, British zoologist and embryologist Walter Heape stated, "it is certain that the Male and Female are essentially different throughout."[168]

Henceforth, woman begins to be studied separately, yet it is also at the time that woman is decoupled from man that her body begins to be seen as truly abnormal. She becomes a being that "is ravaged every month" according to historian Jules Michelet; even in the healthiest woman, "a worm gnaws away at the roots of life" according to pathologist Rudolf Virchow, and she easily succumbs to "nervous hyperagitation" according to physician Adam Raciborski. Removing the clitoris to cure mental ill health and epilepsy becomes a common practice in the latter half of the 19th century, as Carole Groneman observes:

> In a case in 1894, Dr. A. J. Block decided that a thorough physical examination of a nine-year-old girl brought to him by her mother was needed to determine the degree of her perversion (diagnosed as masturbation tending toward nymphomania). He touched the vagina and labia minora and got no response. "As soon as I reached the clitoris," he reported, "the legs were thrown widely open, the face became pale, the breathing short and rapid, the body twitched from excitement, slight groans came from the patient." Block stated emphatically that the child's violent response proved that the clitoris alone was responsible for her "disease." He performed a clitoridectomy.[169]

As long as the clitoris was considered an incomplete penis, removing it was not discussed – it is when it becomes an organ in its own right, unconnected to male genitals, that it begins to be labelled unnecessary and even dangerous.

Both one-sex and two-sex models are patriarchal. As Lacqueur states, they present "a problematic, unruly female body that is either a version of, or wholly different from, a generally unproblematic, stable male body."[170] While one model does not view woman as a human being at all, the other is overtly misogynistic. The first model is milder, but more condescending, while in the second, we have all-out war between the sexes. These two

---

168 Ibid. p. 11.
169 Carol Groneman. (1995). 'Nymphomania. The historical construction of female sexuality'. In Jennifer Terry and Jacqueline L. Urla, *Deviant Bodies: Critical Perspectives on Difference in Science and Popular Culture*, p. 236. Bloomington: Indiana University Press.
170 Laqueur. (1992). p. 36.

narratives of gender continue to co-exist well into our times. The one-sex theory is present in Freud's work, as noted by Luce Irigaray:

> Freud does not see two sexes whose differences are articulated in the act of intercourse, and, more generally speaking, in the imaginary and symbolic processes that regulate the workings of a society and a culture. The 'feminine' is always described in terms of deficiency or atrophy, as the other side of the sex that alone holds a monopoly on value: the male sex. Hence the all too well-known 'penis envy'. How can we accept the idea that woman's sexual development is governed by her lack of, and thus by her longing for, jealousy of, and demand for, the male organ?[171]

It is not until the second half of the 20th century that a new, revolutionary narrative emerges: there are no 'opposite' sexes! Each sex has its own logic, and woman must be understood *without* comparison to man. In the 1930s, scientists discovered that women ovulated and soon the connection between ovulation and menstruation was acknowledged. Yet we have to wait for the 1990s before the clitoris is mentioned in university literature for medical students.[172] Not until this time are its nerve endings described in detail in medical literature, so they can be safeguarded during operations.

From the 1940s onwards, a new narrative influenced by the women's movement begins to emerge. It holds that biological sex is unrelated to social hierarchy and that the sexes should be studied without the purpose of justifying gender roles. The idea that there are two biological sexes that are to be understood based on their respective bodies and not based on morality was a revolutionary insight. The body is not 'binary', rather for the first time the body is allowed to speak for itself, freed from the burden of comparisons to linen fabric and presumptions about hierarchies.

From the 1960s onwards, the notion of equality started making inroads into government policies. In Sweden, equality between the sexes became official policy. Statements about woman's role in society being that of wife and mother all but disappear from official documents. Sex roles become something unwanted, a throwback from a stale, archaic society. In the 1990s, sex roles are renamed gender roles. Gender, it is said, ought not to determine the position of the sexes in social hierarchy. On the

---

171 Luce Irigaray. (1985). *This Sex Which Is Not One*, p. 69. Translated by Catherine Porter. Ithaca: Cornell University Press.
172 Terry and Urla. (1995). p. 241.

contrary, gender is to be abolished, while the sexes are to be left standing in their own right, in their own naked bodies. As Yvonne Hirdman observes: "Seldom has a discourse triumphed so completely!"[173]

---

173 Hirdman. (2001). p. 175.

CHAPTER 11

Return of the One-Sex Theory

It is interesting, and quite disheartening to note that it only took 100 years for gender to reassert its dominance over sex. Twenty-first century gender identity theory contains exactly the same ideological assumptions as the one-sex model dominating from antiquity onwards that social hierarchy constitutes the *real* sex, while biology is rendered less relevant.

The one-sex theory contained narratives of effeminately-behaving men losing their penises, while gender identity theory tells the effeminate man to have it removed. The old theory claimed that men had warmer body fluids than women, while the new one asserts that a more powerful hormone exposure creates a child whose personality will be masculine. Both theories are based on an identical belief in invisible liquids which are said to determine whether an individual becomes dominant or inferior, masculine or feminine. Even the suffix (-er) is the same when describing the sexes: his fluids are stronger, bigger, mightier.

We are told anew that gender roles are innate. While the one-sex theory attributed this to the temperature of body fluids and the wind and shapelessness of the female, gender identity theory puts it down to genes, hormones and the brain. The old theory explained gender using analogies of cloth and wool; the new one has substituted these with analogies from information technology.

Gender is yet again being configured as a spectrum, now with GI Joe on one end and Barbie on the other. It's very simple: the broader one's shoulders, the more interest one has in weapons and consequently the more masculine one is. In contrast, the slimmer one's waist, the more interest one has in dresses – the more feminine one is.[174] Sex no longer exists in its own right, and has again become a personality trait: the more woman you are, the less man, and vice versa.

With this return of idealism, the body has taken on a subordinate significance, as it is now *personality* that determines gender. Gender determines sex, and sex must succumb, and so the body must be adapted. The main difference between today's one-sex model and that of the past is that then, one had to rely on magic to imagine sex changes whereas today we have access to hi-tech medical procedures. Nevertheless, the ideological content remains exactly the same in gender identity theory: it is laden with prejudices about men, women, how they behave and their place in hierarchy. And woman is, again, being relegated to a non-man.

---

[174] <http://www.butterfliesandwheels.org/2019/the-barbie-gi-joe-scale/>.

CHAPTER 12

What Happens to Biological Determinism When There Is No Body?

Despite the fact that gender identity theory is a clear return to biological determinism, it is, astonishingly, its critics who are labelled determinists. Women who criticise gender identity theory from a feminist perspective are often told that we are closet conservatives, or 'bedfellows of the Right'. We are labelled bigots, tyrants, police, judges and are treated harshly, to say the least. Interestingly, those who really *do* take a conservative stance on this matter are not subjected to the same treatment at all, receiving instead a respectful subservience. Philosopher Torbjörn Tännsjö attacks both The Swedish Women's Lobby and J. K. Rowling in an article in Sweden's major daily *Dagens Nyheter*, calling them "conservative feminists" due to their "conventional binary division of the sexes." While Tännsjö accuses feminists of conservatism, he makes no mention of the actual conservative thinkers involved in the trans debate.

Conservative male writers like British author Douglas Murray, Canadian psychologist Jordan B. Peterson, American journalist Austin Ruse and Swedish authors Fredrik Svenaeus and Ivar Arpi have all been extremely critical of gender identity theory. They take issue with the idea that biology no longer matters and that anyone may freely choose their gender, and are particularly opposed to the idea that the new narrative be forced on society at large.

Psychologist Jordan B. Peterson became world renowned for his objections to Canada's Bill C-16, which criminalises addressing a person with anything other than his/her/their preferred pronouns. Peterson denounces the pronoun hysteria as nonsense and equates C-16 to an authoritarian ideology akin to Maoism: "There's a difference [...] between saying that there's something you can't say, and saying that there are things that you have to say."[175] In his book *The Madness of Crowds*, Douglas Murray criticises aspects of gender identity theory, such as the argument that self-identified trans women (men) ought to be permitted to compete in women's sports. This is an area where conservative and feminist thinkers often hold the same opinion. And as feminists are increasingly marginalised from the left wing spaces where we used to belong, conservatism is willing to embrace us, offering freedom of speech and a refreshing break from the word salad that contemporary left wing debates tend to become. With disparaging phrases such as 'woke crowd' or 'social justice babble', conservatives dismiss it all with a laugh. It might be tempting for feminists to adopt these catchwords, which can appear almost like a way to cut the Gordian knot instead of having to untangle it. However, as these conservative thinkers are new to debates on sex, or do not seem to have studied feminist thinking, they often mix up terms and confuse gender, queer, trans, marxism and liberalism to the extent that they believe Judith Butler is a trans activist *and* a radical feminist at the same time (neither is in fact the case) or that marxists are postmodern. They also tend to deliberately ignore feminist opposition to gender identity theory, instead bashing feminists for not speaking out and pretending they were the first to raise their voice, as is painfully shown in the case of filmmaker Matt Walsh, who refuses to acknowledge the existence of feminists like Meghan Murphy and claims the role of women should be to support his project.

And despite their opposition to it, many conservative writers are willing to affirm the biological determinist aspects of gender identity theory. In his book *Det naturliga* (On the Natural, 2019), Fredrik Svenaeus criticises queer and trans activists wanting to "completely overthrow gender roles" and says they should instead "encourage those individuals who by nature were born in the wrong body and who therefore wish to

---

175 Kelefa Sanneh. (26 February 2018). 'Jordan Peterson's gospel of masculinity'. *The New Yorker*.

change this."¹⁷⁶ For Svenaeus then, as long as something is natural – it is fine. Douglas Murray is equally prepared to accept the thesis that people can be born in the wrong body, as long as this reinforces gender roles. He writes about Jan (previously James) Morris:

> For instance, Morris described the fundamentally different viewpoints and attitudes between the sexes. So, as a man, James was far more interested in the 'great affairs' of his time, whereas as a woman, Jan acquired a new concern 'for small affairs'. After becoming a woman Jan writes, 'my scale of vision seemed to contract, and I looked less for the grand sweep than for the telling detail'.¹⁷⁷

Murray adds with satisfaction, "not much of this would satisfy a modern feminist." As long as what a trans person does confirms existing gender roles, it meets with Murray's approval. As long as the status quo around gender roles is maintained, it does not really matter to Murray whether a few people quietly hop over to the other side – in the end, this could even be a good thing. After being treated to Jan's inside information about women lacking the capacity to think about politics as they are more interested in 'small stuff', Murray goes on to happily inform us that Jan didn't dislike male attention, such as when a taxi driver snuck up and placed a not unwanted peck on her (his) lips. Murray makes it clear through his upbeat tone that this is how a real woman should feel.

How are we to interpret all of this? We must understand that while alliances on strategic issues, such as women's sports, can be useful, conservative thinkers actually hold an idea very similar to gender identity theorists. Conservatives want to maintain the union of sex and gender, but believe *sex determines gender*. Thus, women are feminine, men are masculine, and that is the way things are supposed to be. Advocates of gender identity theory also want to keep the two concepts together but conversely hold that *gender determines sex*. In other words: those who are feminine are women, those who are masculine are men, and that is the way things are supposed to be. Same coupling, different order, which amounts to a kind of postmodern biologism. Conservatives and gender identity theory proponents alike believe in gender congruence – the idea that a

---

176 Fredrik Svenaeus. (2019). *Det naturliga. En kritik av queerteorin, transhumanismen och det digitala*, p. 42. Möklinta: Gidlunds.
177 Douglas Murray. (2019). *The Madness of Crowds: Gender, Race and Identity*, p. 194. London: Bloomsbury.

particular body matches a particular personality – but gender identity theory demands that mind should rule over matter. Biology is no longer destiny, instead our minds must mould our bodies according to their wishes: we are the masters of our bodies, not the other way around. It is a very logical evolution, as patriarchy intersects with hi-tech neoliberal capitalism, and the subjugation of nature takes one step further. In a world where man can dominate earth, why should his own body limit him? With gender identity theory, he imprints his ideas on his own flesh, showing it that he is the master, and that his power is limitless. Mind over matter, brains over bodies, technology over nature, gender over sex.

Yet even though the conservative is old-fashioned and the gender identity activist is seen as progressive, when they spot a 'tomboy' or a 'sissy' they both have a similar reaction: they want to change her or him! One wants to change their behaviours, the other wants to change their bodies, but none of their theories has room to tolerate them as they are.

Countering this, feminists have long held that sex ought to be liberated from gender. Sex, say feminists, has nothing to do with the social construct, the oppressive hierarchy, the rotten set of sex-stereotypes that is called gender. For feminists, sex is unproblematic, and gender the culprit that should be abolished. For feminist theory, the tomboy and the sissy do not pose a problem.

CHAPTER 13

How Feminism Started Loving Gender

Something odd has taken place. Suddenly, a part of feminism has begun adopting gender identity theory. How is it that so many feminists can fall for this and how did gender roles become feminism's best friend? How could biological determinists be enemies a few moments ago and allies the next? How is it that Swedish political party Feministiskt Initiativ can embrace the idea that gender is a construct *and* a fixed identity simultaneously, as Sara Edenheim and Malin Rönnblom note – a construct for women, a fixed identity for trans people?[178] How can the Left claim to be materialist while at the same time say that anyone who says they are a woman automatically becomes one?

When we reflect on it, the idea of gender identity being innate is in complete opposition to the core principles of feminism. Feminism and biologism came into being contemporaneously at the end of the 19th century and have, since that time, been in conflict with one another. From Frida Stéenhoff to Virginia Woolf and Betty Friedan, the women's movement has fought for sex to refer to sex organs only and has been adamant that it does not determine one's role in life.

---

178 Sara Edenheim and Malin Rönnblom. 'Representations of equality. Processes of depoliticization of the citizen-subject.' In Hilde Danielsen, Kari Jegerstedt, Ragnhild L. Muriaas and Brita Ytre-Arne (eds). (2016). *Gendered Citizenship and the Politics of Representation*, pp. 75–76. Basingstoke: Palgrave Macmillan.

Since the beginning of the 20th century, feminist thinkers have put forth the notion that the biological differences between the sexes did not automatically lead to inequality and that inequality was instead a consequence of patriarchy. This notion was clarified at the end of the 1970s with the bifurcation of the terms 'sex' and 'gender'. The word gender (from the latin *genus*: origin, sort, kind) henceforth only referred to *preconceptions* surrounding sex. Simone de Beauvoir, writing in the 1940s, never used the term gender, yet the term perfectly sums up her thinking inasmuch as it separates the physical body from patriarchal constructs. Yvonne Hirdman, who introduced the term in Sweden, stated that gender was "cleaner" than the terms 'sex' and 'sex role', as it referred only to the discourse around sex and thereby opened up the possibility of a world where that discourse would be obliterated and sex would only mean – sex.[179] The word gender gave feminism a language which liberated biology from the system created by patriarchy. Sex was a biological reality, no more no less. Sex could thus be declared unproblematic: patriarchy's prisoner was freed. Instead, the culprit was gender, which came to denote a patriarchal social order and all that feminism wished to abolish. (Other, more prosaic reasons to adopt the word gender also existed. As Professor of Literature, Toril Moi, noted, the US women's movement preferred the term 'gender' because the word sex called to mind intercourse.)

When biological determinism made a brief but vocal appearance in the 1990s, it was defeated by a unified feminist movement both inside and outside academia. The '90s was a time when women all over the industrialised capitalist world began seriously challenging men in positions of power. Women who received university education in the '70s had been moving upwards in the labour market and were breaking through the glass ceiling. At the very same time, the market for esoteric theories about the difference between men's and women's brains exploded. In 1993, best-selling titles included *Brain Sex: The Real Difference Between Men and Women*, and *Men Are from Mars, Women Are from Venus*. Poet Robert Bly's book *Iron John* gave rise to a men's movement based in mythology which led to hundreds of thousands of men meeting up in forests to find their lost, wild manhood. Another contributor to this debate, Swedish journalist Maria Borelius – later a rightwing member of parliament –

---

179 Yvonne Hirdman. (2001). *Genus – om det stabilas föränderliga former*, p. 16. Stockholm: Liber.

claimed that new mothers had a lower IQ due to hormone production, and that motherhood thus was incompatible with the rat race of the labour market. Professor Annika Dahlström became a frequent interviewee, spouting opinions about fathers being unsuitable parents and women born in the 1940s being successful due to having received "testosterone in the womb." Delivering these and other clichés about sex became a massive business, to the extent that anyone who worked in a female dominated industry in the 1990s probably attended a conference entitled 'Feminine Style of Management!' and heard speakers address audiences about male order and female chaos and how women are more childlike than men.

1990s biological determinism was a mixture of entrepreneurial spirit, Jungian philosophy and patriarchal counter-revolution. However, it would not be long-lived. Susan Faludi named it and denounced it in her important book *Backlash*, and all over the western world feminist writers tore the idea of a 'natural' female essence to pieces. Perhaps the main reason why biological determinism could not achieve hegemony in the '90s was that it was ill-timed. Postmodernism and neoliberalism fit better with late capitalism, and it was not long before the 1990s would produce a sexual theory much more in accord with its time.

Enter Judith Butler's *Gender Trouble*. An unlikely bestseller, written in an evasive and opaque style, *Gender Trouble* transformed universities and political subculture. The reason? It was postmodernism applied to the topic of sex. Since what characterises postmodernism is the absence of a reference point, and the reference point of sex is – well, sex – material, physical, biological sex all but disappeared.[180] Sex, maintained Butler, does not exist by itself – or at least, we can never perceive of it without being tainted by the notion of gender. Sex, according to Butler, has been gender all along. Ever the poststructuralist, Butler postulated that nothing exists beyond discourse, i.e. that there is no 'pure' material reality outside language. In her thinking, one *becomes* a man or a woman through being referred to as such. In *Gender Trouble*, Butler wrote that the term woman is "a construct that cannot be said to originate or to end," "an ongoing discursive practice" and "the repeated stylization of the body."[181]

---

[180] Victor Malm. (2019). *Är det detta som kallas postmodernism?* pp. 61–62. Malmö: Ellerströms förlag.

[181] Judith Butler. (1991). *Gender Trouble: Feminism and the Subversion of Identity*, p. 43. London: Routledge.

> No longer believable as an interior 'truth' of dispositions and identity, sex will be shown as a performatively enacted signification (and hence not 'to be'), one that, released from its naturalized interiority and surface, can occasion the parodic proliferation and subversive play of gendered meanings.[182]

Chez Butler, gender is primarily an expression, a "corporeal style" – and note here the emphasis on appearance, as opposed to de Beauvoir, for whom being a woman was a material situation. In Butler's understanding, one can never really become a woman or a man, only make constant futile attempts. These attempts are doomed to fail since they subvert themselves, in what was later dubbed 'queer leakage', meaning a persistent effort to appear masculine can give off a self-obsessed vanity that will appear feminine, and vice versa.

In Butler's footsteps followed the queer movement, whose repeated subversion and disruption of gender roles came to be emblematic of the noughties. Drag (dressed-as-a-girl) became the main expression of the queer movement.[183] What is important to note here is that queer theory did not see identities as innate or fixed. There is no essence, nothing 'is', everything is created through language, or at least we can never access an unfiltered reality beyond discourse. As queer theorist and historian Sara Edenheim explains: "No one is guilty of their gender identity, their feelings, their desires. No one is totally innocent either."[184] Despite the fact that Butler later gave a more nuanced account in *Bodies that Matter*, it is the thinking in *Gender Trouble* that became hegemonic.

As the new millennium began, biological determinism had been defeated, but biology itself was thrown out with the bathwater and along with it, material reality. Within academia, this meant fewer and fewer references to women and men: the new generation of students did not write about women's work but about the image of femininity. They wrote not about honour crimes themselves but about contemporary discourses regarding these, not about women's lives but about preconceptions regarding what constitutes a real woman. Empiricism thus gave way to discourse analysis, with discourse taking the place of reality and reality

---

182 Ibid. p. 44.
183 Martin Berg and Jan Wickman. (2010). *Queer*, p. 42. Stockholm: Liber förlag.
184 Sara Edenheim. (1 February 2018). 'Ett samhälle där kroppens begränsningar drabbar alla lika'. *Feministiskt Perspektiv*.

ending up inside quotation marks. In postmodern logic, base and superstructure switch places, meaning ideas are seen as the foundation and matter as the result. This meant that gender was torn away from its foundation (sex), took on a life of its own and began wandering around academia by itself, leaving in its wake labour, reproduction, production and living conditions. Women's Studies was rebranded as Gender Studies and men's violence against women as gender-based violence.

This shift from woman to gender was often explained by assertions that it was high time to start including research on men, or to perform "critical masculinity studies," as it is often called. Of course, this had a flipside: research funds previously reserved for women could from now on also be assigned to research projects about men, as they were also included in the term gender. Gender increasingly came to be referred to as something people *do*, rather than a *system* for classifying people.

And at the turn of the millennium, something occurred with the term gender: it stopped wandering around, froze and turned to stone. Suddenly it was no longer a system to be subverted, but an individual identity – no longer a cultural construct, no longer even something people do. At that point, gender became something a person *is*, an eternal inner essence beyond culture and power structures, even beyond genitalia. Now, gender is said to be something innate that no society on earth can change. We are being told that gender emanates from within us and only we ourselves can know its truth – list your pronouns and I will know who you are! Once you discover your gender, there is no turning back and no doubt – this is the real you. You 'are' woman, man, non-binary, trans or agender and have therefore always been so.

This is a giant step away from queer theory. In fact, postmodernism and queer theory seem rather outdated. They were merely stepping stones that abolished the notion of material sex, whose ruins the new-fangled essentialism was then built on. The grand narrative now returns, claiming to own the truth about gender. Cue the clichés about pink/blue, dolls/weapons, makeup/machines, passive/active.

This ideological transformation from sex, to sex/gender, to gender, to gender/sex, represents a shift from metaphysics to dialectical materialism to postmodernism to postmodern essentialism. However seamless the change might appear, it is important to note that in gender identity theory, we are dealing with an idea that diverges significantly from queer theory in its basic tenets. Whereas queer theory saw everything as discourse and nothing as real, gender identity theory in fact sees gender as very real and innate. Whereas queer theory was engaged in a constant, parodic, satirical subverting of gender, gender identity theory establishes that the discovery of one's true gender is a final verdict – and a deadly serious matter. Whereas Butler postulated that gender was an external system, imposing itself on us through interpellation, making us succumb, gender identity theory sees gender as a truth coming from inside.

This postmodern essentialism is strange indeed, a biological determinism without biology, where the idea of becoming who you want to be is combined with the belief in gendered souls. Yet this is the only possibility for patriarchy to return inside neoliberalism. This way, one maintains notions of individual liberty at the same time as strict rules on gender return with a full blast. (Patriarchy also returns outside the neoliberal paradigm, with a conservative backlash on abortion rights and a clamping down on female sexuality, but this current is unable to fully penetrate ideologically progressive societies and circles.) Biological determinism of old was monolithic and fateful: born in a woman's body, you were told your brain was unfit for higher office. There was no escape. Anyone trying to break the boundaries would hit their head against a wall. As opposed to that, biological determinism of today, gender identity-style, is fragmented: body and soul are said to each have a sex of their own. Thus, an escape route is inbuilt: anyone who feels their gender role is too narrow is given the possibility to change and find a 'truer' self. Both determinisms juxtapose gender and sex, but in reverse order: sex determines gender versus gender determines sex.

Now – and here we come to the baffling part – when biological determinism returns in this guise, it is not met by the same resistance at all! It was self-evident that feminists would oppose *Women are from Venus*, but the prevailing response from feminist political parties, feminist academia and many feminist intellectuals to gender identity theory is one of uncritical praise. Incredibly, it is the very same individuals who were the harshest critics of biological determinism that are now peddling the theory that we are all born with an innate gender identity.

Ulrika Westerlund, former editor-in-chief of the feminist magazine *Bang*, notes that she became a feminist precisely because of the movement's resistance to biological determinism and "statements about the strengths and weaknesses of girls vs boys, women vs men."[185] In the preface to an anthology on biological determinism from 2002, she wrote: "If we accept the notion that our biology limits what we can do and who we are, then capacity for political change is also limited."[186] Fifteen years later, Westerlund was appointed as the government's investigator in its inquiry on transgender people in Sweden which, as discussed earlier, is one long ode to the *new* biological determinism. It maintains that our brains are gendered, that individuals who do not conform ought to be reassigned in order to attain 'gender congruence' and is devoid of any critical outlook on what makes gender in the first place. Why girls who do not want long hair are not girls, how gender is related to patriarchy and whether gender congruence is an ideal compatible with gender equality – these questions are left unasked. In fact, the magazine *Bang* itself has undergone a metamorphosis and now upholds gender identity theory without any debate about it. The same is true of the Left Party and Feministiskt Initiativ, which are the two political parties that have gone furthest in their belief that sex is to be replaced by gender in legislation. Twenty years ago, Brändén's article about men being born to hump and women being born to arch would have elicited howls of derisive laughter, yet now he is seen as an ally – no questions asked. The point is that he is 'in favour of trans rights'. Discussions that were commonplace in the '80s and '90s about beauty myths and sexist stereotypes are curiously nowhere to be seen when the number of young girls who want to be boys is increasing by several thousand per cent.

Even Judith Butler has been criticised for not respecting the idea that gender is innate. Her argument that there is no sex, only gender, rejected *all* innate identities – 'cis' as well as trans. Under continued pressure from the very people who one would think to be her allies, Butler was forced to distance herself from her life's work in an interview:

> *Gender Trouble* was written about 24 years ago, and at that time I did not think well enough about trans issues. Some trans people thought that in claiming that gender is performative that I was saying that it is all a fiction, and that a person's felt sense of gender was therefore 'unreal'. That was never my intention. I sought to expand our sense of what

---

185 Ulrika Westerlund. (2002). *Inledning ur Hjärnsläpp. Bang om biologism*, p. 7. Viborg, Denmark: Bang förlag.
186 Ibid.

gender realities could be. But I think I needed to pay more attention to what people feel, how the primary experience of the body is registered, and the quite urgent and legitimate demand to have those aspects of sex recognized and supported. I did not mean to argue that gender is fluid and changeable (mine certainly is not). I only meant to say that we should all have greater freedoms to define and pursue our lives without pathologization, de-realization, harassment, threats of violence, violence, and criminalization. I join in the struggle to realize such a world.[187]

So the only thing she wanted was to uphold the UN Human Rights Declaration! Butler cannot even make an eloquent retreat based on her own theoretical values, and instead has to find refuge in individualism. Throughout the interview, she battles to consolidate her own theory with gender identity theory. How to stick to her thesis and appease the trans movement at the same time? This proves impossible, as there is no basis in Butler's thinking for gender identity – Butler, as we know, being the author of the notion that gender is created through interpellation, i.e. from outside. She thus lacks the theoretical tools to explain how a person can have a true inner gender. Luckily for her, she is also a master of ambiguity, which now proves to be her salvation. Here is her answer to the question of whether sex and gender are social constructs:

> I think that there are a variety of ways of understanding what a social construct is, and we have to be patient with terms like these. We have to find a way of understanding how one category of sex can be 'assigned' from both and another sense of sex can lead us to resist and reject that sex assignment. How do we understand that second sense of sex? It is not the same as the first – it is not an assignment that others give us. But maybe it is an assignment we give ourselves? If so, do we not need a world of others, linguistic practices, social institutions, and political imaginaries in order to move forward to claim precisely those categories we require, and to reject those that work against us?

What then, is gender, and how is it to be understood? In all ways at once, according to Butler: everyone has the right to think that gender is whatever they want it to be. It is nothing, and yet it is something, both at the same time, if you wish. Though not so for lesbian feminist theorist Sheila Jeffreys, whose opinions Butler labels "feminist tyranny" and a

---

[187] <http://radfem.transadvocate.com/gender-performance-an-interview-with-judith-butler/>.

"moral prison" in the very same interview. Butler also accuses Jeffreys of appointing herself "to the position of judge" and "policing trans lives and trans choices" – Jeffreys seems to hold positions at all levels of the criminal justice system, from police to judge to prison to tyrant, which is quite an impressive achievement for one lesbian feminist author.

Yet it is not only feminist thinkers who are suddenly being viewed as the devil incarnate. The very tenets of feminism itself have now become hate crimes. Any Swedish girl, brought up in the '80s and '90s, remembers Nina Björk's classic introduction to her important *Under det rosa täcket* (Under the pink blanket) from 1996:

> When you go to a public toilet, you choose between two doors. If you were born with a vagina, you choose the door with this symbol: 🚺 This inconspicuous sign contains a statement about what it means to be a woman: women are those who wear skirts.[188]

Björk continues that in fact, "everyone knows what/who a woman is: a person with a vagina and breasts."[189] Her book was a scathing critique of biological determinism, more specifically the idea that a particular body is automatically associated with certain clothing. The quote above is a very clear example of the difference between sex and gender – gender is the skirt, sex is the vagina. The question raised is clear: what have vaginas actually got to do with skirts?

Today, though, the same sentence – "everyone knows what/who a woman is: a person with a vagina and breasts" – is seen by gender identity theory as incredibly controversial. When Kellie-Jay Keen-Minshull from the UK women's movement printed posters and t-shirts with the text "woman: adult human female" in 2018 in order to make the feminist stance on the matter clear, the posters were labelled transphobic "hate speech," and were removed as it was said they made people feel "unsafe."[190] We thus find ourselves in a peculiar situation in which the dictionary definition of a woman is viewed as extremism and hate.

This has led to the odd situation in which large swathes of feminists adopt a form of doublethink: gender is a social construct for everyone

---

188 Nina Björk. (1996). *Under det rosa täcket*, p. 9. Stockholm: Wahlström and Widstrand.
189 Ibid. p11.
190 'Woman billboard removed after transphobia row'. (26 September 2018). *BBC News*.

except trans people, for whom it is an inner essence. According to this notion, trans people would be the only ones with a true relationship to gender, while everyone else is under the influence of social norms. Now, this begs the question: how tenable is it to claim that trans people have a pure relationship to gender *and* oppose gender roles from a feminist standpoint? If trans people have an innate gender identity, doesn't this mean that all people have one? Is it possible to establish that indecision, passivity and vanity are 'feminine' traits without this negatively affecting women's position in society? Julia Serano, trans activist and author, writes in *Whipping Girl*:

> Instead of attempting to empower those born female by encouraging them to move further away from femininity, we should instead learn to empower femininity itself. [...] For many of us, dressing or acting feminine is something we do for ourselves, not for others. It is our way of reclaiming our own bodies and fearlessly expressing our own personalities and sexualities."[191]

Serano puts forward the idea that it is not women but *femininity* that is oppressed. Rather than standing up for women, we should be standing up for femininity. According to Serano, feminism has mainly attracted to its cause masculine women who dislike gender roles and who do not understand that for many, femininity "simply feels right."[192] Serano maintains that so many women "gravitate towards femininity" because it "resonated with them on a profound level."[193]

One wonders why Serano thinks it should be those 'born female' who ought to be encouraged to empower femininity by behaving and dressing in a 'feminine' way. If femininity has nothing to do with women, but is a dressing style like any other, completely independent of sex, such as casual chic or bohemian – why even speak about women? What do we have to do with it? This is a perfect example of how gender identity theory first separates gender from sex, only to bring it crashing back into sex. As Toril Moi observes, "every general theory of gender or 'femininity' will produce a reified and clichéd picture of woman."[194] It is not possible to establish

---

191 Julia Serano. (2007). *Whipping Girl – A Transsexual Woman On Sexism and the Scapegoating of Femininity*, p. 18. New York: Seal Press.
192 Ibid. p. 338.
193 Ibid. p. 339.
194 Toril Moi. (1999). *What is a Woman?* p. 7. Oxford: Oxford University Press.

a connection between femininity and pink dresses without this having negative consequences on women themselves, no matter how much one stubbornly insists that 'femininity' and 'woman' are two different things.

CHAPTER 14

How Patriarchy Incorporated Its Dissidents

> I sure feel like a woman, very feminine, but I'm not a woman. My mother who gave birth to me is a woman, like you and you [points at reporters] but I'm a fag and as gay as they come! Don't try and tell me that those who have had surgery are women because they feel like it, because a woman is my mother, who has a uterus! These girls are men on the inside, no matter how many operations they have![195]

These are the words of the legendary La Veneno, outspoken Spanish transsexual artist and cultural icon with a background in prostitution and one of the first to give trans people a face in Spain. La Veneno's public persona embodied duality: looking like a bimbo with enormous boobs while hollering profane insults in a baritone voice and joking about loving his micropenis. Veneno was truly walking 'on the railroad track' in the spirit of the contemporary song by Spanish band Mano Negra; expanding the limits of what it meant to be a man without ever fleeing manhood; embracing femininity without claiming womanhood. It was a truly liminal life, and a revolutionary stance. In his autobiography, La Veneno writes about his love for extreme femininity and about wanting to be an Übermensch – not an ordinary woman, not an ordinary gay man or an

---

195 La Veneno. (11 November 2016). 'Las 20 mejores frases de La Veneno por las que siempre la recordaremos'. Bekia.es.

ordinary transvestite.¹⁹⁶ It is fascinating to note how the female gender role, so resisted by women, seemed tailor-made for La Veneno, to the point that one wonders if femininity actually is made for gay men and has nothing to do with women at all. Veneno's autobiography is a very important addition to the understanding of gender roles, since it helps us to understand what in men's treatment of women is reserved for women and what is also applied to the male transvestite.

In 2020, four years after La Veneno's death, Spanish TV made a series about his life. However, the Veneno that appears on TV is a cleaned-up, revisionist and boring one. La Veneno is no longer a feminine transsexual gay person with all the complexities that this entails, but a heterosexual woman. Nothing else. Just a heterosexual woman born in the wrong body. None of the old daringness is left, none of the gayness either, instead we are served a politically correct narrative about a woman's brave struggle to be accepted as a woman. "If you are a woman, you'll always be one, it is something you feel inside," says the Veneno character in the series. Irene Montero, Spain's Minister for Equality, hailed the film as being "a decisive factor in getting many people to understand the need for a law that protects your rights. Thank you for fighting."¹⁹⁷ The law Montero is talking about is "Ley Trans," which introduces gender self-identification into Spanish law. According to this proposal, anyone who claims he is a woman, is a woman and should be defined as such by law. This is the *exact opposite* of what La Veneno represented, and so his sister protested: "we always called him Joselito, which is what he wanted, Cristina La Veneno was a public figure!"¹⁹⁸

What is going on here? If someone had claimed 50 years ago that the existence of *trans people* proved that gender identity was innate, most people would have shaken their heads in disbelief: if anything, their existence proved the opposite! If men could behave like women, surely this meant gender roles were a social construct! Even in the mid-90s, trans experience was not said to be characterised by an *essential* or *innate* gender but by the

---

196 Cristina Ortiz, Valeria Vegas. (2016). ¡Digo! Ni puta, ni santa. Las memorias de La Veneno. CEDRO.
197 Comment on Instagram by Irene Montero <https://www.instagram.com/p/CGb-j5-iyZA/>.
198 <https://www.telecinco.es/salvame/hermana-la-veneno-joselito_18_3040545234.html>.

contradiction of this notion. US human rights activist, Leslie Feinberg, put it eloquently and succinctly in 1996:

> I am transgendered. I was born female, but my masculine gender expression is seen as male. It's not my sex that defines me, and it's not my gender expression. It's the fact that my gender expression appears to be at odds with my sex. Do you understand? It's the social contradiction between the two that defines me.[199]

Feinberg makes clear the difference between sex and gender. Sex is biological, gender is social. This is in line with political scientist and feminist Sheila Jeffreys' thinking: "the idea of gender relates to a system in which there are only two genders, masculinity for the male, dominant sex caste and femininity for the female, subordinate sex caste."[200] Jeffreys' and Feinberg's interpretations imply a radical restructuring of the world. Why should women, and not men, wear dresses? Why do women and men have such different statuses in society? Feinberg continues: "Since sex and gender had always been seen as synonymous when I was growing up, disconnecting the two was a very important advance in my own thinking."[201] Being transgender is a deeply revolutionary act, according to Feinberg – it entails not conforming to one's gender. In her book *Transgender Warriors* (1996), Feinberg depicts people throughout history who have challenged gender norms: women dressing as men and going out to war, men dressing in women's clothes, gay people, feminists, 'fags' and 'butches'. Nowhere does Feinberg suggest that this non-conforming means they were born in the wrong body and should now be transferred to the other body in order to conform. On the contrary, she questions patriarchy and the idea that people ought to fit in somewhere at all in the first place.

The gender system has always had its dissidents as well as its refugees, not all of whom have necessarily wanted to overthrow patriarchy. But they have nevertheless been natural allies of feminism due to pointing out the artificiality of a system which forces men to behave in one way and women in another.

---

199 Leslie Feinberg. (1996). *Transgender Warriors: Making History from Joan of Arc to RuPaul*, p. 101. Boston: Beacon Press.
200 Sheila Jeffreys. (2014). *Gender Hurts. A Feminist Analysis of the Politics of Transgenderism*, p. 153. London: Routledge.
201 Feinberg. (1996). p. 102.

However, what was once a progressive movement has become mired in a neo-patriarchal narrative. Rather than criticising stereotypical gender roles, the trans narrative is now aimed at criticising feminism. The previous narrative was about *patriarchy* being too exclusionary, the new one claims *feminism* is. An essentialist narrative about innate gender is now being spun from trans people's experiences, awarding the central part in the new narrative to them. Trans people finally get to be the main characters on stage. The price paid, however, is *patriarchy's appropriation of the trans experience*. In order to get to play this part, the experiences of trans people must follow a pre-written script which reflects deeply patriarchal notions about innate gender. In this script, one can only deviate from the gender system on the system's own terms. The result is that you may deviate – *if* you do it by conforming. Trans people have thus reached a social and media status, which is allotted if and only if they subscribe to the dominant narrative of gender being innate and transition being the solution. The dissidents are thereby brought into the fold and in from the cold to attain a type of *hypernormality*. They are no longer proof that the gender system doesn't hold water, but instead the evidence that it *is* waterproof. Proponents of gender identity theory can finally say that *femininity is natural* and that one is born with it!

But what to do with all those narratives that tell a different story? Those that stubbornly insist on being the dissidents' and refugees' stories? Those whose transitions are more about escaping oppression, homophobia and capital punishment, or for that matter sexuality, autodesire and 'eating the other'? For instance, Swedish author Staffan Beckman, who explores both his gender and ethnicity in his autobiographical novels *Till Jerusalem* (1989) and *Freak* (2013), in which the desire to be the Other is central, writes:

> I can see it clearly now: my images of women are me. On the one hand, libido, the pitch black darkness, vulnerability, on the other strength, resistance, defiance. Woman or Jew, they may as well be the same, though perhaps the strongest image is in the uniting of the two: Jewish woman. [...] And I think of that Staffan, with his happy childhood, and it seems to me that one of the main directions, perhaps the only direction in my life, has been downwards. Step by step down into the abyss of my inner self, toward the Jewish woman that lies there curled up in wait like a small, mean little black knot.[202]

---

202 Staffan Beckman. (1989). *Till Jerusalem*, pp. 207–208. Stockholm: Arbetarkultur.

Beckman, who later changed his first name to Alice, describes how he enters "his large, soft female body."²⁰³ He ties a pillow around his waist with a rope so that it protrudes like breasts and a belly and shifts to writing in the third person:

> He slept in his female body, he cut hedges and raked leaves in his female body, he stood fishing on the jetty in his female body. He knew there was a woman on the other side of the bay who was in the habit of spying on the neighbours with binoculars and he went out on the jetty and cliffs so that she could see him. [...] The novel he wrote told of the dream of resting, of freedom from responsibility; perhaps about the dream of returning to the womb.²⁰⁴

The novel opens with Beckman's wife telling him she feels that he has raped her. This leads him to "try to penetrate through the masks and the role play and see myself. I must grope my way to some kind of answer as to how an unremarkable marital bliss could be dissolved and culminate in rape."²⁰⁵ The writer oscillates between wanting to fully adopt the identity of woman and Jew: "I am after all Jewish in the deepest sense of the word" and being overcome by doubt: "I have no death camp number tattoo! My images are only borrowed!?!"²⁰⁶

Beckman's depiction of his trans experience is about wanting to become the Other, and more specifically, the opposite of a white man. He searches his past for things that could give him an entry ticket: the fact he was born feet first "seems to me a very Jewish beginning" and that his mother bound his hands to stop him scratching his eczema may have resulted in "my sexual fantasies through puberty always involved being tied up, vulnerable, waiting for someone, always the woman."²⁰⁷ By 2013, when he wrote *Freak*, medical science had moved on and Beckman writes that he sometimes fantasises about having bottom surgery:

> Perhaps the most titillating of these fantasies is the thought that I could then go to the public pool [...] and get undressed in front of other naked

---

203 Ibid. p. 259.
204 Ibid. p. 233.
205 Ibid. p. 10.
206 Ibid. p. 36 and p. 228.
207 Ibid. p. 38.

and half-naked women, unambiguously exposing my female body and being one of them ..."[208]

Being seen as a woman by women is a recurring sexual fantasy in many testimonies of the autogynephilic kind, but Beckman also knows that this is exactly what makes him different from women. As demonstrated in these extracts, Beckman's view of gender is not essentialist – he is not claiming that he has a woman's genes – but rather psychological. Gender is a psychological relationship in which the woman is always the losing party. She is powerless, and this is precisely what Beckman wishes to be: freed from responsibility for having raped, he dreams that he "enters his female body" and becomes instead the one who is raped.

In Afsaneh Najmabadi's report on trans people in 1930s Iran, there are various conflicting interpretations. In 1930, Iranian papers carried stories about Munirah, a woman who had decided that "this business of being a woman was no good." She had been married to a man who had not taken care of her, so she said, "I decided to leave womanhood and earn my own living." Munirah changed her name to Abd Al-Ali Khan and found employment as a servant.[209]

Here, the focus is on social standing. Munirah's move is a kind of upward mobility, of achieving freedom through changing gender – but not sex, as her body remains intact. 1930 was, however, also the year Iran's first sex change surgery was carried out. An 18-year-old man walked into the state hospital in Tehran and demanded to become a woman because he had "female desire and no male desire at all."[210] The doctors did as he asked and the papers reported their successful breakthrough as creating this "wonderful creature, who may never have existed previously in the world." In reality, only a few months before, the world's first sex change surgery had taken place in Germany, though it had been unsuccessful and the patient died shortly thereafter. The Iranian 18-year-old, however, is believed to have survived.

These two Iranians describe their experiences in radically different ways. One wants to achieve economic independence while for the other,

---

208 Staffan Beckman. (2013). *Freak*, p. 59. Stockholm: Nomen publishing/Books On Demand.
209 Afsaneh Najmabadi. (2014). *Professing Selves: Transsexuality and Same-Sex Desire in Contemporary Iran*, p. 40. Durham, NC: Duke University Press.
210 Ibid. p. 41.

the issue is one of sexuality. For Munirah, it is a question of class, while for the 18-year-old it is a question of which position one adopts in a heterosexual relationship. For both, rebellion also means capitulation.

For the Swedish journalist Johan Ehrenberg, who recounts his experiences of living as a woman in *Könsbytet* (*My Sex Change*, 1983), it is about understanding the "almost insurmountable wall of fear and contempt that demarcates the boundaries of gender." Ehrenberg describes how he cried on the street as a seven-year-old and was called a girl by an elderly woman, and how this instilled in him a feeling of sorrow that he carried with him throughout his youth. He decides to "try to live as a woman" and his experience gives rise to ground-breaking insights:

> Crossing the no-man's land between the sexes entails experiencing both gender roles and nothing can remain the same afterwards. I smile when I read columnists who write about gender as though it were something 'natural'. I understand why so many try to hide behind talk of chemical substances and genes in order to avoid seeing their own, personal prison and avoid responsibility for the status quo. They want the difference between men and women to be 'natural' because otherwise, their own lives would partly be a failure. But if individuals can change gender, then everyone else can also do away with gender roles. This is what is truly politically revolutionary in all the reporting on sex change.[211]

These kinds of multifaceted stories have become increasingly rare. They are not only seen as outdated, but they are also *abject*, in the Kristevan sense – they embody what no one wants to know as they point to a different interpretation. Gone are the nuances of contradiction and desire, psychology, class and sexuality. Gone is the discussion about patriarchy. Gone also is the trans experience that questions and problematises gender and reveals the arbitrariness of hierarchies. Now, the hegemonic discourse around trans states that the man who feels he is a woman actually is one and has always been one. There is nothing other than this inner essence, and those who have doubts, decide to transition for other reasons, or regret their decision, are said to not be the real deal and therefore do not count. The autogynephile, the scammer, the gay boy and the teen with autism, are all 'trans' the exact same way. It is also claimed that going from a woman to a man is exactly the same as going from a man to a woman

---

[211] Johan Ehrenberg. (2004). *Könsbytet. Mörka berättelser från en annan värld*, p. 109. Stockholm: ETC förlag.

– no gender analysis of this highly gendered phenomenon is attempted any more.

This hegemonic narrative is also applied retrospectively, and thus human history is being reinterpreted at break-neck speed. Patriarchal essentialism is sweeping through the world and dragging with it all cultures and personalities who dared to stand outside gender norms. According to a twisted logic, they are all now simply proof that gender is innate.

"In many Native American cultures, there are more sexes than just male and female," writes molecular biologist Henrik Brändén in a very puzzling sentence. Are we to understand from this that Native Americans can procreate in ways different from other humans? No, in the next sentence he explains what he means: "people with female genitalia who had their hair cut in a similar way to men, went to war carrying bows and arrows and competed with the men."[212] What Brändén is getting at, is that there are women in history who have behaved in a way that *he* does not consider to be typical of women. Brändén is talking about *gender*, not sex. Yet he passes off this and other similar stories as evidence: "the inner feeling of being a man or a woman appears therefore to be largely innate."[213] Brändén thus assumes that the Amazon warrior women *felt like men from birth*. How does he know this? If short-haired female warriors were an unremarkable sight amongst Amazons, perhaps fighting in wars was not considered to be a particularly male undertaking in the first place? Nor does Brändén provide a reason for why it is precisely amongst the Amazons that there should be significant numbers of women with an 'innate' male identity. We might also ask: are women who fight in wars not real women? Why must Brändén exclude them from his definition of female – why can't he broaden his *own* ideas about what women can do and have done in history?

Where biologists such as Brändén get on with the business of discovering the eternal and natural gender identity in the brain, social scientists attempt to discover it in history and culture. Upon a re-reading, notorious cross-dressing Swedish thief Lasse-Maja, Norse god Thor and

---

212 Henrik Brändén. (2020). *Själens biologi och vår fria vilja*, p. 276. Lund: Celanders förlag.
213 Ibid. p. 277.

Greek goddess Athena are shown to be trans people.[214] We discover that Swedish Queen Kristina was actually a man since such a strong and powerful person could surely not have been a woman.[215] Joan of Arc is described in the same way: the woman who led a mediaeval army to victory at the age of 17 and was killed because she wore 'men's clothing' is now said to have been a man. Seeing as she wore trousers and was so warring, and also perhaps interested in women, she must have been a man, despite the fact she referred to herself as "the Maid."[216] The Swedish soldier Elisa Servenius is listed on Wikipedia under "LGBTQ History in Sweden," even though she was a woman married to a man, for the sole reason that she went to war wearing trousers. Artist Elisabeth Ohlson Wallin claims to have realised that many lesbian women "were and are of course not lesbian women but trans men."[217] The idea that individuals ought to be allowed to define themselves does not appear to apply to history anymore.

Researcher Sam Holmqvist questions why we call eminent women in history women – if they wore men's clothing, should we not say they were trans men or perhaps just men?

> Did the person say anything about being a man or that they felt like a man? Did the person make any attempts to change their body or how it was perceived? Did the person live as a gender different to the one assigned at birth, or were attempts made to hide their assigned gender? If we answer in the affirmative to these questions we can, according to Cromwell, view a person as trans regardless of the fact that they lived long before this term existed.[218]

Thus, anyone who has failed to conform to restrictive gender norms can be reinterpreted as 'actually' having been born in the wrong body and thereby be written out of the history of their sex. Women's history immediately

---

214 For such a reading, see for example Sam Holmqvist. (2017). *Transformationer:1800-talets svenska translitteratur genom Lasse-Maja, C.J.L. Almqvist och Aurora Ljungstedt*, p. 29. Göteborg: Makadam Publishing Company.
215 Loretto Villalobos. (3 March 2017). 'Transmannen Kristina får liv'. *Aftonbladet Kultur*.
216 Emilia Philomena Sanguinetti. (2016). *Joan of Arc: Her Trial Transcripts*. USA: Little Flower Publishing.
217 Elisabeth Ohlson Wallin. (28 February 2018). 'Transpersonen är Guds gåva till mänskligheten'. *Expressen Kultur*.
218 Sam Holmqvist. (2016). 'Att skriva transhistoria. Cisnormativitet och historiens könsöverskridare'. *Tidskrift för Genusvetenskap*, Vol. 37, No. 4.

becomes a lot poorer on such a reading because all valkyries and queens, all thinkers and inventors, all pioneers and lesbians lived 'as men' to some degree. Does it follow that they actually were men? If we answer in the affirmative, the history of eminent women becomes men's history.

In the Spanish TV series *Chicas del cable*, set in the 1930s, we follow the lives of a group of women working as switchboard operators. Two of them fall in love with each other and the viewer thinks there will be a representation of lesbian love. This lasts for all of one episode, however. In the next episode, a man called Miguel is introduced and he then begins a relationship with both women – cue hot threesome scenes. And then just when Miguel succumbs to substance abuse, disappears from the series and the viewer thinks the lesbian love affair will be revived, one of the women discloses that her name is not actually Sara but Óscar. She begins binding her breasts and dressing in men's clothes, explaining that now she and Carlota can marry because "you aren't marrying Sara, you're marrying Óscar." No sooner was the lesbian storyline introduced than it vanished. In this way, lesbians are posthumously erased from history. The stale moral of the story, which poses as progressive, is that lesbian women are actually men.

We are witnessing a revision of history, in which widely differing traditions and cultures are swiftly engulfed by a patriarchal narrative about eternal, innate gender roles. Non-western cultures are often used, partly to legitimise the story (due to the frequent conflation of non-western cultures and the 'natural'), and partly to show how western countries are at the forefront when it comes to human rights. There's just one problem: journalists often find something completely different to be the case. Those cultures which have institutionalised full sex change as a cultural practice are in fact often the most patriarchal societies in the world, and not those which have come the furthest in terms of feminism and gay rights, as shown by the fact that sex change is most common in Iran and Thailand.

Iranian doctors had long been at the forefront when it came to this kind of surgery, and following the Islamic Revolution, Iran became the country that carried out the second largest number of sex change surgeries in the world.[219] Gay people are often forced to undergo sex change

---

219 Neha Thirani Bagri. (19 April 2017). '"Everyone treated me like a saint" – in Iran, there's only one way to survive as a transgender person'. *Quartz*.

operations, if they don't, they risk a flogging or even capital punishment.[220] Homosexuality is seen as a disease with a cure: sex change. This practice brutally restores the heterosexual order – we are no longer dealing with a man who desires a man but a woman who does so – and points to an extreme readiness of the individual to submit to this order, to the extent that they sacrifice their fertility. A man who confides in a mullah that he dreams of having sex with other men is often sent to a sex change clinic.[221]

In a country where morality police patrol the streets and arrest or even kill women who show their hair, films about trans people are aired on state TV. A man who changed his sex to become a woman says, "Everyone treated me like a saint. They adore me so much and they admire me so much for doing such a courageous thing – they respect me on a whole different level."[222] An Iranian LGBTQ organisation interviewed 100 gay people and reported that "dozens" of them were forced to undergo sex change operations against their will. Many do so in order to be able to get married, but then have to hide their previous identity. It is also common that people forced to undergo surgery commit suicide.[223] Many western journalists seem to have frequently overlooked what is actually going on here: that a state is 'curing' homosexuality by sterilising gay people. On the contrary, Iran is often portrayed in many articles on the subject as a "trans paradise," a country that looks after trans people's rights, never mind the fact that "stigma is still widespread."[224] "Iran's transgender rights are unique," claims the US magazine *Quartz*.[225] There is also often a mix-up between the treatment of trans and gay. Johanna Nilsson's young adult novel *Om vi bara kunde byta kroppar med varandra* (If only we could switch bodies with each other) turns history on its head. In the novel, Queen O comes to Sweden because in Iran "you get the death penalty for being like

---

[220] Mohammadrasool Yadegarfard. (20 May 2019). 'Are Iranian gay men coping with systematic suppression under islamic law? A qualitative study'. *Sexuality and Culture*.
[221] Ali Hamedani. (5 November 2014). 'The gay people pushed to change their gender'. *BBC News*. <https://www.bbc.com/news/magazine-29832690>.
[222] Thirani Bagri. (19 April 2017).'"Everyone treated me like a saint" – in Iran, there's only one way to survive as a transgender person'. *Quartz*.
[223] Johan Bergendorff. (6 December 2019).'Transparadiset Irans mörka baksida'. Sveriges Radio.
[224] Thirani Bagri. (19 April 2017).'"Everyone treated me like a saint" – in Iran, there's only one way to survive as a transgender person'. *Quartz*.
[225] Ibid.

her, being born in a body with the wrong gender." The character explains: "I'll probably be hanged, but only after they've raped and tortured me for months."[226] None of the reviewers seems to have noticed this blatant revisionism, but then Nilsson also confuses Shia and Sunni muslims without repercussions.

In Afghanistan *bacha posh*, or girls who are dressed as boys for a few years, is a relatively common phenomenon. A family who requires help in their shop or with weaving carpets can simply decide that their daughter is a son; she is then allowed to change her name and clothing. This allows her to move around more freely. Journalist Jenny Nordberg, who investigated the phenomena in her book *The Underground Girls of Kabul* (2015), writes that *bacha posh* arose as a form of resistance to rigid patriarchal rules and is partly a practical solution to escape these rules. However, it is also a way for a mother to salvage her honour, since she who 'only' gives birth to daughters is judged harshly by society. In addition, it serves as a ritual to increase one's chances of birthing a boy since it is believed that those who make their daughter a son are more likely to give birth to a son. Nordberg interviewed a mother who explained:

> There was one additional reason for the transition. Azita says it with a burst of low laughter, leaning in a little closer to disclose her small act of rebellion. 'I wanted to show my youngest what life was like on the other side'. That life can include flying a kite, running as fast as you can, laughing hysterically, jumping up and down just because it feels good, climbing trees to feel the thrill of hanging on. [...] To speak up without fear and to be listened to, and rarely have anyone question why you are out on your own in comfortable clothes that allow for any kind of movement. All unthinkable for an Afghan girl.[227]

Basically, being human. All this is only possible until she reaches puberty, though. From the moment pregnancy becomes a possibility, she must be locked up and protected like other girls while they await marriage. Nordberg reports that many girls find it hard to readjust to this life cut-off from the outside world. Some refuse and claim that they are boys. Others benefit from their time living as boys: they'll keep on enjoying an

---

226 Johanna Nilsson. (2018). *Om vi bara kunde byta kroppar med varandra*, p. 9. Stockholm: Rabén och Sjögren.
227 Jenny Nordberg. (2015). *The Underground Girls of Kabul: In Search of a Hidden Resistance in Afghanistan*, p. 15. New York: Crown Publishing Group.

increased self-confidence compared to other girls. Afghan society does not disparage women who have lived as boys or their families. It is an accepted phenomenon that has existed in the region longer than Islam.[228]

In Albania, a similar phenomenon used to exist, albeit not as widespread. 'Sworn virgins', or *burrnesha*, are referred to in the *kanun*, the set of Albanian traditional laws from the 15th century. By swearing an oath in front of village elders, a woman could take on a man's status and privileges. She was thus permitted to do business, smoke, use a watch and use swear words. She would dress in men's clothes and would be viewed as a man throughout her life in all aspects but one: sexually. She must swear never to have intercourse and to remain a virgin to her death.[229]

In Iran, Afghanistan and Albania, these permitted transgressions of gender norms become a way to incorporate the exception to the rule in society's moral code without questioning the status quo – a way of making rebellion palatable. It thus doesn't matter if a man has sex with a man if he does it *as a woman*. It's okay for a girl to play football and fight as long as she does it *as a boy* since she therefore does not threaten the ban on women's sports. The fact that the phenomenon is accepted, indicates that society is in fact fully aware that girls *can* fight and play football – they are simply not permitted to do so *as girls*. Thus, the combination girl + freedom of movement remains forbidden and the combinations woman + status and woman + rights continue not to exist. According to Afghan patriarchal values, a woman cannot do business unless she renounces her identity as a woman. These examples also highlight how a change in gender identity *must be located outside the sphere of reproduction* – either prior to it as in Afghanistan, or instead of it, as in Albania. But why should this be the case? Why must *burrnesha* remain virgins and why can't *bacha posh* continue in the role of a boy once menstruation begins? The answer to this is that reproduction is central to creating that which we call gender – the culture of women's oppression.

Gender is a patriarchal system predicated on allocating one status to those who give birth and another to those who impregnate. In fact,

---

228 Zarifa Sabet. (2 March 2018). 'Bacha posh. An Afghan social tradition where girls are raised as boys'. *The Newsminute*.
229 Emilienne Malfatto and Jelena Prtoric. (5 August 2014). 'Last of the burrnesha: Balkan women who pledged celibacy to live as men.' <https://www.theguardian.com/world/2014/aug/05/women-celibacy-oath-men-rights-albania>.

patrilineage is a central tenet of patriarchy: that inheritance flows from father to son. This is clearly linked to the emergence of private ownership and to families' ownership of assets. If the man has the power and wants to pass on his property to his son, the woman's fertility must be controlled. Patrilineal societies have made use of many ways of doing this, among them foot binding, genital mutilation, abortion bans, capital punishment for adultery and, above all, pre-marital chastity, something that has never been the case for men. These are all local flavours of a global rule: man must know his child is his. A matrilineal society has no inherent need to control men, as a woman would naturally know her child is hers, and could thus pass on her name and property without needing to tie her man down. But since patrilineal society is based on the illogical principle of valuing the one connection that is invisible (father-son have no umbilical chord) ownership is transferred *through* woman and thus man has to know who she has been with. Therefore, norms surrounding female sexuality have not arisen independently, and are not a result of some irrational 'jealousy' of men, but are a clear function of patrilineal societies. Restricting women's access to the public sphere, classifying them as whores and madonnas where only the latter are granted marriage and to give birth to children eligible for inheritance of a man's name and property, are not arbitrary rules but global rules which logically follow in patriliny's footsteps.

These restrictions are, however, very impractical. To imprison half the population in their houses, unable to leave without a male guardian, creates all sorts of everyday problems. Women and girls can, for example, not work outside the home and a family with only daughters has a hard time surviving. Gender 'changes' for women have thus arisen as a tool to address problems created by the system's own rules. The stricter the rules, the harder it is for an entire society to abide by them. *Bacha posh* or *burrnesha* are not about finding one's 'real' identity, or about tolerating deviance. They are about allowing exceptions for practical reasons while maintaining patriarchal rules. And they do not come without a high price for the women – an Albanian woman had to sacrifice both sexuality and reproduction entirely, only to be able to have the little freedom to own a little shop or wear a watch, a choice that no man ever had to make.

Today, in contrast, these traditions are being held up as evidence of gender roles being innate. It is argued that these women acquired a male identity in the womb and that their cultures simply 'acknowledged' this. Even a BBC journalist contends that the existence of *bacha posh* provides a progressive sign that shows how "the notion of gender has escaped any such constricting boundaries for centuries."[230] Gender is here portrayed as some kind of unwavering natural force that stands against culture and oppression all on its own. Some researchers argue that *bacha posh* can be seen as an example of "trans subjectivity,"[231] while the British documentary filmmaker Isla Badenoch mourns the decline of *burrnesha* as a "vanishing transgender tradition."[232] But why have *burrnesha* largely disappeared while *bacha posh* live on? Surely, this is because in modern-day Albania, women are allowed to do business, wear trousers and move freely, while in Afghanistan this yet again remains impossible. As one of the last burrneshas says in an interview with the *Guardian*: "Nowadays, women have more freedom. They don't need to become burrneshas to escape their condition." Albanian women's chromosomes are unchanged, but society has changed and with it, the understanding of what a woman is.

According to contemporary gender identity theory, deviance from gender roles is no longer a way of destabilising the sex-gender connection, as Butler says. Nor is it an act of rebellion against oppression. Rather, it is a person's true identity – one does not perform one's gender but *is* one's gender – and gender identity is fixed and cannot be changed. One is born with it and it remains intact for the rest of one's life, unaffected by puberty, life or culture. Even a several thousand per cent increase in young girls wanting to transition to boys is not accepted as meaning anything. Proponents of gender identity theory claim, with a straight face, that the number of people who feel this way have always been the same, they were just not visible before.

This is a classic example of a metaphysical worldview – everything that exists today has always existed, nothing can be created or changed. Everything can only be visible or hidden, permitted or forbidden and human nature is immutable. Friedrich Engels described the metaphysical worldview thus:

---

230 Catriona White. (7 March 2018). 'A gender mindbender'. *BBC*.
231 Julienne Corboz, Andrew Gibbs and Rachel Jewkes. (2019). 'Bacha Posh in Afghanistan. Factors associated with raising a girl as a boy'. *Culture, Health & Sexuality*. Doi: 10.1080/13691058.2019.1616113.
232 <http://www.islabadenoch.com/burrneshaarchive>.

> Observing nature's objects and processes in their isolation, apart from their connection with the whole [...] of observing them not in motion but at rest; not as essentially changeable but as fixed substances, not in their life but, in their death.[233]

This is in contrast to the dialectical worldview, which focuses on change to answer the question: where is the world headed? The metaphysical worldview is incapable of understanding changes and therefore it does not recognise its own role in them either. Rather, it consolidates the status quo as eternal.

---

233 Friedrich Engels. (1982). 'The Development of Socialism from Utopia to Science', p. 10. Translated from German for *The People*, official journal of the Socialist Labor Party of America by Daniel De Leon. <http://www.slp.org/pdf/marx/dev_soc.pdf>.

PART 2

ONE PILL MAKES YOU A GIRL, ONE PILL MAKES YOU A BOY – THE 71 GENDERS BECOME TWO

CHAPTER 15

When States Reassign Their Citizens' Sex

Kamratposten is a popular Swedish magazine for children approximately 8 to 13 years of age. In its Q and A section 'Body and Mind', readers can pose questions to a psychologist on puberty, bullying or anything they are afraid to ask their parents. The following appeared in June 2018:

> Hiya! I've felt like a boy in a girl's body for the entire 12 years of my life. I want clothes from the boys' department and want to play the role of a boy in different situations. I try to hide my breasts and feel distress at the thought of my period. I feel psychologically unwell about being born a girl but don't dare to tell anyone this. How will I be able to tell people that I'm trans? *Hasselfäll is my name*

A person called Fox Foxhage, *Kamratposten's* agony uncle, answers:

> Hiya!! I understand that you want to tell people you're a boy, because it's hard for you to have a girl's body now that puberty is around the corner. And maybe you also want to be seen by others the way you feel about yourself. Be brave! Tell someone who you believe will support you. Remember that you have the right to be who you are and to be respected for it. Tell your parents when you're ready. They can help you to access the school health service and then trans health care. This way you'll be able to get help to be the boy you are, in the way you want to.[1]

---

[1] Fox Foxhage. (2018). 'Kropp och knopp, Fox Foxhage svarar på läsarnas frågor'. *Kamratposten*, No. 6, p. 18.

Suddenly they are everywhere: children and young people who want to transition. In the US, several new clinics are being opened each year and they are still struggling to meet the demand for puberty blockers, hormone injections and surgery. In Sweden, the number of children and youngsters being diagnosed with gender dysphoria has increased by several thousand per cent in the last decade. Those diagnosed are also younger than ever. Whereas fifteen years ago, barely one person a year in the ten to 12-year-old age group received the diagnosis, now there are several each week.[2]

Nearly all of those diagnosed are girls. This did not use to be the case – in the past, those who said they wanted to transition were primarily older men; in fact, most people still conjure up the image of an older man when they hear the word transsexual. It was transvestites and later MtF transsexuals who blazed the trail and, most importantly, that most trans research is based on. Indeed, as recently as 1999, Professor of Literature, Toril Moi, wrote that we should ask ourselves why so few women want to change sex.[3]

The fact that a majority of those accessing trans clinics are now girls in their early teens signals a major shift. There are currently more girls than boys in the 13 to 19 age bracket being prescribed testosterone in Sweden.[4] Applications to Sweden's Tax Agency to change legal sex are up 4000 per cent – from ten to 15 applications a year in the year 2000 to 446 in 2018.[5] The rise is most prominent in large cities: in Stockholm, the number of girls aged between 15 and 19 diagnosed with gender dysphoria has risen by 8250 per cent since 2006.[6] In Great Britain, the number of young girls being treated for gender dysphoria has increased by 4400 per cent in the last decade.[7] The same phenomenon is apparent in other parts of the world too.

---

2   Socialstyrelsens statistikdatabas, Diagnoser, Endast specialiserad öppen vård, Antal patienter, F64 Könsidentitetsstörningar, Riket, Ålder: 10–14, 2006–2019.
3   Toril Moi. (2019). *What Is a Woman?* p. 116. Oxford: Oxford University Press.
4   'Läkemedelsstatistik antalet patienter G03BA03 testosteron, Stockholms län, ålder 15–19', *Läkemedelsverket*.
5   <http://www.anova.se/TM3.htm>.
6   Socialstyrelsens statistikdatabas, Diagnoser, Endast specialiserad öppen vård, Antal patienter, F64 Könsidentitetsstörningar, Stockholms län, Ålder: 15–19, 2006–2019.
7   Stella O'Malley. (2019). 'Trans kids. It's time to talk'. In Michele Moore and Heather Brunskell-Evans (eds). *Inventing Transgender Children and Young People*, p. 153. Newcastle upon Tyne: Cambridge Scholars.

Some might argue that this is merely an indication that society has become more diverse and tolerant. After all, perhaps the number of individuals wanting to change sex has remained constant over the years, forced to live in denial and stigmatised, unable to disclose their wishes? This is undoubtedly the case for some – yet can it explain all the cases?

US doctor and researcher Lisa Littman's studies of cases where children and young people accessed trans health care found they had a lot in common. 82.8 per cent were girls and, contrary to what the diagnostic criteria stipulate (namely that the person ought to have "felt they belong to a sex other than that assigned at birth for a long time") the gender dysphoria these girls presented with often arises out of the blue. Families were frequently surprised by their sudden wish to change sex. In a 2019 anthology, 13-year-old Anna's parents recount their experience:

> When she was 11 Anna got her own smartphone and stopped being sporty, stopped going out, stopped having friends on visits. When the smartphone came, she spent more and more time in the room with the phone. She became in a way 'not present'. We don't know what happened but she went through a comprehensive change of behavior in a short space of time. She began to be interested in Japanese comics, Cosplay, made new online friends. Then soon after, one evening, she said, 'Mom, I'm a boy'.[8]

Her parents explained that they did not know what to think, as Anna had never displayed any dissatisfaction with being a girl before. Anna then sent a text message to her parents in which she said that they must refer to her using 'he' from then on, despite them being 'cis' – meaning they didn't really understand her circumstances. After this, events began unfolding very rapidly: Anna bought a binder to hide her breasts and independently got in touch with health care services. Her parents thought she'd be in good hands there and explained to staff that their daughter's issues may be a result of being bullied at school. In response, they were informed that they did not in fact have a daughter, but a son called Jaako. The solution to Jaako's problems was for his puberty to be blocked with injections.

> We begged gender clinicians to look at what Anna had been going through that might give insight about why she changed so rapidly and

---

8   Michele Moore. (2019). 'Rapid Onset Gender Dysphoria'. In Michele Moore and Heather Brunskell-Evans (eds). *Inventing Transgender Children and Young People*, p. 242. Newcastle upon Tyne: Cambridge Scholars.

decided she was a boy. No one had expected this; this girl, who loved dolls, dresses, glitter and ribbons, was no longer identified as 'she' but suddenly became a dark and gloomy 'he' binding her chest with duct tape. We were not heard.

Not only does gender dysphoria often begin quickly – treatment is right around the corner, too. Services for individuals with gender dysphoria have gone from being cumbersome, frustrating and lengthy to the complete opposite. In Stockholm, it used to take an average of seven months from the first appointment to puberty blockers and hormone treatment being prescribed. In the 2010s, Swedish health care began adopting lobby group World Professional Association for Transgender Health's (WPATH) standards of care and their idea that 'affirming care' is the only way forward. This basically entails confirming the patient's worldview – should the patient want treatment, the healthcare provider must under no circumstances question this. Even in cases where a patient hesitates or has doubts, many clinics in the US recommend that treatment be initiated while the patient reflects. There are now very few places a young person can turn to which do not follow this affirming approach, as illustrated by the correspondent of the agony uncle column at the beginning of this chapter. The 12-year-old who feels she is a boy because she prefers clothes from the "boys' department" is not advised to take her time and think things through, nor is she told that clothes for different sexes do not actually exist. Rather, she is told to contact the transgender health service directly to get help becoming "the boy you are."[9]

Over the course of the new millenium, gender identity services have opened in several Swedish cities. 2016 saw the inauguration of Anova, the medical service for trans people in Stockholm at Karolinska Hospital. "A star is born," Karolinska proudly reported and a live band played as the rainbow ribbon was cut by the county councillor for health care, the Liberal Party's Anna Starbrink. The premises had purposely been built off the hospital site, as the "aim is to send a signal about leaving behind stigmatisation and marginalisation, opening the service in fresh, new

---

9   'Kropp och knopp, Fox Foxhage svarar på läsarnas frågor'. (2018). *Kamratposten*, No. 6, p. 18.

premises."[10] A special department, known as the Kid-team, was also established to treat children and young people.

Anova quickly became known all over Sweden as the place where it was easiest and quickest to get treatment. The clinic operated on a 'turn no one away' principle, explaining on their website that, "during the assessment stage, we try never to question or challenge an individual's feeling of their gender."[11] The purpose of assessment has gone from trying to work out the extent to which a patient was 'actually' transsexual, to the complete opposite today, with the patients diagnosing themselves, regardless of age, and the health service following suit.

Anova's explanation of what they treat is also contradictory. On the one hand, they state that gender identity is biologically determined: "Increasingly, research supports a biological determinist model, which finds that gender identity is established in the fetal stage." On the other hand, they do not locate this identity in the body, nor do they appear to know what the diagnosis they are treating is caused by: "We do not know what causes gender dysphoria. The research that exists to date indicates that something happens in the brain during fetal development." No sources are given for this statement, nor is there any mention of the big body of research that contradicts this claim. What this 'something' might be is not described in further detail, nor do they have any scientific methods capable of determining it: "It is likely that transsexualism is a normal variant of human behaviour that is established early on in development."[12]

The Anova clinic also claims it is ignorant of the reason for the dramatic increase in requests for its services over recent years. One reason given on its website is that people suffering from a mental health condition must no longer be denied treatment, which is described as "a positive development." Another may be that "Sweden's population is increasing and the birth rate between 1988 and 1991 was unusually high" and that "since the mid-1980s, large numbers of diagnoses of Transsexualism [sic] in Taiwan and Iceland" have been observed. What Iceland and Taiwan have

---

10 'En stjärna föds' – Invigning av ANOVA. <https://nyheter.ki.se/en-stjarna-fods-invigningen-av-anova>.
11 <http://www.anova.se/TM3.htm>.
12 Louise Frisén et al. (11 October 2019). 'Multidisciplinärt samarbete har gett bättre kunskapsläge'. *Läkartidningen.se*. <https://lakartidningen.se/klinik-och-vetenskap-1/artiklar-1/klinisk-oversikt/2019/10/multidisciplinart-samarbete-har-gett-battre-kunskapslage/>.

to do with each other, or, for that matter, with Sweden, is unclear. Equally confusing is why the increase in the number of children born at the end of the 1980s (seven per cent) should explain a several thousand per cent increase in the numbers of people (actually born in the 2000s) applying for gender reassignment today.[13] Anova is certain about one thing, however: "gender dysphoria entails great suffering for the individual and gender affirming therapy is an effective treatment." We will soon find out to what extent this is the case.

---

13   SCB, Befolkningsutveckling – födda, döda, in- och utvandring samt giftermål och skilsmässor 1749–2018. (Statistics Sweden. Births, deaths, immigration and emigration, marriages and divorces for the years 1749–2018.)

CHAPTER 16

"Doctors are Salivating at the Prospect of Applying Puberty Blockers"

In 2015, Sweden's National Board of Health and Welfare issued a recommendation for medical intervention to block puberty where a child about to go through puberty reports an increased sense of discomfort over their sex.[14] The Board claimed that since puberty entails "a large degree of psychological strain," blocking it can "decrease suffering." The Board cautioned that the process should happen swiftly, usually before the age of 12 in girls, as it "is harder for the individual to be recognised as being congruent with their gender identity in adulthood" if the process is begun too long after puberty. The Board therefore recommended that measures be put in place prior to the development of breasts or growth of the penis, in the form of "puberty blocking hormone treatment with Gonadotropin Releasing Hormone analogues (GnRHas) in order to decrease suffering and the risk of mental ill health."

Blocking puberty is described as risk-free – just giving the child some breathing space to think about which gender they want to be. Astonishingly, the Board advised that hormone treatment be started even in cases where gender dysphoria has not been definitively diagnosed. The fact that breasts and penis have not developed was portrayed as "good grounds" for a later decision since

---

14 National Board of Health and Welfare. (2015). 'God vård av barn och ungdomar med könsdysfori. Metodbeskrivning och kunskapsunderlag'. *Socialstyrelsen*, pp. 33–34.

the young person thus gets a chance to further explore their gender identity. Should the young person's gender dysphoria not continue (which would be unlikely), they can stop the medication, at which point the body's natural puberty development is restarted.

The Board of Health and Welfare neglected to mention that the medication they recommended has not been approved for treating gender dysphoria in children – it is, in fact, a medication used for treating prostate cancer which results in 95 per cent of the body's production of male sex hormones being stopped. The only approved use in children and young people is for those extremely rare cases of early onset puberty, defined as development of secondary sex characteristics before the age of nine. In such cases, GnRH analogues can be used to delay puberty, though only for limited periods of time and only exceptionally for longer than a year. Even in these cases, professionals normally recommend "waiting first to see if the condition persists."[15] Dosages are also the lowest possible: 3.75 milligrams, with children weighing under 30 kg to be given half this dose.[16]

Yet all across the western world, this medication is now being used off-label on children with gender dysphoria. 'Off-label' is a term denoting a drug used on a condition or on a group of people that it has not been licensed for. The term does not imply a prohibition – doctors are allowed to use the drug – but pharmaceutical companies are not allowed to advertise it for off-label use since it has not been proven to be safe and effective for that specific purpose. Consequently, neither pharmaceutical companies nor national licensing agencies collect data on the drug's effects when used off-label. Data on adverse effects are also not reported, nor are patients covered by insurance. Drug manufacturers are not responsible for this application of their product and do not respond to questions about patient groups, despite making money from them. When I contacted Ipsen, manufacturer of Pamorelin (one of the most common GnRH analogues in Sweden), the company denied having any knowledge of how this product is used with children and young people with gender

---

15 Mats Halldin, 'För tidig pubertet'. <www.netdoktor.se>.
16 Läkemedelsverket, Produktresumé (Patient Information Leaflet). Pamorelin 3.75 mg pulver och vätska till injektionsvätska, depotsuspension, L02AE04, Triptorelin.

dysphoria since "gender dysphoria is not an indication" for the drug and "we have not undertaken any research in gender dysphoria."[17]

In a presentation held for Swedish school doctors, Olle Söder (Anova's head of hormone treatment) informs participants that the clinic prescribes Pamorelin injections of 11.25 milligrams to children with gender dysphoria.[18] The Swedish Medical Products Agency strongly advises against using amounts this large when treating children and states in its medicine information leaflet:

> Safety and effects have not been established in newborns, infants, children and young people. Pamorelin 11.25mg must therefore not be used on these age groups.[19]

Furthermore, the agency advises that the drug has only been tested on "20–22 year old male volunteers" and "is not indicated for use by women".

How, then, did this drug come to be used so widely as a treatment for gender dysphoria? Interestingly enough, it began in Holland. In the 1990s, two Dutch endocrinologists were trying to come up with a solution to the problem that many of those who transitioned never fully 'passed' as the opposite sex. Having gone through puberty, features such as height, voice, hand and feet size or Adam's apple would always be visible. What if one could start earlier?[20] By stopping puberty before it ever started, the patient would be given the chance to pass as the desired sex. Boys would thus never develop an Adam's apple or shoot up in height and girls would never begin to menstruate or develop breasts. Henriette Delemarre-van de Waal and Peggy Cohen-Kettenis experimented using GnRHas on a 13-year-old girl who later underwent a sex change operation at the age of 18. Their results were published in a high-profile study and it was not long before people across Europe began referencing the 'Dutch protocol' for treatment of transsexualism in children.

---

17 Email correspondence with Erik Sandberg, Ipsen Nordics, 20 December 2019.
18 Olle Söder. (2017). 'Könsidentitet ur endokrinologiskt perspektiv'. Lecture at Skolläkarföreningen in Gävle. <www.koxxnsdysfori-gaxxvle-feb-2017.pdf (slf.se)>.
19 Läkemedelsverket, Produktresumé (Patient Information Leaflet). Pamorelin 3.75 mg pulver och vätska till injektionsvätska, depotsuspension, L02AE04, Triptorelin.
20 First Biennial Conference, 'Transgender health care in Europe'. EPATH 2015, pp. 16–17.

Delemarre-van de Waal and Cohen-Kettenis founded the world's first 'gender identity clinic' for young people, and, in so doing, started something of a revolution as individuals' *identity* had never before been the object of a clinic's attention. Specialist clinics for sex change had existed in the US in the 1960s, though these were clinics specialising solely in plastic surgery for adults.

A new industry was born. The Dutch protocol entails prescribing puberty blockers at the age of 12, hormones at 16 and a full sex change at the age of 18.[21] British TV aired a programme about British children travelling to The Netherlands and envying Dutch children who did not have to go through puberty.[22] Cohen-Kettenis also took up a position at the lobby group WPATH, which publishes guidelines on healthcare for transsexuals.

The pharmaceutical industry soon began opening its eyes to the enormous potential brought about by this revolution. Ferring Pharmaceuticals, owned by Swedish 'pill billionaire' Frederik Paulsen, sponsored conferences at which Delemarre-van de Waal and Cohen-Kettenis gave keynote speeches.[23] Ferring had pioneered hormone research in the 1950s and, as they manufactured GnRHas, the company quickly saw this was their chance to make the first move. They even began sponsoring Delemarre-van de Waal and Cohen-Kettenis's research, which explains why the pair are the authors of the majority of papers on the topic: the financial support from Ferring allowed them to publish papers at breakneck speed.

The studies have two things in common. Firstly, nearly all find that puberty blockers have a positive effect, and secondly, the majority include a special thanks to Ferring Pharmaceuticals for facilitating the research. Furthermore, Ferring is lead sponsor of the American College of Obstetricians and Gynecologists' conference, sponsorship which led to a

---

21 Paul W. Hruz, Lawrence S. Mayer, Paul R. McHugh. (Spring 2017). 'Growing pains: Problems with puberty suppression in treating gender dysphoria'. *The New Atlantis*.

22 Michael Biggs. (July 2019). 'The Tavistock's experiment with puberty blockers', p. 2. Oxford University. <https://www.transgendertrend.com/tavistock-experiment-puberty-blockers/>.

23 Peggy Cohen-Kettenis and Henriette Delemarre-van de Waal. (2006). 'Clinical management of gender identity in adolescents. A protocol on psychological and paediatric endocrinology aspects'. *European Journal of Endocrinology*, p. 155.

declaration by the conference that trans health care ought to be publically funded,[24] and has donated over £250,000 to the British Liberal Democrats. Three years after the donation, the party demanded trans children be given the 'right' to be prescribed puberty blockers,[25] though Ferring in an email to me claims the donation was made to support a no vote for Brexit.[26] Ferring's competitors would not be outdone by this performance: Pfizer, AbbVie and others joined in and sponsored studies and conferences on the topic of medical interventions on gender development.[27] In the absence of this significant support and sponsorship, equally rapid developments would have been unlikely.

Enter American endocrinologist Norman P. Spack, who sees himself as father of the trans revolution and holds TedTalks entitled "How I help transgender teens become who they want to be." To others, he is known more prosaically as evangelist-in-chief for early medical intervention. Spack immediately realised the immense potential of puberty blockers, began using them on his patients at the Children's Hospital in Boston and progressed from there to found America's first children's clinic for sex change in 2007. Currently, there are 80 such clinics. He recounts how his motto of "Why wait?" had parents flocking from near and far to access treatment for their children. The sooner one implements hormone treatment, the better the results, according to Spack, who often boasts he has succeeded in shortening the predicted height of a young person from six foot four inches to five foot ten inches.[28]

In Spack's view, a more thorough diagnostic assessment of children and young people with gender dysphoria is unnecessary, as the treatment itself *is* the assessment:

---

24 <https://annualmeeting.acog.org/sponsors/ and https://www.acog.org/About-ACOG/News-Room/Statements/2019/Physicians-Urge-Trump-Administration-to-Protect-Transgender-Patients-andWomens-Health?IsMobileSet=false>.
25 <https://nationalfile.com/pro-trans-liberal-democrats-receive-300k-frompuberty-blockers-firm/>.
26 Email correspondence from Ferring Pharmaceuticals, 10 February 2020.
27 <https://www.eurospe.org/news/item/12555/First-ESPE-ScienceSymposium-%27The-Science-of-Gender%27>.
28 Pagan Kennedy. (30 March 2008). 'Q&A with Norman Spack. A doctor helps children change their gender'. *Boston Globe*.

> If a girl starts to experience breast budding and feels like cutting herself, then she's probably transgendered. If she feels immediate relief on the [puberty-blocking] drugs, that confirms the diagnosis.[29]

Spack claimed in 2008 that the real obstacle was the cost of the medications and complained that few parents could afford them:

> [doctors are] salivating at the prospect of applying the Dutch protocol for pubertal suppression, yet without permission from health insurers to pay for the expensive drugs.[30]

Spack soon remedied this situation himself, however, as he was appointed to the board of The Endocrine Society, along with Cohen-Kettenis and Delemarre-van de Waal. They were thus able to include the recommendations for puberty blockers in the guidelines for care of transsexual children.[31] Unsurprisingly, their own papers feature heavily among the studies they cite as proof of the efficacy of puberty blockers. The trio did not stop there: as Cohen-Kettenis also sat on the board of the lobby group WPATH and partook in rewriting their guidelines, puberty blockers and the papers authored by the group found their way into these as well.

Moreover, Cohen-Kettenis acted as a consultant when the fifth edition of the Diagnostic and Statistical Manual of Mental Disorders, the DSM-5, was edited to include gender dysphoria in children as a specific category in the early 2000s. The manual details eight criteria that must be met for a child to be diagnosed with gender dysphoria; five of these relate to gender roles and include playing with friends of the opposite sex or toys that are considered to 'belong' to the opposite sex, and dressing in clothing considered to be for the opposite sex.[32] Following these new guidelines, states and insurers began financing treatment.

Henceforth, received wisdom was in favour of early intervention, while in the past, caution was advocated with a 'wait and see' approach based on

---

29 Ibid.
30 Norman P. Spack. (2008). Foreword in *Brill and Pepper*, p. xi.
31 Wylie C. Hembree, Peggy Cohen-Kettenis, Henriette A. Delemarre-van de Waal, Louis J. Gooren, Walter J.III Meyer, Norman P. Spack, Vin Tangpricha and Victor M. Montori. (1 September 2009). 'Endocrine treatment of transsexual persons. An endocrine society clinical practice guideline'. *The Journal of Clinical Endocrinology & Metabolism*, Vol. 94, No. 9.
32 <https://www.psychiatry.org/patients-families/gender-dysphoria/what-is-gender-dysphoria>.

evidence that the majority of those who experience gender dysphoria in their early teens grow out of it. Differences in sex characteristics between children are insignificant; it is with the onset of puberty that physical differences between the sexes become tangible, which can also entail a fair share of psychological turmoil. Yet Spack and his group of pioneers claimed gender identity was immutable: if we can see its manifestation in the teenage years, it will likely remain unchanged.[33] Their own studies demonstrated that all the children who had been treated with puberty blockers progressed to cross-sex hormone therapy and sex change and that none of the participants abandoned the treatment over the course of the studies. Should some children change their mind, there was no harm done, Spack et al. argued; the effects of puberty blockers were completely reversible.

The reversibility of puberty blockers was repeated so often it became a mantra. Claims about puberty blockers being safe, harmless and reversible were written into WPATH's and the Endocrine Society's guidelines, from where the information was then copied and disseminated. A BBC documentary explained didactically that puberty blockers were akin to pressing pause (cue the image of a pause button), to then later, when one wanted to start puberty again, pressing play (cue image of play button).[34]

In 2008, Cohen-Kettenis and Delemarre-van de Waal asserted that several reasons existed for starting treatment early.[35] They had noted that the age of individuals accessing clinics was decreasing and that "these youngsters are no longer willing to wait for many years" but want treatment immediately. They are well-informed, aware and supported by their parents and if they can avoid developing breasts or facial hair, they will experience fewer problems passing as a member of the opposite sex in the future. Starting treatment early is portrayed as a way of addressing violence and discrimination, with the justification that the easier it is for young people to pass as their chosen sex, the less likely they are to be subjected to

---

33 Peggy Cohen-Kettenis, Henriette Delemarre-van de Waal et al. (2008). 'The treatment of adolescent transsexuals. Changing insights'. *The Journal of Sexual Medicine*, Vol. 5, pp. 1892–1897.
34 Michael Biggs. (July 2019). *The Tavistock's Experiment with Puberty Blockers*, p. 8. Oxford: Dept of Sociology, Oxford University.
35 Peggy Cohen-Kettenis, Henriette Delemarre-van de Waal et al. (2008). 'The treatment of adolescent transsexuals. Changing insights'. *The Journal of Sexual Medicine*, Vol. 5, pp. 1892–1897.

discrimination and violence. Granted, there were disadvantages to starting early, such as the fact that if a penis never fully develops, the remaining tissue is not sufficient to create a vagina. But concerns about functioning organs were seen as inconsequential in the face of the important matter at hand: being able to pass in the eyes of others.

Matters have gained traction since 2008, with the British NHS deciding in 2010 to conduct a puberty blocker trial on 50 children. The results indicated that fewer behavioural problems were experienced and that self-esteem increased. Simultaneously, however, participants displayed greater suicidal tendencies and increased physical and psychological distress. Notwithstanding these rather confusing results, it was decided in 2014 that puberty blockers be prescribed regardless of age.[36] This remained so until 2022, when after widespread criticism and lawsuits, the Cass report to the NHS advised caution when prescribing puberty blockers to children with gender dysphoria, due to lack of knowledge about their effects and risks of disruption to brain development.[37]

Swedish gender clinic Anova still provides similarly reassuring information to its patients and the public: "treatment is safe and well-tested."[38] Most recently, some endocrinologists have begun voicing the opinion that all children ought to be prescribed puberty blockers until they decide which puberty, male or female, they would rather experience.[39]

Yet no long-term studies exist on the consequences of completely stopping a child's puberty, as the studies involving children are in fact about individuals who have had puberty *delayed*. The physical effects of preventing the process by which a child becomes an adult remain unknown and the majority of studies on GnRHas are of adults. They show that GnRHas are a far cry from the safe and reversible treatment that trans clinics claim them to be. Common side effects for men include "fatigue, hot flashes, decreased

---

36 Michael Biggs. (2019). 'Britain's experiment with puberty blockers'. In Michele Moore and Heather Brunskell-Evans (eds). *Inventing Transgender Children and Young People*, p. 46. Cambridge Scholars Publishing.
37 Hilary Cass. (February 2022). 'Independent Review of Gender Identity Services for Children and Young People'. Interim report.
38 Olle Söder. (2017). 'Könsidentitet ur endokrinologiskt perspektiv'. Lecture at Skolläkarföreningen in Gävle. <www.koxxnsdysfori-gaxxvle-feb-2017.pdf (slf.se)>.
39 Transgender 201: Advanced Practice in the Care of Gender-Diverse Youth, AACAP Annual Meeting, 18 October 2019.

libido, decreased quality of life, obesity, diabetes mellitus, coronary artery disease, decreased bone mineral density, and increased risk of fractures." According to the Swedish Medical Products Agency, sustained use of the drug leads to "atrophy of sex organs," or penile and testicular shrinking.[40] Over one in ten women suffer hemorrhaging, while particularly those women who take the drug in early puberty report osteoporosis, tooth loss and suicide attempts.[41] Another common adverse effect is loss of libido – in fact this is the reason for the drug's use on US sex offenders. The US Food and Drug Administration's (FDA) statistics on deaths connected to reports of GnRH analogues have increased dramatically since 2010, though the reason is difficult to ascertain. Furthermore, since only cases in which the drug was used as indicated are listed, children and young people with gender dysphoria are not included in the statistics.[42]

Prescribing hormone suppressants to an adult who has already gone through puberty is one thing. Completely obstructing the natural process of puberty is another. It entails penis and breasts never developing, one's voice not breaking, internal and external sex organs and skeleton never fully developing, hips not widening and menstruation never starting. In a Swedish case, puberty blockers were given to a young girl for a full four years – double the amount of time recommended by international guidelines – and after she complained of extreme back pain, it was discovered that the girl suffered from osteoporosis, that her skeleton was porous and that her growth had stopped.[43] Treatment with puberty blockers can even impede brain development. Studies on animals show that puberty blockers can worsen memory and other brain functions and that long-term memory does not improve when treatment is ceased.[44]

---

40 Läkemedelsverket, Produktresumé (Patient Information Leaflet) Pamorelin 11.25 mg pulver och vätska till injektionsvätska, depotsuspension, L02AE04, Triptorelin.
41 Christina Jewett. (2 February). 'Drug used to halt puberty in children may cause lasting health problems'. *Statnews*.
42 FDA Adverse Advents Reporting System: Lupron (P), Lupron Depot-Ped (P), 30 June 2019. <https://fis.fda.gov/sense/app/d10be6bb-494e-4cd2-82e4-0135608ddc13/sheet/45beeb74-30ab-46be-8267-5756582633b4/state/analysis>.
43 Uppdrag granskning avslöjar: Flera barn har fått skador i transvården. (2021). SVT News.
44 D. Hough et al. (2017). 'Spatial memory is impaired by peripubertal GnRH agonist treatment and testosterone replacement in sheep'. *Psychoneuroendocrinology*, Vol. 75, pp. 173–182.

A Brazilian case study of a boy given puberty blockers for two years and four months concluded that his IQ had diminished:

> A Global IQ reduction is observed. At the end of 28 months of treatment, speed processing and memory remain lower than before GnRHa treatment.[45]

Shockingly, the boy's mental development did not simply stagnate – it actually deteriorated.

The Medical Products Agency does not recommend off-label use of medicines, but states this can be done in the absence of alternatives. Should there be a lack of proven scientific evidence, use ought to occur within clinical trials. This involves testing the drug on groups of healthy individuals in four phases and thoroughly following up on results. Upon more widespread prescription, the agency emphasises the importance of adequate safety follow-ups and reporting of suspected adverse effects.[46] We must therefore ask: how does the Swedish national health service monitor children and young people with gender dysphoria who have been prescribed GnRHas? The distressing answer is they do not.

---

45   Maiko A. Schneider et al. (14 November 2017). 'Brain maturation, cognition and voice pattern in a gender dysphoria case under pubertal suppression'. *Frontiers in Human Neuroscience*, Vol. 11, p. 528. <doi:10.3389/fnhum.2017.00528>.

46   Sweden's Medical Products Agency's view on off label-prescribing, Läkemedelsverket, 24 September 2020.

CHAPTER 17

They Will Probably Become Infertile, But That's the Price You Pay – The New Era of Sterilisations

The issue with puberty blockers is not only their adverse effects, but the fact that the majority of those who are prescribed them proceed to cross-sex hormones. Earlier research demonstrates that 80 per cent of individuals expressing a desire to change sex in their teens who are left without intervention, no longer express this desire once adulthood is reached. Remarkably, the results are reversed among those who *are* prescribed puberty blockers, with the majority of individuals in this cohort moving on to hormone treatment and later surgery.[47] A mere 1.4 per cent of those taking puberty blockers abandon treatment.[48] This is precisely what was observed by Cohen-Kettenis and her colleagues: that so few in this group change their minds. She argues that this is proof they have been correctly diagnosed, i.e. that individuals on puberty blockers

---

47 Karolinska Institutet. (2018). Comment regarding motion 'Ändring av det kön som framgår av folkbokföringen' (Changing legal sex), Ds. Departementsserien (Government briefing papers) 2018, No. 17. <https://www.regeringen.se/remisser/2018/05/remiss-ds-201817-andring-av-det-kon-som-framgar-av-folkbokforingen/>.
48 Annelou L. C. de Vries. (October 2020). 'Challenges in timing puberty suppression for gender-nonconforming adolescents'. *Pediatrics*, Vol. 146, No. 4. <e2020010611; DOI: 10.1542/peds.2020-010611>.

are in fact transsexual; were they not, she claims, they would abandon treatment. Most transgender care professionals share this reasoning.

Yet as we have noted, an alternative possibility exists, namely that puberty blockers themselves impede the option of choosing a different path. This explanation would account for the significant difference between the group prescribed puberty blockers and the cohort which experiences puberty. A 13-year-old who remains a child while their classmates begin to develop has rooted their entire identity in their body. The body becomes a project, and that project is sex change. The ongoing contact with health services, the injections and appointments, are a constant reminder of the young person's identity as a trans teen, which in most cases is complemented by membership of an online community founded on trans identity. Since an increasing number of schools in the western world have adopted a policy of changing trans youths' names even before an official sex change, the youngster assumes their new identity fully. The more one invests and sacrifices, the harder it usually is to backtrack.

Whatever the reasons may be, results are clear: those who start puberty blockers will continue on to cross-sex hormones and surgery. Thus, puberty blockers are not just an opportunity to explore one's identity in peace and quiet. Contrary to claims, they become a way of expediting the journey down a specific path.

While the effect of puberty blockers can be reversible when stopped in time (despite the adverse effects already mentioned), this is not the case when testosterone or estrogen are prescribed immediately after. This sequence is highly likely to lead to life-long infertility.[49] Since sexual maturity is never reached, the body cannot produce egg cells or sperm. One US study of young people prescribed puberty blockers found that none of the participants had preserved fertility.[50] Endocrinologists are well aware of this – even hormone evangelists like Norman P. Spack acknowledge it, though they claim it is a price worth paying:

> When young people halt their puberty before their bodies have developed, and then take cross-hormones for a few years, they'll probably be infertile.

---

49 <https://transcare.ucsf.edu/article/information-estrogen-hormone-therapy>.
50 John F. Strang et al. (2018). 'Transgender Youth Fertility Attitudes Questionnaire: Measure Development in Nonautistic and Autistic Transgender Youth and Their Parents'. *Journal of Adolescent Health*, Vol. 62, No. 2, pp. 128–135.

> You have to explain to the patients that if they go ahead, they may not be able to have children. When you're talking to a 12-year-old, that's a heavy-duty conversation. Does a kid that age really think about fertility? But if you don't start treatment, they will always have trouble fitting in. And my patients always remind me that what's most important to them is their identity.[51]

Consequently, children who first access clinics aged ten to 12 and are informed it is completely harmless to hit the pause button on puberty while they explore their identity, are highly likely to begin a journey down a path leading to infertility. Rather than being a chance to stop and catch one's breath, this supposedly innocuous break from puberty is in fact a fast forwarding to sterilisation. *Kamratposten* magazine's advice to its young readers to approach trans health care clinics thus has far reaching consequences, which children are not informed about.

In fact, a young person searching for information regarding effects of hormone treatment will find nothing about its most serious consequence: infertility. Indeed, this is not mentioned at all on RFSL Ungdom's site (youth arm of The Swedish Federation for Lesbian, Gay, Bisexual, Transgender, Queer and Intersex Rights), which is regularly consulted by young people wanting information on the topic. On the contrary, young people are led to believe they can simply "stop hormone treatment and wait for the body's own hormone production to restart."[52] Neither Anova nor Sweden's equivalent of NHS Direct list infertility among the side effects, although one can guess at this consequence by reading between the lines due to sentences like the following: "Before you begin treatment, you'll be asked whether you want to preserve your sperm or egg cells so that you may be able to have children you are genetically related to in future,"[53] though such subtleties may not be easy for a 12-year-old to understand.

Sterilisation of trans people is often referred to as a crime of the past, but is in fact occurring as we speak, with sterilisation not of adults but of children and teenagers. Sweden's National Board of Health and Welfare stated in 2015 that hormones can be prescribed regardless of age,

---

51 Pagan Kennedy. (30 March 2008). 'Q&A with Norman Spack. A doctor helps children change their gender'. *Boston Globe*.
52 <http://www.transformering.se/vardhalsa/hormoner>.
53 <https://www.1177.se/liv--halsa/konsidentitet-och-sexuell-laggning/konsdysfori/>.

provided the young person "understands the effects and consequences of treatment."[54] This is rather a tall order, for how can a ten-year-old possibly make an informed decision about a procedure whose implication is life-long infertility? How can they decide at this early age that they will never want to experience fetching a child from nursery, or seeing a grandchild graduate? The age limit on voluntary sterilisation for the general public is 25 for this very reason – not even at the age of 18 are our brains sufficiently developed to contemplate the consequences of such a decision. The Board contends there is a lack of scientific research concerning nearly all aspects of fertility in young trans people, yet holds that children be informed regarding the possibility of freezing their sperm or egg cells – this despite the fact there are often no sperm to freeze in cases where puberty blockers have been prescribed early on.

The tone adopted in the Board's methodological framework is nonchalant and breezy, as though they were discussing hypothetical medical experiments. One option, they claim, is to harvest egg cells and freeze them, which can be achieved through "hormone stimulation and transvaginal ultrasound-guided aspiration of the ovaries" of a 14-year-old! Another is to "freeze ovarian tissue from which it may be possible to extract mature eggs for IVF." This procedure is flanked by a caveat: "results thus far have been disappointing."[55] The procedure entails a girl receiving hormone stimulation with extremely high doses of estrogen and progesterone in order to increase egg cell production. Subsequently, she would be given high doses of testosterone to masculinise her body. What are the physical and psychological effects of this on a teenager? No one appears to know.

This significant decrease in fertility following use of puberty blockers and hormone treatment has opened up a new market for endocrinologists: IVF for trans people. Several US clinics have already specialised and offer young women the option of freezing their egg cells prior to commencing

---

54 Socialstyrelsen (National Board of Health and Welfare). (2015). 'God vård av barn och ungdomar med könsdysfori. Metodbeskrivning och kunskapsunderlag', pp. 33–34.
55 Ibid. p. 93

testosterone treatment. Once they feel ready to have children, the same clinics provide embryo transplants using surrogates.[56]

It is not only childbirth which is denied to individuals on puberty blockers and hormone treatment. Sexual function and pleasure can both potentially be seriously damaged, too. A boy prescribed puberty blockers at 11 followed by hormones will retain the penis of an 11-year-old for the rest of his life, should he wish to keep it. Many teenagers report that their libido disappears completely after these interventions.[57] What happens to these teenagers as adults? Five to ten years later, it is not uncommon to find them at fertility clinics.

In late 2020, I interviewed a physician in the IVF sector, who reported having noticed the effects in his field of treatment for gender dysphoria over the course of the previous year. One of his patients was a woman in her 20s who had been unable to conceive. Tests revealed her ovaries contained a higher than expected proportion of connective tissue including several small cysts. Blood tests showed ovarian activity was extremely low and it was unlikely that she would ever be able to conceive. On hearing this, the woman broke down and disclosed she had been treated as a teen by the Anova clinic with puberty blockers and testosterone. She had subsequently decided to return to living as a woman and had been informed by the clinic that the treatment she had undergone would not result in any risks to her fertility. The physician contacted the Board of Health and Welfare, from where he was directed to Anova. He inquired as to their follow-up procedures for patients and was told they undertook no long-term tracing at all. "It is completely illogical," he said. "A drug with equally drastic side effects would not be prescribed without long-term follow-up of patients under any other circumstances. Gynaecology and oncology departments remain in contact with their patients for five to ten years post-treatment. It cannot be claimed that the treatment is harmless when no attempts are made to ascertain whether this is the case."

The list of adverse effects continues. When it comes to long-term estrogen treatment of men, they are five times more likely to suffer

---

56 Sarah Marie Winther. (16 August. 2017). 'Egg-freezing is giving young trans men hope for starting a family'. *Vice Magazine*.
57 S. Nikkelen and B. Kreukels. (2018). 'Sexual experiences in transgender people. The role of desire for gender-confirming interventions, psychological wellbeing, and body satisfaction'. *Journal of Sex & Marital Therapy*, Vol. 44, No. 4.

from cardiovascular disease.⁵⁸ A Danish study of all individuals who had undergone sex change treatment in Denmark between 1978 and 2010 corroborated this, finding an increase in cardiovascular disease. In addition, 9.6 per cent of the participants had died at an average age of 53.5 years.⁵⁹ Other common complications of estrogen therapy include depression, anxiety, mood swings and insomnia, which are experienced by over one in ten users.⁶⁰ Swedish trans woman Vanessa Lopez reports:

> I have plenty of regrets. My health has deteriorated, I've got brittle bones and my doctor said I've got the body of a 93 year old. I've got back pain and they still don't know how the drugs affect your heart. I'm on medication for the rest of my life.⁶¹

Upon discovering that the hormone could aggravate mental health issues, the mother of a boy with depression prescribed estrogen by the Anova clinic decided to confront the clinic and record the phone conversation. In it, Anova director Cecilia Dhejne and psychologist Annika Johansson are heard minimising the risks:

> Cecilia Dhejne: No, generally speaking estrogen doesn't cause depression.
>
> Parent: But it *is* a common side effect?
>
> CD: No.
>
> Parent (consulting medication information leaflet): Estradot common side effects may occur in one in ten users, so that's like ten per cent: depression, anxiety, mood swings, insomnia. This is off the FASS database.⁶²
>
> CD: Mmh. But Estradot is a medicine and it's what we prescribe, which we both use in a lot of cases, especially for menopause, over long periods of time.
>
> Annika Johansson: There are a number of issues to explore in more depth. And how one assesses well-being, I mean in treatment of gender

---

58 M. S. Irwig. (September 2018). 'Cardiovascular health in transgender people'. *Reviews in Endocrine and Metabolic Disorders*, Vol. 19, No. 3, pp. 243–251. <doi:10.1007/s11154-018-9454-3>.

59 Rikke Kildevæld Simonsen et al. (2016). 'Long-term follow-up of individuals undergoing sex-reassignment surgery. Somatic morbidity and cause of death', *Sexual Medicine*, Vol. 4, No. 1, pp. e60-8. <doi:10.1016/j.esxm.2016.01.001>.

60 <https://www.fass.se/LIF/product?userType=2&nplId=20011130000260>.

61 Malin Aunsbjerg. (5 April 2019). 'Vanessa om könsbytet: "Jag har ångrat mig många gånger"'. *Allas*. Article since removed.

62 FASS is the Swedish equivalent of the EMC (Electronic Medicines Compendium).

dysphoria compared to the slightly raised risk from estrogen and I mean, gender dysphoria itself is really depressing, not being able to express yourself the way you want, or experiencing that constant body dysphoria and so on. So if you can get some kind of respite from that then you could feel better once the gender dysphoria is treated.

Parent: But what about these side effects on the medicine information leaflet for Estradot – the depression and that? Don't they apply to people with XY chromosomes?

CD: Yes, well, it doesn't really matter whether one has XY or XX chromosomes, but among endocrinologists and gynaecologists prescribing this medication there isn't any clinical evidence of significant numbers of patients getting depression.[63]

The clinic managers thus deny the very risks which are so well-documented they appear on the medication information leaflet.

The mother of another girl who received treatment at Anova began asking questions critical of hormone therapy in a meeting for family members, questioning the extent to which it had in fact undergone reliable tests. She was promptly informed her questions were unsuitable for the meeting and was denied entry to future meetings, with the justification that she had behaved "aggressively." The clinic offered her a private meeting with the physician-in-charge, during which she was presented with a monologue about treatments, but was not permitted to ask any questions. Her requested second meeting for questions was cancelled – the reason given by the physician-in-charge was that it was "beyond our remit"[64] to answer questions from family, and she was advised to contact one of the "relevant national authorities."

---

63 Recording of call between Cecilia Dhejne, Annika Johansson, mother 'M' and patient, 17 January 2020.
64 Email from Cecilia Dhejne to mother 'T': "Acting PFC Katarina Görts Öberg and I have considered your request and decided to withdraw our initial offer of yet another meeting. We are therefore unable to receive you on 1 October. We judge that the purpose of this meeting is beyond our remit. Regarding your queries about treatment and information about the risks involved, we confirm the information we supplied earlier, i.e. that we follow the National Board of Health and Welfare's guidelines, science and proven experience. Patients are informed about risks and side effects of treatment. Regarding your more general questions, it is beyond our remit to respond to them and we therefore suggest you contact one of the relevant national authorities."

In the place of factual information regarding risks, parents are fobbed off with statements about "new ground being broken" and, should they disagree with hormone prescription for their child, that the child is a suicide risk.[65]

In 2015, the first large-scale study on effects of puberty blockers and hormones on children with gender dysphoria was announced.[66] The endocrinologists conducting the study are already familiar to us and have been selected directly from the industry. Our friend Norman P. Spack, famed for salivating over the prospect of prescribing pubertal blockers, is among them. The hormone enthusiast Robert Garofalo, Division Head of Adolescent and Young Adult Medicine at Lurie Children's Hospital and recipient of large pharmaceutical company grants, is also present. UCSF Child and Adolescent Gender Center founder Stephen Rosenthal is included. He is a long-standing advocate for use of Lupron in treating gender dysphoria and has received sponsorship from Lupron manufacturer AbbVie. Last but not least, the list of authors includes Johanna Olson-Kennedy, director of the Los Angeles Center for Transgender Health and Development Children's Hospital and former employee of both AbbVie and Endo Pharmaceuticals.[67]

Olson-Kennedy maintains that hormone therapy is always the right option and when deciding, it is not necessary for a physician to be certain of their decision as "compassion is more important than safety."[68] She has personally treated children as young as 12 and proudly reports never having prescribed puberty blockers to anyone who did not subsequently progress to hormone therapy. Removing young girls' breasts is not a big deal, she claims, since "if you want breasts later in life, you can just go and

---

65 <https://vettigt.blog/2018/05/30/foraldrar-skrams-till-tystnad-avtransvarden-i-brist-pa-vetenskapligt-stod/>.

66 Juliana Bunim. (17 August 2015). 'First U.S. study of transgender youth funded by NIH'. University of California.

67 AbbVie information in David A. Klein. (July 2015). 'Care of a transgender adolescent'. *American Family Physician*, Vol. 92, No. 2, p. 229. Endo Pharmaceuticals information in Murray (2019).

68 <https://www.healio.com/endocrinology/pediatric-endocrinology/news/online/%7Ba2eedc18-0009-4682-80dd-b259bc13b45a%7D/care-fortransgender-children-starts-with-affirmation-safety> and <https://www.gendergp.com/gender-affirmative-johanna-olson-kennedy/>.

get another pair."⁶⁹ Moreover, Olson-Kennedy believes the hippocratic oath of 'above all, do no harm' (primum non nocere) is a relative concept:

> [First do no harm] is really subjective. Historically we come from a very paternalistic perspective ... [in which] doctors are really given the purview of deciding what is going to be harmful and what isn't. And that, in the world of gender, is really problematic.⁷⁰

---

69 Douglas Murray. (2019). *The Madness of Crowds: Gender, Race and Identity*, pp. 223–225. Bloomsbury.
70 Johanna Olson. (November 2014). Speech to medical students. <http://theshortcoat.com/tag/johanna-olson/>. Post later removed at Olson's request. Transcript of lecture available on <https://www.gendertrending.com/2014/11/11/skipping-the-puberty-blockers-american-transgender-children-doctors-are-going-rogue/>.

CHAPTER 18

When States Convert Homosexuals

At first glance, one might think that the patients of youth trans clinics only have one thing in common: that they are trans. However, several studies show a much more complex picture.

The vast majority of young people seeking treatment at trans clinics are homosexual or have one or several neuropsychiatric diagnoses. Most come from a highly educated family background and 41 per cent previously identified as gay or bisexual. 62.5 per cent of girls in a British study had previously been diagnosed with a psychiatric or neuropsychiatric illness.[71] Anorexia is especially common, as are ADHD, depression and trauma. The figures are nearly identical in other countries: 60 per cent of patients at transgender clinics in Sweden and Norway suffer from complex mental health needs.[72] Similarly, a US study found 44 per cent of girls aged three to 12 diagnosed with gender dysphoria who did not undergo hormone treatment turned out to be lesbian or bisexual in their teens.[73] A 2011 Dutch study followed up 77 children referred to a gender dysphoria clinic when they were aged eight and obtained similar results: the majority

---

71 Lisa Littman. (16 August 2018). 'Parent Reports of Adolescents and Young Adults Perceived to Show Signs of a Rapid Onset of Gender Dysphoria'. *Plos One*, 13(8): e0202330.
72 SVT. 'Tranståget och tonårsflickorna'. (April 2019). 'Uppdrag granskning'. Presenter: Karin Mattisson.
73 K.D. Drummond, S.J. Bradley, M. Peterson-Badali et al. (2008.) 'A follow-up study of girls with gender identity disorder'. *Developmental Psychology*, Vol. 44, No. 1, pp. 34–45.

later turned out to be gay or bisexual. This was overwhelmingly true for boys, 46 per cent of whom no longer had gender dysphoria in their teens. Around half of the participants later identified as gay and, of those whose gender dysphoria persisted, all were in gay or bisexual relationships. The researchers, Cohen-Kettenis among them, were obliged to draw conclusions in complete contradiction of their previous work:

> Most children with gender dysphoria will not remain gender dysphoric after puberty. Children with persistent GID are characterized by more extreme gender dysphoria in childhood than children with desisting gender dysphoria. With regard to sexual orientation, the most likely outcome of childhood GID is homosexuality or bisexuality.[74]

Several of the male participants had been taken to the clinic due to their feminine behaviour in childhood. Investigations into their gender identity consisted of parents being questioned regarding their children's play habits and their gender role behaviour patterns. The children were observed at play and required to respond to questions like "Do you think it's better to be a boy or a girl?" Forty-four boys were identified as 'feminine'. The study showed that only one of the boys treated continued to identify as a girl, while the others (who never underwent gender reassignment) proved to be gay or bisexual. "Of these 44 feminine boys, only one youth was gender dysphoric at the age of 18" meaning "80% of the feminine boys were either homosexual or bisexual."

The studies mentioned were all conducted prior to the tremendous increase in teen gender dysphoria. A fundamental flaw is that around 30 per cent of participants did not respond to follow-up questionnaires. Therefore, it is impossible to state with any certainty how they felt and why. Yet one thing is clear: it is above all gay children and teenagers who are taken to gender reassignment clinics. Through injections and later surgery, they are made to resemble members of the opposite sex. In other words, made to look heterosexual. The boy who behaves 'effeminately' and is taken to a clinic at age eight, is made into a girl and probably sterilised in the process. Here are the words of a mother of an 11-year-old boy:

---

[74] M. S. C. Wallien, P. T. Cohen-Kettenis. (2008). 'Psychosexual outcome of gender-dysphoric children', *Journal of the American Academy of Child and Adolescent Psychiatry*, Vol. 47, No. 12, pp. 1413–1423.

We gave him the idea. He liked wearing dresses and then we read in the paper that one could be born in the wrong body. We thought we were helping him. We didn't understand that it would lead to this. We confused being feminine with being a girl.[75]

Pressure can also be exerted by schools and wider society, as experienced by the parents of this US primary school pupil who loved princess dresses, swords, pokemon and his long blond hair. They received a phone call from the school's principal in which they were informed that "Sam needed to choose one gender or the other, because kids could be mean. He could either jettison his pink Crocs and cut his hair or socially transition and come to school as a girl."[76] Society appears provoked in particular by boys behaving 'effeminately'. While girls who play with boys are often considered strong and independent, there is apparently something unsettling about unmasculine boys.

Advocates of gender reassignment in children often liken their campaign to the struggle for gay rights, since this provides a ready-made narrative about an oppressed sexual minority fighting for recognition. As the narrative goes, the oppressed minority meets resistance from conservative and religious groups, but tolerance eventually triumphs and society at large understands all people must be accepted as they are. Fifty years of struggle by the gay rights movement has paved the way and trans people are thus merely the next group in line expected to tread the same path. What gay people went through in the past, the reasoning goes, trans people are going through now. This is merely history repeating itself. With the discourse thus presented, the crux becomes about being on the right side of history – and there is no doubt what that entails: upholding everyone's right to 'be themselves'.

Despite initial resistance from transsexual organisations to joining gay rights organisations, fearing, as one Swedish transsexual group put it, being 'associated with transvestites' and 'sexualised language', the analogy between gay and trans has been successfully ingrained into our collective

---

75 Quoted in Jannika Häggström. (30 October 2019). 'Blandar vi ihop två alldeles diametralt motsatta idéer?' Anhöriga berättar. < https://genid.se/personligt/blandar-vi-ihop-tva-alldeles-diametralt-motsatta-ideer/>.

76 Margaret Talbot. (11 March 2013). 'About a boy. Transgender surgery at sixteen'. *The New Yorker.*

consciousness.⁷⁷ Remember the gay rights struggle? This is exactly the same! Questioning hormone treatment for children is thus equated with opposition to Stonewall, Pride marches and marriage equality! Journalist Ulrika Stahre writes that criticising surgical interventions on children contains "echoes of homophobia."⁷⁸ The term "echoes" swiftly associates one thing with another without having to actually perform an analysis. Stahre continues:

> It is particularly ironic to be reminded of this considering it is 40 years since the occupation of the National Board of Health and Welfare by LGBTQ-activists, an action which led to homosexuality being depathologised [in Sweden].

One is thus supposed to equate GnRHas with homosexuality: what they fought for then, we fight for now!

However, whereas the gay rights movement fought for the right to be oneself *against* pathologisation and medicalisation, transactivists now struggle *in favour of* medicalisation – most often of the very same gay people. Thus, what is being portrayed as one and the same struggle are in many instances in fact polar opposites. When three-year-old Jazz Jennings' parents who took him to a doctor because he liked wearing dresses, were told he ought to start hormone treatment soon and later have his penis removed, he was not being 'accepted as he is'. Rather, he was being labelled as flawed on the basis that a boy should not wear dresses. Thus feminine, possibly gay, boys are being transformed into heterosexual girls. Gender incongruence is currently considered a medical condition in need of treatment. 'Feminine' young boys who like wearing dresses, experimenting with different hairstyles, putting on dance performances at home and do not take an interest in football are being sterilised. Girls who are disinterested in cosmetics, like football and fixing cars and sit with their legs uncrossed are, in turn, being rendered infertile.

Is this not in reality a form of gay conversion therapy? Where medical practitioners diagnose gay and lesbian people as deviant and reassign them as heterosexual – the price being sterilisation? What if history really is repeating itself, only the other way around, with the activists of the past

---

77 'Ändrad könstillhörighet'. (2007). p. 38.
78 Ulrika Stahre. (2 September 2019). 'Nej det finns ingen transmaffia', *Aftonbladet Kultur*.

doing a 180 degree turn? What if lazy thinking, guilt-by-association and intense lobbying has made the gay rights movement fight against – gay people themselves?

CHAPTER 19

What is a Man without a Penis?

On the road to gender reassignment, surgery normally follows puberty blockers and hormones. Anova clinic's website explains: "Demand for gender affirmation chest, genitals, vocal cords and Adam's apple surgery, including procedures for voice therapy, fertility preservation, hair removal and hormone treatment is increasing."[79]

Yet despite the fact that even the extremely far-reaching Dutch protocol does not recommend surgery on minors, it is occurring ever more frequently. The first stage for young girls is generally mastectomy, or breast removal. Around 80 per cent report satisfaction one to two years following surgery,[80] though the procedure leaves permanent scarring and makes breastfeeding impossible. Lobby group WPATH does not recommend a specific age limit for mastectomies, saying only that they can be performed on individuals of any age provided they have been taking testosterone for one year.[81] Several US states impose no age limit either, requiring the signature of only one parent for the surgery to be performed.[82] In Sweden, mastectomies have been carried out on at least

---

79 <http://www.anova.se/TM3.htm>.
80 'God vård av barn och ungdomar med könsdysfori. Metodbeskrivning och kunskapsunderlag', Socialstyrelsen (Swedish Board of Health and Welfare). (2015), p. 51.
81 The World Professional Association for Transgender Health. (n.d.). 'Standards of care for the health of transsexual, transgender, and gender nonconforming people, No 7', p. 21.
82 UPDATE: Transgender Healthcare in Oregon. (14 August 2015). TransActive Health Project.

one 14-year old – the exact figures are difficult to come by since clinics are unwilling to disclose them. Per-Anders Rydelius, former director and physician-in-chief at Anova's Kid-team, explains:

> If breasts are a source of distress for a person to the extent that they cannot show themselves in public, socialise with their peers, attend school and have a good time, then it makes sense in this situation (if parents, professionals and the young person perceive this to be the case) to help her get rid of her breasts.[83]

In cases where operations are not covered by public health care funding, young people turn to crowdfunding in order to afford them and employers post encouraging messages on social media.[84] Breast removal is euphemistically referred to as 'top surgery' or 'chest surgery' – note the word 'breast' has already turned into a taboo and been removed in language – and is marketed by clinics as the road to happiness. Canadian provider McLean Clinic goes so far as to promise breast removal will lead to freedom from depression, to self-love, making friends, and even finding love:

> In addition to the overall mental benefits of FTM top surgery, there are also emotional benefits. This can include a wide range of positive effects from decreased risk of depression to increased feelings of self-worth and confidence.
>
> To live a happy and full life, whatever that may look like to you, involves self-love and healthy self-worth. While this doesn't happen overnight, FTM top surgery can definitely help you start on the path to loving and appreciating yourself so much more. Having greater confidence can help to lead to building genuine and long-lasting relationships with your friends, family members, and work colleagues. This can also include finding a partner to share it all with.[85]

It is relatively unusual for girls to have surgery to reconstruct their genitalia to that of a male, since it is as yet not possible to create a functioning penis. Using skin from a leg, surgeons can create the resemblance of a penis in

---

83   *SVT Nyheter.* (3 April 2019). 'Sveriges största könsmottagning har opererat bort bröst på minst en 14-åring'.
84   Jared Lawthorn. (19 July 2019). 'Transgender man's mastectomy surgery dubbed "mutilation".' *BBC Wales.*
85   <https://www.ftmtopsurgery.ca/blog/ftm-surgery/positive-effects-ftm-top-surgery/>.

order to achieve the desired bulge, but it will not be able to have erections. Most FtM transsexuals therefore retain their female genitalia, however those who change legal sex no longer receive invitations to cervical screening appointments. Very little is ever said about this conundrum: the female who wishes to become a male cannot achieve what is touted as the ultimate symbol of manhood: a phallus. She will look like a man, but only up to a certain level of intimacy. In sexual relationships, there will always be a moment when she will have to reveal that despite looking like a man, there is no penis. For females, changing sex is therefore a procedure which mainly involves the upper body.

Genital surgery is far more common in MtF transsexuals; a procedure known as vaginoplasty which turns the penis inside out to create a closed vault. The main purpose of the vault is to resemble a vagina and facilitate penetration, as it is unable to give birth or release menstrual blood. The procedure is complex and can result in various complications: 27 per cent of patients contract infections, 15 per cent suffer blood loss and, in 21 per cent of cases, the resulting vault is not deep or wide enough.[86] Other common adverse effects include hair growing on the inside of the vault, rectovaginal fistulas and urinary tract infections.[87] Vaginoplasty has also resulted in loss of life. Furthermore, regular, life-long use of a dilator is necessary in order to ensure the vault does not close up. In many cases, this is too tiresome and I have heard testimonies of more than one former gay man turned transsexual whose vault simply has closed, and who therefore, in order to have sex with men, has reverted back to anal sex. The dilator manufacturers explain the vault should be considered a wound and that

> dilation therapy is an absolute must to keep your neo vagina functional […] Usually, MtF transgender patients start using vaginal dilation a few days after surgery and continue to use vaginal dilators, to some degree, for the rest of their lives.

---

86   S. Cristofari et al. (February 2019). 'Postoperative complications of male to female sex reassignment surgery. A 10-year French retrospective study'. *Ann Chir Plast Esthet*, Vol. 64, No. 1, pp. 24–32. <doi: 10.1016/j.anplas.2018.08.002. E-pub. 27 September 2018>.
87   Toby Meltzer. (17 June 2016). 'Vaginoplasty procedures, complications and aftercare'. <https://transcare.ucsf.edu/guidelines/vaginoplasty>.

For those concerned about quality of life following surgery, the manufacturers offer these reassuring and encouraging words: "It takes genuine inner strength to become who you are and we want to congratulate and celebrate you, wherever you are on your journey."[88]

---

88 'After your surgery'. (n.d.). *The Pelvic Hub*. <https://www.thepelvichub.com/conditions/sr-surgery>.

CHAPTER 20

Younger, Faster, Happier?

The current lower age limit for genital surgery in Sweden is 18. Internationally, however, it is not uncommon for surgeons to operate on younger patients, especially when it comes to boys. A 2018 legislative proposal put forward by the then Ministers for Social Affairs and Culture and Democracy (Annika Strandhäll and Alice Bah-Kuhnke), suggested lowering the age limit to 15 without the requirement of parental consent.[89] Furthermore, the bill proposed that children from the age of 12 be able to change their legal sex with parental consent and from the age of 15 without. A 12-year-old would not even require consent from both parents – if one objected, Social Services could overrule him/her:

> In cases where one parent or guardian does not consent, it is suggested that Social Services be given the power to decide regarding applications for change of legal sex, where this is deemed in the child's best interests.[90]

Currently, minors in Sweden are not even permitted to change their surname without both parents' signatures. Even a parent with sole custody cannot remove the other parent's surname from the child if that parent does not give consent. Thus, if you are a single mother with sole custody of your child whose surname is Johnson like his father, you cannot remove

---

89 Socialdepartementet, Regeringskansliet. (2018, No. 11). 'Vissa kirurgiska ingrepp i könsorganen', Departementsserien (government briefing papers).
90 Annika Strandhäll and Lars Hedengren. (30 August 2018). 'Vissa kirurgiska ingrepp i könsorganen och ändring av det kön som framgår av folkbokföringen'. Lagrådsremiss (Council on Legislation).

Johnson without district court proceedings.[91] Compare this situation to that proposed in the above bill: a mother could change the child's legal sex without the consent of the father even if they had shared custody! The bill further suggested: "For the best interests of the child, it is important that the parents' perspective in these cases does not interfere."[92] It goes so far as to threaten parents who do not give their consent with being investigated: "Lack of consent from a parent or guardian ought to lead to a report of concern to Social Services."[93]

If the bill had been approved, changing legal sex would have been possible without the need for any medical certificate whatsoever. On the other hand, changing it back was not to be so easy. Those wishing to change back to their original sex would have to undergo a comprehensive assessment to prove "they can be expected to continue living in that gender in future."[94] Thus, an outcome which a 12-year-old can obtain through nagging and a decision a 15-year-old can make overnight, would be significantly more onerous to reverse. This risks trapping very young people in circumstances with immense consequences. The bill stipulates that a 15-year-old ought not "be prevented from having genital surgery on the sole grounds that one or both parents/guardians withhold consent." The government even stated that removing sex organs may be the *only* way a young person could feel normal:

> The suffering involved may lead to absence from school, being unable to socialise, start relationships, and feeling uncomfortable about their body or about having sex. At times, genital surgery is the only way in which a young person is able to live in alignment with their gender identity and enables them to experience 'normal' teenage years.[95]

The bill contains no reflection regarding the underlying causes behind a teen's desire to remove their sex organs. No questions are asked about whether the organ itself is somehow faulty, whether the problem in fact is the gender role, or whether something entirely different is occuring,

---

91 <https://www4.skatteverket.se/rattsligvagledning/edition/2018.1/361282.html#h-Namnbyte-for-barn-som-har-fyllt-12-ar>.
92 Annika Strandhäll and Lars Hedengren. (30 August 2018). 'Vissa kirurgiska ingrepp i könsorganen och ändring av det kön som framgår av folkbokföringen'. *Lagrådsremiss*, p. 32.
93 Ibid. p. 41.
94 Departementsserien (government briefing papers) 2018, No. 17, p. 8.
95 Departementsserien (government briefing papers) 2018, No. 11, p. 75.

such as teen angst or bullying. And to claim that a teenager who has barely reached the age of consent will attain a 'normal' sex life through extremely complicated and risky organ surgery, with possible scarring and damage to nerve ends, is simply unfathomable. A 15-year-old may not even have started using their natural sex organ! And why is it so important to the government that a 15-year-old can have a sex life?

It is astonishing enough that one of the reasons given for removing sex organs of minors is to enable them to have intercourse, but it is utterly unbelievable to presume that an operation which risks seriously damaging the capacity to have sex and has notable life-long consequences is the only solution to a teenager's problems. What is also bewildering is that the government does not seem to have an understanding of what these surgeries entail. The fact that genital surgery for girls who wish to become boys, for an overwhelming majority is not even possible, makes this bill even more perplexing.

The bill is particularly eye-catching in a country like Sweden, where minors cannot even start therapy without both parents' approval. The proposal was developed "in consultation with" Cecilia Dhejne (physician-in-chief at Anova and the person performing the operations), The Swedish Association for Sexuality Education (RFSU) and The Swedish Federation for Lesbian, Gay, Bisexual, Transgender, Queer and Intersex Rights (RFSL and RFSL Ungdom). No women's rights organisations were invited to collaborate or comment, nor were any organisations working on children's and young people's rights.

In fact, the proposal was heavily criticised by experts. In their comment, Karolinska Hospital's DSD (Disorders of Sex Development) team states that it is "completely inappropriate" to change the legal sex of a person under the age of 15. They further note that approving sex change operations on young people cannot be considered in line with "science or proven experience," since research shows the opposite: that 80 per cent of people wanting a sex change in puberty later change their minds and continue to live in their original sex.[96] Considering the fact that the mental ability to judge the consequences of a decision does not fully develop until age 20-25, it is noteworthy that the proposal retains the 12-year age limit

---

96 Karolinska Institutet. (2018). Comment on bill 'Ändring av det kön som framgår av folkbokföringen', Departementsserien (government briefing papers) 2018, No. 17.

despite the DSD team's stern counsel against it prior to the proposal. Furthermore, the team also notes that it is common for young people who approach transgender services to have other psychiatric diagnoses and that it is difficult for young people to foresee the consequences of their decisions.

The bill received criticism from several other stakeholders, including The Swedish Paediatric Society and The Swedish National Council on Medical Ethics, which held that genital surgery on minors ought not even be contemplated. Further criticism came in the form of a research review by Västra Götland region's Health Technology (HTA) centre, which evaluates methodologies and techniques in health care. They concluded:

> The available literature includes only observational studies of mostly poor quality, comparative studies are few and data from long-term follow up are lacking. The certainty of evidence for the benefits of genital, facial, and body gender affirmation surgery is generally very low [...] while major surgical complications probably are frequent after genital gender affirmation surgery.[97]

The most severe criticism came from the Council on Legislation, which stated that the bill contravened the European Convention on Human Rights.[98] Letting a child's will supersede parents' right to decide meant, according to the Council, that "in practice, parents' right and duty to decide in the best interests of their child in these matters is removed and they can even be denied access to the process in which interventions are made." Notably, no organisations working on gender equality between the sexes were among those selected to comment on the proposal.

The bill may very likely have become law, had it not been for investigative journalist programme *Uppdrag Granskning*'s broadcast "Tranståget och tonårs flickorna" (The Trans Train and Teenage Girls) (2019),[99] coincidentally produced at precisely the same moment that the bill was being debated. The programme was fiercely critical of sex

---

97 K. Georgas et al. (2018. No. 102).'Gender affirmation surgery for gender dysphoria – effects and risks'. Health Technology Assessment. *HTA report*, p. 5. Västra Götalandsregionen Sahlgrenska Universitetsjukhuset.

98 Extract from protocol of meeting 23 October 2018: 'Vissa kirurgiska ingrepp i könsorganen och ändring av det kön som framgår av folkbokföringen', Lagrådet (Council on Legislation).

99 SVT. 'Tranståget och tonårsflickorna'. (April 2019). 'Uppdrag granskning'. Presenter: Karin Mattisson.

change operations on young people: in it, two girls who had undergone irreversible procedures and later regretted these, spoke out about their disappointment with a healthcare system that had turned their back on them. In the second part of the program, the recently appointed Minister for Social Affairs, Lena Hallengren, was questioned following the discovery of several factual errors in one of the documents the government had relied on when compiling its bill. Hallengren suddenly tasked the Board of Health and Welfare with reviewing their advice regarding surgery on young people. Miraculously, the Board made an about-turn. In 2018, they had supported the government's recommendations fully – two years later, in March 2020, their report held that "there is currently more evidence against than in favour of enabling surgical interventions on individuals under 18."[100]

Two changes were thus made to the bill: changing legal sex would only be possible with parental consent, and genital operations would only be permitted from the age of 18. Yet the rest of the bill stands, and the Social Democratic government promised that in the year 2022, it would be submitted to a parliamentary vote. As a new right-wing government was formed after the September 2022 elections, nothing has yet been said about a possible date for the vote. Several political parties want to go even further, removing age limits on sex change operations altogether. The Liberal Party, The Left Party, the Pirate Party and Feministiskt Initiativ (FI), along with RFSL and RFSU, would like there to be no age limit whatsoever on gender affirmation surgery, including on procedures that remove sex organs.[101] FI believes a child's wish and one parent's consent to be sufficient. The Left Party refrains from mentioning the parents at all, instead apparently viewing the matter as one physicians should decide on. In a 2015 bill, then party leader Jonas Sjöstedt wrote that it is "problematic to impose a lower age limit on interventions by healthcare providers" since "decisions must be made on a case by case basis and an age limit would therefore not serve any purpose."[102] In 2018, the Left Party hardened its

---

100 Socialstyrelsen (Board of Health and Welfare). (31 March 2020). 'Åldersgräns för vissa kirurgiska ingrepp i könsorganen och socialnämndens roll vid ändring av det kön som framgår av folkbokföringen--Redovisning av regeringsuppdrag'.
101 RFSU comment to SOU (Official State Enquiries). (2017 No. 92). 'Transpersoner i Sverige. Förslag för stärkt ställning och bättre levnadsvillkor'
102 Jonas Sjöstedt et al. (Left Party). (2015/16 Motion No. 49). 'Förstärkta rättigheter för transpersoner'. Motion to Parliament.

stance further by demanding age limits be abolished altogether for sex change surgeries, with the explanation that "all individuals should have equal rights."[103] In a bill from 2017, the Liberal Party contended that "there is no objective reason to establish a lower age limit in law," with the reason given that access to gender reassignment ought to be "assessed in the same way as access to all other forms of health care."[104] Even the Conservatives (Moderaterna) and The Green Party (Miljöpartiet) want to lower the age limit, although it is unclear by how much. The latter hold the view that lowering the age limit for medical interventions could "empower young people" and lead to shorter waiting times.[105] The Pirate Party apparently sees no role for parents in the decision-making process either, believing children of all ages are competent individuals who know their own mind: "We also want to remove the age limit for gender reassignment treatments, since we believe physicians, psychologists and patients are better equipped than politicians to know when the time is right."[106] One cannot help but wonder: why have age limits for anything? Following this reasoning, age limits could be removed entirely for all activities and procedures, such as voting, driving, drinking and getting a tattoo.

The antagonism which normally characterises politics is wholly absent here. The Conservatives and the Left both agree – the extent and the speed at which the changes should be implemented being the only divergence in opinion. The Conservatives want to lower the age limit while the Left Party wants to abolish it altogether. The easy-going breeziness which characterises the parties' respective proposals is noteworthy, while the fact they are often signed by party leaders is evidence the matter is considered significant. Yet none of the parties appear to consider the issue a complex one. Their tone is one of 'onward and upward, the faster, the better!' No consideration appears to have been given to the fact that removing children's sex organs is a matter requiring serious ethical reflection. It is as though the people known as 'trans' are no longer being seen as humans of flesh and blood, but have instead become symbols of

---

103 <https://www.vansterpartiet.se/politik/hbtq/>.
104 Jan Björklund et al. (Liberal Party). (2017/18 Motion No. 3578). 'Liberal politik för hbt-personers rättigheter'. Motion to Parliament.
105 Åsa Lindhagen et al. (Miljö Partiet – Green Party). (2018/19 Motion No. 2297). 'Nya reformer för hbtq-personers rättigheter'. Motion to Parliament.
106 <https://www.qx.se/samhalle/sverige/27335/partiernas-svar-om-transpolitiska-fragor/>.

modernisation. Most parties are not advocating for an age limit of ten years, nor five nor even of one year. They are proposing to *do away with* the age limit completely.

Do these political parties really understand what they are suggesting? Do they understand what they are opening the flood-gates to? How can they, often in the very same bills that demand official apologies for adults who have been forcibly sterilised, propose children be sterilised for life?

CHAPTER 21

Hormone Evangelists in the Pharmaceutical Industry

One might wonder why the WHO and various governments around the world are recommending comprehensive procedures that have not been subjected to scientific scrutiny. One could also question the blithe attitude with which political parties are making decisions on the trans issue.

It is often noted that the most striking aspect of the debate around gender reassignment is the speed at which changes have occurred. While other groups, such as women and homosexuals, have had to fight for decades just to witness slight improvements in their circumstances, changes in laws pertaining to gender identity have made it onto the agenda and been prioritised without anyone really knowing how this happened. The trans issue has had a breakthrough over the course of only ten years, whereas homosexuals had to fight for 50 years just to be able to register their partner with the authorities. In some countries, for example Chile or Argentina, individuals were free to choose their gender while abortion was still illegal.

What one tends to forget when comparing these struggles is that gender reassignment is a market. A completely new customer base has emerged for the pharmaceutical industry: in the US, this demographic is approaching one per cent of the country's young people. It is the ideal consumer group: they come of their own volition, beg for medication and once they have begun, remain on it throughout their lives. Puberty blockers alone cost US$775 a month which, if the patient stays on them for five years, totals US$27,000. Gender reassignment surgery costs US$300,000. Add to this hormones, hair removal, facial surgery, Adam's Apple or breast removal and we are in the region of half a million US dollars. Repeat customers are every company's dream and here is a patient group that has no choice but to continue. A financial analysis by *Global Market Insights* describes the market for gender reassignment as a very good investment, since it is predicted to grow by 25 per cent in the six year period 2020-2026:

> Sex Reassignment Surgery Market size was more than USD 316 million in 2019 and will witness 25.1% CAGR [compound annual growth rate] during 2020 to 2026. Increasing awareness related to transgender problems, availability and accessibility to gender reassignment surgical centers are some of the significant factors augmenting the sex reassignment surgery industry growth. Also, inclination of patients towards changing sex as well as increasing number of gender reassignment surgeries are some of the factors driving the market growth.[107]

Particularly lucrative is the market for girls who want to become boys: it is estimated to account for 73 per cent of profits. The fact an increasing number of clinics now specialise in mastectomies and hysterectomies will "[boost] more customers across the regions that in turn will propel the market growth." *Global Market Insights* thoroughly analyse different parts of the world and identify the US, Germany and South East Asia as the most promising markets to invest in. Those idealists who thought the world was moving beyond sex and gender will be disappointed, for the market analysts paint a very binary picture of the future indeed. According to a 2018 report by *Transparency Market Research*

> … the market can be bifurcated into male to female and female to male. The male to female segment can be classified into facial, breast, and genitals. The female to male segment can be categorized into facial, chest, and genitals."[108]

---

107 Global Market Insights. 'Sex reassignment surgery market size by gender transition (Male to Female {Facial, Breast, Genitals}, Female to Male {Facial, Chest, Genitals}, Industry Analysis Report, Regional Outlook, Application Potential, Price Trends, Competitive market share and forecast, 2020–2026'. (March 2020).

108 Transparency Market Research. (2018). 'Sex reassignment surgery market. Global industry analysis, size, share, growth, trends, and forecast 2018–2026'.

There is, however, a prerequisite for investments paying off: States must be convinced to fund treatments. Poor countries where healthcare does not cover the costs of sex change operations and hormone treatment are unprofitable investments. The two factors that "drive the global sex reassignment surgery market [are] rise in prevalence of gender dysphoria" and "favorable government policies"[109] according to the 2018 report. Thus, for the market to grow, increasing numbers of people must be diagnosed with gender dysphoria and states must foot the bill for treatments and surgery. Anyone and everyone unsatisfied with their body is a success story in waiting for this industry.

The industry's game plan is clearly laid out in a very revealing strategy document published by the world's largest law firm, Denton, and the news conglomerate Thomson Reuters Foundation, with support from the EU and LGBTQ organisation IGLYO (The International Lesbian, Gay, Bisexual, Transgender, Queer and Intersex (LGBTQI) Youth & Student Organisation).[110] The document is entitled 'Only adults? Good practices in legal gender recognition for youth' and begins by explaining that "there are certain techniques that emerge as being effective in progressing trans rights in the 'good practice' countries."

They recommend linking the issue to human rights, as detractors will then experience "the political stigma of a human rights violation." References to the "right to health" in UN declarations should be interpreted to include gender reassignment procedures, the "right to respect for private and family life" to encompass a right to gender self-identification and the phrase "best interests of the child" should be interpreted to mean that the child has the right to decide about undergoing treatment.[111] Changes in the law should not come across as being in the interests of pharmaceutical companies and clinics, but as young people's right to not have to "be ashamed of who they are."[112] Thus, it is not a child's right to safe and evidence-based care but the right to receive gender reassignment without parental consent that is being advocated. Parents are considered

---

109 Ibid.
110 IGLYO, Dentons, Thomson Reuters Foundation och Nextlaw. (November 2019). 'Only adults? Good practices in legal gender recognition for youth. A report on the current state of laws and NGO advocacy in eight countries in Europe, with a focus on rights of young people'.
111 Ibid. p. 19.
112 Ibid. p. 8.

an obstacle: "It is recognised that the requirement for parental consent or the consent of a legal guardian can be restrictive and problematic for minors."[113] The report further counsels that the word 'surgery' is best avoided, as it can sound alarming. Instead, operations should be referred to as "the right to be yourself." The key to success is to tie campaigns to more popular reforms, such as the campaign for marriage equality, since they provide "a veil of protection, particularly in Ireland, where marriage equality was strongly supported, but gender identity remained a more difficult issue to win public support for."[114] The most effective practice is to directly lobby young politicians, though public debate about the issues is best avoided:

> Another technique which has been used to great effect is the limitation of press coverage and exposure [...] many believe that public campaigning has been detrimental to progress, as much of the general public is not well informed about trans issues, and therefore misinterpretation can arise. In Ireland, activists have directly lobbied individual politicians and tried to keep press coverage to a minimum in order to avoid this issue.[115]

This is precisely what happened with the Swedish government's bill: it was hastily introduced, comments and responses were limited to two months over the summer vacation, there was no time for debate, and there was a heavy emphasis on decreasing suffering of a vulnerable group over mentions of medical procedures and surgery. No discussion regarding market interests was undertaken.

While the industry is invisible, LGBTQ oganisations appear to be behind the changes. One such organisation is IGLYO, whose board is comprised of idealistic youth between the ages of 21 and 29 who list their proudest achievement as founding an "anti-fascist drumming troupe in Croatia in support of animal rights."[116] Drum-toting animal lovers would find it difficult to achieve legal changes alone, however. For this, resources and access to funding are required.

On closer inspection, it is the same individuals who own clinics and conduct research who also make the decision to fund interventions

---

113 Ibid. p. 16.
114 Ibid. p. 20.
115 Ibid. p. 20.
116 <https://www.iglyo.com/wp-content/uploads/2018/09/Board-Applications-2018.pdf>.

through taxes. An often-cited example is the Pritzker family, one of the wealthiest in the US. The Pritzker Group is based in Chicago and owns hundreds of companies, among them the Hyatt hotel group and others within the data, AI, and pharmaceutical industries.[117] They own the University of Chicago medical faculty, Pritzker School of Medicine, where research on gender dysphoria is conducted.[118] Among the school's research collaborators is AbbVie, manufacturer of puberty blocker Lupron.[119] The family is one of the main investors in clinics for children with gender dysphoria and 'LGBTQ-clinics'– a somewhat misleading moniker since homosexual, bisexual and queer people do not require special health clinics. The Pritzker group has also endowed professorships in trans studies at the university.[120] Their investments include several clinics for gender affirmation treatments of "gender incongruent children" as well as

> $6.5 million to the Program in Human Sexuality at the University of Minnesota; $5.99 million to Palm Center, an LGBTQ think tank, for a study on trans people in the military; $2 million for the world's first chair of trans studies at the University of Victoria, British Columbia; $1 million to Lurie Children's Hospital of Chicago for a Gender and Sex Development Program; and $50,000 for the first trans-study course at the University of Toronto.[121]

They are also long term financiers of lobby group WPATH, which publishes guidelines on what they believe to be best practice procedures in trans health care. In 2018, WPATH received US$250,000 from Pritzker, earmarked for the development of their new SOC8 guidelines which are used globally by states, governments and healthcare professionals.[122] WPATH lobbies intensively to get company health insurance to cover hormone treatment and surgery and has entered into a partnership with

---

117 <https://www.pritzkergroup.com/venture-capital/portfolio/>.
118 <https://www.plasticsurgery.theclinics.com/article/S0094-1298(18)30014-2/abstract>.
119 AbbVie News Center. (20 April 2016). 'AbbVie, University of Chicago collaborate to advance cancer research'.
120 <https://thefederalist.com/2018/02/20/rich-white-men-institutionalizing-transgender-ideology/>.
121 <https://www.vanityfair.com/news/2019/06/why-billionaire-republican-donor-jennifer-pritzker-is-abandoning-trump-after-coming-out-as-trans>.
122 <https://www.wpath.org/media/cms/Documents/History/Awards/2018/Awards%20Information%20Page.pdf>.

Starbucks, which offers free breast removal for female staff and free of charge implants for male staff – though it does not offer the procedures the other way around.[123] Pritzker family members also sit on boards of university institutes for sexuality and trans studies. Apart from the lucrative investment opportunity offered by an industry with 25 per cent predicted growth, it is possible that a genuine personal motivation exists in this specific case. Colonel James Pritzker, Republican, paratrooper and billionaire founder of war museums became Jennifer Natalya Pritzker in 2013 and thereby appeared on America's richest women list overnight.[124]

Jennifer's cousin is Illinois governor J. B. Pritzker, who decreed the state's healthcare would cover hormone treatment and gender reassignment surgery.[125] Thus, the same group that funds clinics not only finances studies on their activities but also passes laws making taxpayers foot the bill for it all. "Healthcare is a right, not a privilege," the governor proudly declared. He has further presided over making all Illinois toilets gender neutral, requiring all public schools in the state to teach history that includes the contributions of transgender people, as well as setting up a trans task force of 25 staff, handpicked by the governor, whose remit is to ensure that trans and non-binary people's rights are respected.[126]

These could be considered positive steps. The problem is that what are being referred to as 'rights' are not what is ordinarily understood by the term, such as the right to not be bullied or subjected to discrimination, but a full-scale ideological change of course. Merely a year after its foundation, the task force has ensured that all school staff understand gender identity is "… unrelated to the person's sex assigned at birth. Gender identity is an innate part of a person's identity" and has required schools to establish Gender Support Plans and hire Gender Support Coordinators whose role it is to acknowledge and support individuals in their gender identity. Disclosing an individual's gender identity is not permitted as it "violates state and federal privacy laws," though this can be a difficult balancing act

---

123 <https://www.wpath.org/media/cms/Documents/Public%20Policies/2018/6_June/Transgender%20Medical%20Benefits.pdf>.
124 <https://www.vanityfair.com/news/2019/06/why-billionaire-republican-donor-jennifer-pritzker-is-abandoning-trump-after-coming-out-as-trans>.
125 Ethan Conley-Keck. (7 April 2019). 'Pritzker changes state's Medicaid policy to cover sex reassignment surgery' WQAD-TV.
126 Dan Petrella. (26 July 2019). 'Gov. J.B. Pritzker signs law requiring one-person public bathrooms be gender-neutral'. *Chicago Tribune*.

since staff must simultaneously not misgender as "persistent misgendering is a form of bullying and harassment." Should parents or guardians not support a student in their transitioning, a Gender Support Coordinator ought to intervene and establish a support plan with the student. All students who request one must be supplied with a personal Gender Support Plan, documenting their wishes regarding preferred changing rooms, pronouns and possible future measures. Finally, students must not be asked to use the changing room for their sex, as gender self identification is the determining factor. These provisions extend beyond school staff: all contractors hired by the school are required to sign up to them.

For idealists fighting for LGBTQ rights this is a progressive revolution. For clinics and pharmaceutical companies it is nothing more than business. Somewhere along the line, these two stakeholders – who could easily have clashed and become adversaries – have merged into one. The activists are fighting for everyone's right to be themselves while the clinics' main focus is transforming people, yet instead of fighting one another, they have entered into a curiously symbiotic relationship. What would otherwise be considered a cynical business that sterilises young people to turn a profit, is instead considered one that saves lives, increases tolerance and subverts gender boundaries. Sales and profits are being passed off as humanitarian assistance. The line between industry and activism is blurred, and suddenly the industry has become a human rights hero.

The Pritzker Group is a good example, among many, of capitalists who invest in gender reassignment of children and at the same time are no strangers to exerting political pressure. With one hand, these capitalists open clinics, with the other, they lobby office holders to ensure taxpayers cover the costs, all the while paying lip service to equal rights by declaring they simply want to help people be themselves. Pioneers in the field have been awarded acknowledgements and prizes in honour of their work for human rights, despite the fact they often work for the very industry profiting from the clinics and pharmaceuticals sold. Diane Ehrensaft is a case in point. The author of a series of books about gender variance in children and young people, she has been awarded numerous prizes by psychology associations. While writing the books, she worked at pharmaceutical company AbbVie.[127]

---

[127] Curriculum vitae, Diane Ehrensaft, Ph.D. <https://files.eqcf.org/wp-content/uploads/2016/09/35-Doe-MPI-UNDER-SEAL.pdf>.

A similar development is discernible in Sweden where physician-in-chief at Anova, Cecilia Dhejne, was named "Trans Hero of the Year" at the 2017 Pride Festival. The fact that a doctor responsible for converting several homosexuals into heterosexuals receives an LGBTQ award is undeniably a historic twist. Yet it also exemplifies a peculiar phenomenon: researchers and physicians are increasingly acting as lobbyists.

Cecilia Dhejne is in the habit of engaging in activism and prompts discussions on Facebook groups regarding trans issues. Following investigative journalist programme *Uppdrag Granskning* showing young people with mental health issues accessing trans services, Dhejne posted the following in a trans activist Facebook group:

> Is there anyone in the group or does anyone know someone who can do a write-up with scientific references on 'social contagion'? What's the evidence it exists and how does it work? I think this is going to be needed. There's another ug [Uppdrag Granskning] programme coming out this autumn.[128]

In the thread, Dhejne discusses matters with young trans activists, and constantly uses the words "us" and "them." "Us" consists of her – head physician at Karolinska Hospital's trans unit – and the young trans activists, many of whom are her patients, while "they" are all those critical of the services her team offers. She writes that, "they are claiming people commit suicide due to regretting their transition. They don't understand that such research does not exist."

In other countries, key roles are played by British organisation Mermaids and Spanish Chrysallis, founded by parents of trans children. Mermaids has received £500,000 in lottery funding under buzzwords such as 'tolerance' and 'respect'. The organisation has an aggressive stance on medical interventions on children, with speakers at conferences supporting their arguments with statements like "in other countries twelve-year-olds are considered old enough to fight in wars."[129] Thus, the fact that children in Sudan are maimed is being used as a yardstick for procedures to be performed on children in peacetime. In July 2019, Chrysallis succeeded in winning a case in the Spanish constitutional court

---

128 Cecilia Dhejne. (12 June 2019). Comment in the group 'Tankesmedja – transpersoner och transexkluderande feminism'.
129 Julian Vigo. (27 December 2018). 'Pseudo-scientific hokum and the experimentation on children's bodies'. *Forbes*.

where it was decided that a parent would have the right to change their child's legal sex regardless of age and without the other parent's consent.[130] Chrysallis now intends to go even further to remove the requirement for a child to be assessed by a physician beforehand. In Sweden, RFSL has adopted a similar policy, advocating removal of the age limit, albeit without resorting to war metaphors.

RFSL (The Swedish Federation for Lesbian, Gay, Bisexual, Transgender, Queer and Intersex Rights) has come a long way since October 1950, when 36 people converged to listen to gramophone records and form an organisation for the rights of homosexuals. Nowadays, it is a major power player receiving millions of Swedish krona every year in public funds: now that legal equality for homosexuals has been achieved, the trans issue has become the organsiation's top priority. In fact, the issue has given RFSL continued relevance: it is charged with creating materials for training on trans issues and selling courses with LGBTQ certifications to businesses, public service providers and schools. It is consulted by the government as an expert on trans-related matters and investigators for government inquiries have been selected directly from the organisation's ranks.

RFSL has gone from defending homosexuals' right not to be pathologised to being the most vocal campaigner for the medicalisation and surgical remaking of people. Their youth site, transformering.se, sells chest binders to teenage girls and explains, "flattening your breasts with the help of a binder can be a form of self-care."[131] Readers are assured that hormone treatment is risk free

> … there is no danger in taking hormones as long as they have been prescribed to you by a physician and you take them according to their instructions, any risks are by and large the same as those which occur when the body itself produces hormones.[132]

If a young person's parents do not approve hormone treatment, they are advised to turn to social services as "being denied gender affirming care can result in serious consequences for the health of the child."[133] RFSL

---

130 J. J. Gálvez and R. Rincón. (19 July 2019). 'Los menores transexuales podrán registrar su nuevo sexo en el DNI'. *El País*.
131 <http://transformering.se/vard-halsa/hjalpmedel/binders-och-binding>.
132 <http://transformering.se/vardhalsa/hormoner>.
133 <http://transformering.se/ratt-och-fel/nar-vardnadshavare-vagrar>.

representatives have even contacted detransitioners to encourage them to be mindful of the way they express themselves to the media.[134]

RFSL constantly downplays the risks of hormone treatment and medical interventions and counters research findings in the field. When researcher Lisa Littman published her study on the increasing numbers of teenage girls who suddenly became gender dysphoric, RFSL commented that they took issue with Littman's term 'Rapid Onset Gender Dysphoria'. The organisation claimed that it is "very common for gender dysphoria to manifest in connection to puberty" and that "children's gender identity and reflections on gender must be respected." 'Respect for children' is the kind of vague terminology plucked directly from law firm Dentons strategy document – after all, very few would oppose children *reflecting* on gender.

In May 2019, the WHO changed the classification of gender dysphoria in their diagnostic manual ICD-11, moving it from the section on psychiatric diagnoses to sexual health and renaming it *gender incongruence*.[135] This revision has considerably enlarged the patient group. We have gone from the old diagnosis of transsexualism, which focused on an individual having felt like the opposite sex his entire life, to gender dysphoria (with its focus on suffering here and now) and on to gender incongruence. The focus now is on identifying "play, toys, games, or activities and playmates that are typical of the experienced gender rather than the assigned sex."[136]

When diagnosing *transsexualism*, physicians were concerned with establishing that a person had behaved in alignment with opposite gender roles *throughout his life*. This was replaced with gender dysphoria, which focused on suffering: the patient had to feel unwell to the point that an intervention or surgery was deemed necessary. Consistency was no longer important, which opened up for ROGD patients. *Gender incongruence*, on the other hand, is above all about deviating from gender roles. Despite this, in theory, being insufficient for a diagnosis (according to criteria, gender-incongruent behaviour alone does not suffice for a diagnosis), the term can be applied to even very young children. The individual's psychological well-being no longer forms part of the definition.

---

134 Conversation with X, trans person, October 2020.
135 ICD-11, International Classification of Diseases 11th Revision. (2019). The global standard for diagnostic health information.
136 ICD-11, HA61 Gender incongruence of childhood.

This change is of utmost importance for the pharmaceutical industry. It enables early diagnosis of an extremely large number of children and young people, thereby creating a steady customer base. Moreover, it means that a person accessing care for gender dysphoria is referred to an endocrinologist instead of a psychologist and hormones can be prescribed directly without the need for a psychological consultation first. The change was negotiated in close partnership with lobby group WPATH.[137]

RFSL welcomed the change, calling it an excellent solution: on the one hand, it means trans people are no longer pathologised, on the other hand, medicalisation ought not be removed entirely, since "a diagnostic code is required to ensure access to care."[138]

Removing the diagnostic code would entail individuals having to pay for their own operations, while retaining it would be an admission that something may not be right and the patient may need psychological support. This presents a dilemma: how to access free hormones without having to go through a psychologist?

Endocrinologists provide the solution in the statement "a diagnosis does not have to be a disease." The Swedish Board of Health and Welfare included this exact statement in their 2015 recommendations.[139] In 2018, identical wording appears in the government's bill regarding surgery on sex organs. The bill also proposes renaming the diagnosis gender incongruence, stating that "it is worth mentioning that a diagnosis does not necessarily have to be a disease."[140]

What this means in practice is that gender roles are being codified in law. There is such a thing as being congruent and non-congruent. There are now officially toys for boys and toys for girls. A three-year-old boy who plays with cars is normal – a three-year-old girl who does is not. According to the government's new guidelines, she can be diagnosed as gender incongruent.

---

137 'WPATH consensus process regarding TRANSGENDER and TRANSSEXUAL-RELATED DIAGNOSES in ICD-11'. (31 May 2013).
138 FAQ om könsdysfori som diagnos, RFSL. (14 February 2019).
139 "God vård av vuxna med könsdysfori: nationellt kunskapsstöd," Socialstyrelsen (Board of Health and Welfare). 2015.
140 Socialdepartementet, Regeringskansliet. (2018). 'Vissa kirurgiska ingrepp i könsorganen'. Ds Departementsserien (government briefing papers), No. 11, p. 32.

CHAPTER 22

Tumblr, Trans and Trauma – Testimonies from Teens

Testimonies from the current generation of young women reveal a picture far more complex than that presented by trans health care clinics. Their stories are not the classic transsexual tales of always having felt as if one was born in the wrong body. Mainly, they are about being a teenage girl and not fitting in. Through interviews, YouTube clips, blogs and autobiographies, young women speak about their transition journeys. The backgrounds and life experiences may differ – some had happy childhoods while others felt maladjusted; some refer to themselves as tomboys while others report having never thought about gender until their teens – yet the narratives follow a remarkably similar framework, both among those who claim gender reassignment saved their lives and those who say it was the worst mistake they ever made.

After a period of feeling lost at the beginning of their teens, with loneliness as a result of bullying and loss of friendships, sometimes coupled with experiences of assault and anorexia, what followed was a sense of not belonging and not being able to live up to others' expectations of how to be a girl. As a result, they turned to online communities. Tumblr is often mentioned and several girls tell of how they created a non-binary, agender or tri-gender avatar for themselves only to later 'go all the way' and become trans men. The role of the internet is fundamental: it features in the vast majority of accounts. Indeed, it is through online searches and joining forums that the girls report 'realising' that they were trans. One user specifies: the videos which began appearing in the "recommended stream" were what "gave a name to [my] discomfort."[141]

Gina from Sweden recounts:

> At that stage, I had started watching more and more YouTube videos where young trans people told their stories, showed how hormones and surgery had changed their lives and transformed them into their real selves. I would become very emotional as I watched these videos and could sit in my bed for hours on end just crying. I felt I *was* the person in the video, that my story was theirs and that I needed the same help they had got. It felt somehow awful that I had not received this help before. The assessment and diagnosis took just over a year and after that I was ready for a mastectomy.[142]

"TUMBLR! Oh my God! TUMBLR! Youtube too. That's how I found out that I was trans – it was from a YouTube video."[143] "I would never have discovered my true gender without Tumblr," says a teenager who has started testosterone treatment. "It was after I started reading about trans and other gender identities that I discovered I was a boy," says 18-year-old Eirin on the website of a young people's sexual health and wellbeing organisation.[144] Another describes her realisation happening just after she had come out on Tumblr: "The more I posted, the more I found that anytime I reblogged a post with a 'trans' tag, the post would go viral," while a third youth observes, "I actually learnt about agender and all the other genders from Tumblr."[145] "I tend to think that, in many ways, I began life as my real self online," says Mikael Hansén Goobar in an anthology of young trans people. "Online, I could come out of my body and into something else – a virtual body, a personality based on my words, an image of myself

---

141 Jesse Singal. (July/August 2018). 'When children say they're trans'. *The Atlantic*.
142 'Upptäcker trans'. (10 February 2018). *En annan typ av kvinna*. <https://enannantypavkvinna.wordpress.com/2018/02/10/en-detransitioners-resa/>.
143 Quoted in Dianna T. Kenny. (2019). 'Gender development and the transgendering of children' in Moore and Brunskell-Evans (eds). *Inventing Transgender Children and Young People*. Newcastle upon Tyne: Cambridge Scholars. p. 102.
144 <https://www.umo.se/umo-podden/umo-podden/umo-podden-5.Jag-ar-kille-men-kanner-mig-som-tjej/>.
145 see <http://theconversation.com/theres-something-queer-about-tumblr-73520> and Harsin Drager. (2012.). 'Transforming cyber space and the trans liberation movement. A study of transmasculine youth bloggers on Tumblr.com'. Undergraduate Honors Thesis. Bolder: University of Colorado. <https://scholar.colorado.edu/concern/undergraduate_honors_theses/v979v348j>.

that more accurately reflected my feelings."[146] Researchers have termed Tumblr 'trans technology', since it differs from, for example, Facebook, in that it encourages use of pseudonyms and alternative identities.[147]

In 2013, Tumblr was the most popular website among 13 to 25 year olds: it was there that they revealed their innermost secrets, learnt about politics and created their identities.[148] Gender identity was a central element of user profiles: a typical profile might feature 'they/them' as preferred pronouns and 'biromantic pansexual' as gender identity. The informal yet ultimately very strict rules read: everyone defines their own gender; sexual and romantic orientation are unconnected to gender identity; gender identity is an inner essence while gender expression varies day to day; and gender boundaries can be crossed while ethnicity remains fixed. On Tumblr, users could follow each others' transitions day by day and it was here that users started posting photos of their mastectomy scars accompanied by captions reading "Free at last!" showered with comments like "So brave!" and "wow, goals!" Several blogs featured donate icons, where readers could crowdfund surgeries. Tumblr was the birthplace of debates which would later move onto Twitter and thus onto adults' radar – there was even a saying doing the rounds on Tumblr that quipped: "Twitter is everything Tumblr was three years ago."[149]

Tumblr's popularity peaked between December 2013 and February 2014.[150] 2014 was also the year in which the number of referrals for gender identity assessments sky rocketed: increases of this magnitude

---

146 Mikael Hansén Goobar. (2011).'På mina villkor – en inloggning bort' in Veronika Berg and Edward Summanen. *Det är vår tur nu! Att vara trans i en tvåkönsvärld*, p. 29. Stockholm: RFSL(Swedish Federation for Lesbian, Gay, Bisexual, Transgender and Queer Rights).
147 Oliver L. Haimson and Gillian R. Hayes. (2017). 'Changes in social media affect, disclosure, and sociality for a sample of transgender Americans in 2016's political climate'. Department of Informatics. Irvine: University of California Press.
148 Harsin Drager. (2012). 'Transforming cyber space and the trans liberation movement. A study of transmasculine youth bloggers on Tumblr.com', p. 18. Boulder: University of Colorado.
149 'Tumblr: A call-out post'. (4 February 2019). Helena/The Pique Resilience Project.
150 <https://hackernoon.com/tumblr-is-tumbling-d6deb3bb831e>.

were unprecedented.[151] In fact, 2014 was named the "Transgender Tipping Point" by *Time Magazine*.[152]

The other central theme in young people's stories is loathing of the female body. Time and again, these young women express with what disgust and horror they relate to their bodies. While some report having never felt at ease in their body, for the overwhelming majority, these feelings did not arise until puberty. Special revulsion is reserved for breasts. Dagny, a 23-year-old from the US, says:

> I remember being so emotionally destroyed by the knowledge that I had this female body. It was crushing. I've talked elsewhere about the self-harm that I did when I was 15-16-17 before I got on hormones. And I was just, it was like waging war with my own body, seething down the walls where I just wanted to break it down. You know, that was when my body was developing, when I was getting all these things I didn't like, breasts and my period was such a source of distress for me, self-harming became a way to lodge an attack against it. I think that is where my gender dysphoria primarily manifested, this really extreme hatred for my body and for the idea that it was a female body.[153]

She initially identified as trigender – "it meant that I was more than just a girl" – and later demanded her parents agree to allow her to start hormone treatment, which they did after two years.[154] Timo Hedberg recounts the following in an autobiographical series:

> I didn't feel at home in my body after puberty hit. There was something wrong with it, only I couldn't articulate what. I felt like a consciousness unattached to a body, it was as though I had the wrong mind for my body.[155]

---

151 Louise Frisen, Per-Anders Rydelius and Olle Söder. (2017, No. 9–10). 'Kraftig ökning av könsdysfori bland barn och unga'. *Läkartidningen*.
152 Katie Steinmetz. (29 May 2014). 'The Transgender Tipping Point'. *Time*. <https://time.com/135480/transgender-tipping-point/>.
153 'Dagny of The Pique Resilience Project on detransitioning' (26 March 2019). *Feminist Current* podcast.
154 Ibid.
155 Timo Hedberg. (2011). 'Trangst – en självbiografisk serie' in Berg och Summanen. *Det är vår tur nu!, att vara trans i en tvåkönsvärld*, p. 54. Veronica Berg and Edvard Summanen (eds.). Stockholm: RFSL.

On *A Transman's Blog*, Mike writes:

> I loved swimming as a child but then my teenage years came and I started feeling extremely uncomfortable with it. Being mostly naked was not fun at all! I didn't know back then that it was because I didn't feel at home in my body.[156]

A cartoonist on Tumblr describes similar feelings:

> So I was content enough living as a girl until around puberty. Puberty was uncomfortable and scary for me, but I still didn't suspect anything yet. I mostly wore baggy and comfortable clothes, sweatshirts and tshirts and jeans. [...] I made use of the incognito window on my laptop and did some research of my own, learning some basic terminology. I started learning about different trans identities.[157]

YouTuber BrotherWarrior XXX posted the following, which was swiftly removed again, after four years of clips about a supposedly successful transition:

> When I decided to go on hormones it seemed like the most logical choice for me. I was in a very bad place emotionally. I hated myself a lot. I hated my body. I didn't identify with it, and I felt very separate from my body. And finding YouTube videos of other people who were transitioning and finding out it was an option to do so kind of deeply affected me. [...] My parents were really cool with it. They were not cool with me being a lesbian at all ... [now] they didn't have to say, "I have a lesbian daughter. [Instead they could say] I have a son who's straight."[158]

Others report that the trigger was assault. "I knew I didn't want to be a woman because bad things happen to women" says an anonymous ex-trans man in an anthology.[159] "I developed a very masculine sense of self after being raped, and it was absolutely to dissociate myself from the pain." Since she had been subjected to violence and hatred targeted at her female body, she wanted to rid herself of it – a male body could not be raped.

---

156 TransMan's Blog. (19 August 2018). <https://mikael-nc.tumblr.com>.
157 <https://a-trans-comic-by-me.tumblr.com>.
158 'The trans-kid honeymoon is sweet – while it lasts'. (19 February 2016). *4th Wave Now*.
159 Carey Maria Catt Callahan. 'Unheard voices of detransitioners'. (2018). In Brunskell-Evans and Moore (eds). *Inventing Transgender Children and Young People*, p. 177. Newcastle upon Tyne: Cambridge Scholars.

Solveig, who took testosterone as an 18-year-old and lived as a man for several years, says it was the female role that she could not stand:

> I was fleeing from being a woman. I couldn't stand the fact I had to live in this role that was assigned to me. You were meant to be a certain way, look a particular way and behave like this or like that. As a teenager, I experienced unrequited love and I started living a kind of fantasy life with this boy I was in love with, so much so that I became a boy myself. I discovered that if I toughened up a bit and dressed more like a boy then I could be part of the gang.[160]

Solveig preferred to "be free and strong, go horseback riding and not have to deal with people's comments about her body." After the assault, she could no longer live with her female body. It was not until the age of 59, when she watched a TV programme about a woman who regretted transitioning, that she realised she was not alone.

Being attracted to girls but not being able to contemplate the idea of being lesbian is another common theme in testimonies. Nele from Belgium remarks:

> I really had this image that I would be this disgusting woman, and that my friends wouldn't want to see me anymore because they'd think I might hit on them ... I watched some YouTube videos of trans guys who take testosterone, and they go from this shy lesbian to a handsome guy who is super-popular.[161]

For 22-year-old blogger Lucas Fabray, the feeling that she did not want to be a woman began one day in a supermarket as she looked around at the older female shoppers: "They were casually pushing carts, holding their baskets, sorting coupons [...] and I realized that I didn't want to grow old as a woman."[162]

In addition to breasts, menstruation is experienced by many as particularly unpleasant. In a newspaper interview, Benjamin says: "When I bleed, I feel dirty and like my body is completely out of sync with me as a

---

160 <https://www.svtplay.se/video/24001219/uppdrag-granskning-nar-solveig-angrade-sig>.
161 Linda Pressly and Lucy Proctor. (10 March 2020).'Ellie and Nele. From she to he – and back to she again'. *BBC News*.
162 Jessie Ellison. (24 December 2012). 'For transgender youth, a home on Tumblr'. *The Daily Dot*.

person."[163] Similarly, Skylar Kergil describes in her autobiography *Before I Had the Words: On Being a Transgender Young Adult*, how she had a breakdown during a car trip when she noticed blood between her legs.[164]

Anna Bohlin of the University of Gothenburg has interviewed trans people about menstruation. While some trans women express curiosity, trans men's accounts are overwhelmingly angst-ridden and describe complex relationships with this function of the female body.[165] Nearly all feel the word menstruation is so shrouded in taboo and shame that they find paraphrasings and employ strategies like buying shaving foam at the same time as pads so they can pretend the latter are for someone else. Several of them use dramatic turns of phrase: "I felt utterly naked and exposed […] like it'd be the end of the world if others realised it was me." One interviewee, called A, tells of how her hatred toward her period began with anorexia: "I think it's slightly connected to eating disorders […] when I realised I was trans, it sort of slid over to that in a way."

Very few describe a desire to actually be a boy. Instead, it is not wanting to be a girl which clearly dominates the accounts, with the most unpleasant part being the transformation of the body from that of a girl to a woman and the confrontation with the world during this process. Briton Charlie Evans says:

> I've always been a scruffy, gender non conforming, truck loving, short haired, soft butch. And, as a teenager, like almost all girls, I hated my breasts – this new part of my body that suddenly drew male gaze. New hips, new shapes, that now made me an object. I was no longer able to run around in mud and have fun, instead, I had to think about crossing my legs, covering my chest, not provoking the men three times my age. Not 'distracting' the male teachers with my shoulders. At the age of 12, maybe 13, I told my best friend I fancied her. It spread around the school quickly. I was kicked out of the changing rooms for PE and had to change alone in the toilets. The other girls started to like boys – they'd text them, hold their hands in the corridor. And I desperately wanted a girl to look

---

163 Tindra Englund. (27 April 2016). 'P-pillren minskar Benjamins ångest och smärta'. *Helsingborgs Dagblad*.
164 Skylar Kergil. (2017). *Before I Had the Words*. New York: Skyhorse Publishing.
165 Beatrice Berg. (2017). 'Transgendering menstruation. En kvalitativ studie av uppfattningar kring menstruation i relation till transidentitet i Sverige'. University of Gothenburg, School of Global Studies, Bachelor's thesis in Global Studies, p. 22.

at me the way they looked at those boys. I cropped my hair short, wore cologne, took science subjects for GCSEs. Every role model I had was a man – Albert Einstein, epidemiologist John Snow. I had posters of them. And then someone said something that changed my life. 'Could you be a boy born in the wrong body?' Yes. Yes! This was it – it's exactly that. I have a boy brain! That's why I love science, and guns, and mud, and trucks, and mechanics, and cars, and girls. I am a boy. That is why I hate my body! I was meant to be a boy. I had the answer. Everything fell into place, and I knew shaving my head, tightly binding my chest, and changing my pronouns was how I could find peace at last. I just needed to pass as the man I knew I was. My doctor confirmed my gender dysphoria, and I knew with certainty that I would have a mastectomy when I turned 17, and then phalloplasty. It's all I thought about, all day every day, and I ordered illegal testosterone gel to help get ready for my transition. My 17th birthday came and went, 18 came and went, never having the funds or the time between my studying to have the treatment I wanted to 'fix' my body to 'match' my brain. And then I started university. Science distracted me. I stopped correcting people when they said she, I stopped wearing a binder so I could breathe properly in class. My gender dysphoria never went away. It's still here. But I accepted I could never really have changed sex – I would have something that resembled a penis, it would hurt, I would have to pump it up from a balloon in my leg. The mastectomy would cause nerve damage. More pain. But most importantly, for me – transitioning because I was taught by men to hate my female body, transitioning because I didn't 'feel' like a woman, was propping up the gender binary.[166]

Protests against puberty are part and parcel of being a woman and of the female narrative. Earlier generations have starved and cut themselves, saved up for breast enlargements and cultivated depression as an expression of youth culture. Nine out of ten teenage girls report being unhappy with their bodies and wanting to change them – this compared to only four out of ten boys.[167] For many teenage girls, it is a deeply shocking experience to suddenly find themselves in an unfamiliar body which others observe and judge and which seems to belong to the world more than to oneself. The representations of women they are surrounded

---

166 <https://www.mumsnet.com/talk/womens_rights/3674531-i-have-a-retraction-to-make-last-year-i-tweeted-this-in-response-to-getthelout-in-london>.
167 'Reklamera!'. (2013). Sveriges Kvinnolobby. Swedish Women's Lobby campaign against sexist advertising.

by offer no alternative view: the female form is portrayed as alienated, a product to buy and sell. The dissociation from one's body is already present, albeit latently. A female body is not something a woman is, but something she has – that much is clear. And sometimes she feels like she doesn't even have it, but that it belongs to others – she just happens to inhabit it. It is something unfamiliar that she must become accustomed to, yet this body is already colonised by the gaze of others. Gone is the stripey unisex fashion of the 1980s – those growing up in the new millennium are faced with an unprecedented form of gender fundamentalism. The girls' department in clothing shops is an explosion of pink glitter, while the boys' section is a military battlefield. Teenagers no longer encounter porn through magazines leafed through secretly but on their phones, where the teen who curiously types in a search for 'sex' or 'boobs' can be plunged into a world of misogynistic sadism and torture. Women in music, film and social media can be as 'strong' as they like, but their bodies are supernatural creations which no teen can identify with. Gender divisions in the labour market may slowly be becoming a thing of the past but our body images have never been this divided: each single part of the female body, from nails to asses, lips to eyelashes, is the subject of massive marketisation – which is not the case for men.

Psychologist Lisa Marchiano has questioned whether "adopting a transgender identity has become the newest way for teen girls to express feelings of discomfort with their bodies."[168] Often, it is the same individuals who initially struggle with anorexia, that later express a desire to become boys. In becoming 'boys', all the previous hatred for femaleness, rejection of womanhood, alienation, dissociation and body/mind split, all so common in women under patriarchy, find an outlet. The difference is that this new way of battling the female body is state sanctioned.

It is noteworthy that few public bodies – healthcare systems, authorities, government investigators, let alone LGBTQ organisations – seem to have any explanation for what is unfolding. In 2019, SBU (the Swedish Agency for Health Technology Assessment and Assessment of Social Services) concluded:

---

168 Lisa Marchiano. (2017). 'Outbreak. On transgender teens and psychic epidemics'. *Psychological Perspectives*, Vol. 60, pp. 345–366.

> We have not found any studies addressing the question of whether prevalence of gender dysphoria has changed over time, nor any studies on potential factors that might explain the increase.[169]

There appears to be a complete lack of awareness of the internet in these remarks. Social media and its attendant subcultures are not even mentioned as causes for the dramatic increase of several thousand percent. The fact that Tumblr and YouTube have provided rich fodder for academics who make their living studying identity formation speaks for itself, as does the plethora of academic publications with titles combining 'cyber', 'trans', 'identities', 'post' and 'space'.[170] Nevertheless, western authorities often appear entirely ignorant of these developments.

Nor is the central issue mentioned, namely that this is about gender and sex. It is striking that so few provide a gendered analysis about a phenomenon which is de facto about gender. Official projects and proceedings in many countries now require Equality Impact Assessments – urban planning, foreign affairs and education are all examples of sectors which must undergo assessments based on gender equality, meaning how it affects men and women respectively, based on an understanding that women are discriminated against. For some reason, this is not a requirement when the issue is gender itself. How does gender dysphoria and the treatments for it affect men and women? That question is not asked. The subject of gender is thus exempt from a gendered analysis. Healthcare, public inquiries, government ministers and LGBTQ organisations all claim to be listening to what trans people *want*, yet no one appears to be listening to what they are actually *saying*. The common explanation for the increase in gender dysphoria from researchers, politicians and healthcare professionals is that 'visibility' and 'tolerance' have increased. Rather than interpreting the increase as an alarm bell, the above reasoning makes it appear as an improvement: the numbers of women who are 'in fact' men have remained constant over the years, they were just hidden until now.

---

169 SBU (Swedish Agency for Health Technology Assessment and Assessment of Social Services). (20 December 2019). 'Könsdysfori hos barn och unga. En kunskapskartläggning', p. 74.

170 Harsin Drager. (2012). 'Transforming cyber space and the trans liberation movement. A study of transmasculine youth bloggers on Tumblr.com'. Undergraduate Honors Thesis. Boulder: University of Colorado. <https://scholar.colorado.edu/concern/undergraduate_honors_theses/v979v348j>.

In 2004, then Minister for Social Affairs in Sweden, Berit Andnor, launched a campaign to counteract gender roles and low self-esteem among young girls, titled 'Flicka' (The Girl Project). It was publicly funded and focused on highlighting the damage caused by beauty ideals in contemporary advertising, questioning gender roles and cultivating strong self-esteem in young girls. Nowadays, in stark contrast, as gender dysphoria in young women increases by several thousand percent, no such projects are on the horizon. Instead in 2019, Sweden's Minister for Social Affairs, Annika Strandhäll, wanted to remove obstacles for young people to access gender reassignment, believing the process should be quick and easy. When female handball player Loui Sand ended her career in sports to await gender reassignment, Strandhäll tweeted: "Good luck with everything that lies ahead for you. Courageous and meaningful that you're so open."[171] That a female sports star quits sports due to severe dysphoria is not seen as a problem, but as a brave decision. Sand made an attempt to play in men's handball, but quit after one game.

The fact that over 50 per cent of young trans people report having a problematic relationship to food is interpreted by the Publich Health Agency in Sweden as evidence of discrimination against trans people – not as a sign of oppression of women. Thus, a large group of girls with anorexia neatly becomes a non-issue.[172] They are no longer referred to as 'girls' and any problems they have are chalked up to their trans identity. The crucial question – What is it about our present that is making young women flee womanhood en masse? – is not being posed.

---

171 <https://twitter.com/strandhall/status/1082406960547487744?lang=en>.
172 'Hälsan och hälsans bestämningsfaktorer för transpersoner: En rapport om hälsoläget bland transpersoner i Sverige'. (2015). *Folkhälsomyndigheten*, p. 37.

CHAPTER 23

Mastectomy or Death: Harnessing the Threat of Suicide

The message from healthcare and wider society to young people who feel ill at ease in their bodies is take hormones and have surgery – you will feel better and fit in. You'll achieve gender congruence, that is, your physical appearance and inner emotions will be in alignment and you'll be normal. Because if you don't fit in as a girl, you *will* as a boy.

Interviews with happy trans people who say surgery is the best thing that happened to them abound in the media, with headlines proclaiming, "Now Amanda can finally be herself."[173] The message also claims it is easy to change sex and language is wielded in very precise ways to ensure the message has its desired effect: breast removal is known as 'treatment', sterilisation as 'care', and blocking the body's sexual development is referred to as 'taking time out to think'. These euphemisms are contrasted with a far more dramatic message: if you do *not* opt for these interventions and procedures, you risk death. In the absence of scientific evidence of the efficacy of treatments, clinics and their advocates present an argument which is difficult to counter: children risk suicide if we prevent them from having hormone treatment and surgery.

Diane Ehrensaft, chief psychologist at the UCSF Benioff Children's Hospital Child and Adolescent Gender Center Clinic, reassures skeptical parents with these words: "having the gender affirmation interventions is

---

173 Håkan Öberg. (30 March 2016). 'Nu kan Amanda äntligen vara sig själv'. *Piteå-Tidningen*.

as life-saving as the oncology services for children who have cancer."[174] She goes so far as to claim that failure to implement puberty blockers and hormone treatment is akin to child abuse: "We might even consider the denial of the service a form of child abuse – there's a life jacket right there, we're watching, and we're letting the child drown."[175] Joel Baum, head of education at US organisation The Gender Spectrum, opts for this wording to convince parents to provide consent for hormone treatment:

> You can either have grandchildren or not have a kid anymore because they've ended the relationship with you or in some cases because they've chosen a more dangerous path for themselves.[176]

Agreeing to sterilise a 15-year-old would make most parents think twice, especially in cases where this idea appears out of the blue. Yet if the alternative is that the child commits suicide, the situation is immediately cast in a very different light. This assertion about young people being at risk of suicide if gender reassignment procedures are not performed has even made it into several state-commissioned inquiries. In the Swedish 2014 inquiry 'Juridiskt kön och medicinsk könskorrigering' (Legal sex and medical gender reassignment), it is claimed that the existence of a natural sex organ in particular is the cause of suicide in young people:

> It is particularly important to realise the existence of cases of young transsexuals committing suicide while awaiting surgery due to the suffering caused by gender dysphoria. Parents and medical professionals are on occasion undoubtedly constrained by the age limit and thus cannot use what in some cases is a powerful tool to help the young person, namely a (surgical?) intervention in the individual's sex organ or removal of their reproductive organ.[177]

This information made a considerable impression on politicians and it was not long before proposals were submitted demanding to lower the age limit for removal of sex organs to 15 years without parental consent.

---

174 Quoted in Lisa Marchiano, 'Outbreak. On transgender teens and psychic epidemics', *Psychological Pespectives*, 2017, Vol. 60, No. 3, p. 358.
175 Diane Ehrensaft. (2017). *The Gender Creative Child. The Experiment LLC*, p. 13. New York: Workman Publishing.
176 Quoted in Lisa Marchiano. 'Outbreak. On transgender teens and psychic epidemics', *Psychological Pespectives*, 2017, Vol. 60, No. 3, p. 358.
177 SOU (Official state enquiries). (2014 No. 91 p. 161). 'Juridiskt kön och medicinsk könskorrigering'. Betänkande av Utredningen om åldersgränsen för fastställelse av ändrad könstillhörighet.

Social Affairs Minister Lena Hallengren captured politicians' panic: "This child, this young person, cannot even cope with living their life – if we look at the prevalence of suicide and so forth, we find it is overrepresented in this target group."[178]

Despite the frequent repetition of this causal link, its source remains unclear. The government inquiry does not cite a source and when Sweden's public service broadcaster SVT tried five years later to get to the bottom of the matter, the investigators who had worked on the inquiry could only lament that it

> is unfortunate that it is phrased incorrectly […] I cannot answer that – how we wrote it and why it came out phrased in this particular way. It should have said that young trans people take their own lives due to their living conditions.[179]

In fact, Louise Frisén from Anova's Kid-Team reports that none of the clinic's patients have committed suicide: "We would know if one of our patients had committed suicide because they would not turn up at appointments or we would be contacted by the referring psychiatrist."[180] In any case, a child committing suicide is extremely unusual.

Yet the erroneous information continues to circulate. In summer 2019, RFSL claimed that "91 per cent of attempted suicides were carried out prior to receiving gender affirming treatment. Therefore, gender affirming treatment saves lives." This figure was then re-quoted in *Amnesty Press*.[181] Attempts to locate the source of the statistic resulted in my being directed to an ongoing study conducted by a Norwegian professor who happened to also be one of Norway's most prominent trans activists, who pleaded confidentiality when I emailed him, as the study had not yet been published. As of October 2022, the study has *still* not been published. Despite no one having set eyes on a statistical basis for these figures, the statement circulates as fact. In a popular Swedish magazine for young women (*Vecko Revyn*) it is claimed that parents who fail to change their child's name and who use incorrect pronouns could be found responsible

---

178 <https://www.svt.se/nyheter/granskning/ug/ug-referens-transtaget-del-2>.
179 'Självmordsrisk används som argument för underlivskirurgi på unga transpersoner – saknar stöd'. (9 October 2019). *SVT Nyheter*.
180 Ibid.
181 Jennie Aquilonius. (31 July 2019.) 'PRIDE2019: Självmordstankar vanligt bland transpersoner'. *Amnesty Press*.

for the child's death. In the article, entitled 'Calling trans people by their correct name decreases suicide and depression', the authors maintain that "inadequate trans health care and the public's lack of understanding through misgendering and deadnaming are considered causes of [suicide and depression]."[182]

Are any of these assertions based on fact? Several studies have indeed proven that trans people experience suicidal ideation to a higher degree than the population at large. It is also true that this appears to have worsened over the years: in a 2007 study by the predecessor to Sweden's Public Health Agency, 67 per cent of trans people reported having good mental health, against 12 per cent who said their mental health was poor. At the time, 21 per cent had attempted suicide but trans people in fact reported better mental health than lesbian women, of whom 60 per cent reported having good mental health.[183]

Eight years later, in 2015, the figures for poor mental health were significantly higher. Eighteen per cent of trans people reported suffering mental health issues according to a Public Health Agency report and suicidal ideation had increased markedly: 33 per cent had attempted suicide and 57 per cent of 15 to 19-year-olds had seriously contemplated taking their own life over the previous year.[184] Granted, definitive conclusions cannot be drawn from self-selected web surveys and contemplating suicide is not the same as attempting it. Nevertheless, the difference is significant enough to warrant attention and the question arises: what happened over the course of these eight years?

The Public Health Agency's report states that trans people's health has not improved over the previous ten years despite "changes in discrimination laws to cover gender expression and identity, children under 18 having the right to transgender health care and social services without having to secure consent from both parents" as well as other improvements. The conclusion drawn does not question whether these changes are in fact capable of improving trans people's mental health – the

---

182 Irena Pozar. (13 April 2018). 'Att kalla transpersoner vid rätt namn minskar självmord och depression'. *VeckoRevyn*.
183 Regina Wintzer and Gunnel Boström. (2001). 'Psykisk ohälsa, självmordstankar och självmordsförsök bland homosexuella, bisexuella och transpersoner (hbt) – resultat från två svenska undersökningar'. *Suicidologi*, No. 1.
184 'Hälsan och hälsans bestämningsfaktorer för transpersoner: En rapport om hälsoläget bland transpersoner i Sverige'. (2015). *Folkhälsomyndigheten*, p. 40.

report's authors merely reassuringly surmise that it presumably takes a long time for the effect of the improvements to be seen.[185]

Yet the question remains: if it is easier to get treatment nowadays, why do trans people feel worse? Why is suicidal ideation increasing? What if trans healthcare services have engulfed a group of young people who are in fact grappling with altogether different issues? What if the procedures which promise better emotional health are actually making people feel worse? What if the increased prescribing of puberty blockers and hormones is exacerbating the situation for many?

One of the most comprehensive and most-cited long-term studies of people undergoing sex reassignment surgery is the 'Long-term follow-up of transsexual persons undergoing sex reassignment surgery. Cohort study in Sweden'. It found that deaths from suicide are much higher among those who have undergone sex reassignment surgery than those who have not.[186] The study is of 324 Swedish people who had sex reassignment surgery between 1973 and 2003. Fifty-nine per cent are MtF which can be explained by the fact that the study was conducted before the significant increase in gender dysphoria among teenage girls. Results show that suicide attempts begin to increase ten years after surgery; the same is true for psychiatric illness. The study concludes that sex reassignment is not beneficial in decreasing suicides among transsexuals.[187] (It must be added that it is difficult to draw comparisons between people who have had sex reassignment surgery and and the population at large.) In 2004, the University of Birmingham reached the same conclusion in a review of 100 medical studies of people who had undergone sex reassignment, namely that no robust clinical evidence exists that sex reassignment leads to improved mental health.[188]

---

185 Ibid. p. 48.
186 Cecilia Dhejne et al. (2011). 'Long-term follow-up of transsexual persons undergoing sex reassignment surgery. Cohort study in Sweden'. <https://doi.org/10.1371/journal.pone.0016885>.
187 The study's author, Cecilia Dhejne is employed in trans health care as physician in chief at the Anova clinic and has on several occasions attempted to explain the study's findings by arguing that suicide can occur as a result of an individual not passing and that, in these cases, the surgery was carried out "too late." In addition, she has suggested that suicides may depend on factors entirely unrelated to the sex reassignment. Yet these conclusions are not supported by the data in her study.
188 David Batty. (30 July 2004). 'Sex changes are not effective, say researchers'. *The Guardian*.

One individual who took his life following sex reassignment surgery was Jonatan from Uppsala in Sweden, whose case is recounted in the magazine *Filter*.[189] Jonatan had not shown signs of gender dysphoria as a child or teenager. His parents describe him as a happy, sociable, caring boy with a good relationship with them and others. His best friend from high school and ex-girlfriend also state they never noticed signs of gender dysphoria when he was in his teens. It was in his 20s that Jonatan began displaying signs of a psychosis: he became indifferent about his studies, preferring to play 'World of Warcraft' for days on end. His parents describe him "wandering around the house and talking to himself" when he came to visit them. He stopped adhering to his routines and eating.

Following four appointments with the student psychiatric service at Lund University, he was referred to Lund's gender identity clinic due to his "uncertain desire to change sex." The clinic concluded that he suffered from borderline, narcissistic and schizoid personality disorder and anxiety. At this point, Jonatan had become involved with the online trans community and turned instead to the Anova clinic in Stockholm. After two meetings with them, he was referred to an endocrinologist and for surgery to remove his sex organs. His parents desperately tried to contact the clinic by phone and in writing to ask that they delay the surgery due to Jonatan's displaying severe psychotic traits, a diagnosis which had been confirmed by Professor Jan Ivar Røssberg, a schizophrenia specialist. The parents' attitude was described as a "concern" by the head physician at Anova and they were asked to support and respect 'Jennifer's' wishes.

Five months after the surgery, Jonatan was taken into police custody having been found wandering around the city of Lund. He had entered a house, left blood in his trail and spoken about agents whose voices he could hear in his head. He risked eviction due to causing noise disturbances at night, had dropped out of university and his parents were transferring money to the local supermarket every month so he could buy food. The day after he admitted himself to a psychiatric unit in Lund, a second surgery was scheduled at the Anova clinic. Jonatan travelled by himself to Stockholm and, despite the fact that staff at Anova noted he was wearing sandals in mid-winter and talking to himself, the surgery was performed. This was now the second time Anova had carried out an operation on

---

189 Madeleine Pollnow, Oskar Sonn Lindell and Mattia Göransson. (Dec/Jan 2019–2020).'Fartblinda'. *Filter*.

Jonatan while he was in a psychotic state. The clinic's notes state Jonatan's studies were going well, that his finances were fine, that he was leading a healthy social life and had several friends.

One month later, Jonatan was again taken into police custody when he was found at Copenhagen airport without money or a passport saying he was a diplomat on his way to India. Not long after this episode, he smashed the windows at Lund's botanical gardens, claiming to be the goddess Shakti. In July 2017, Jonatan was found dead – he had hung himself in his flat.

When I spoke to his parents, they recounted their lengthy, unsuccessful battle to obtain the understanding of healthcare services. They have reported the hospital to the police, engaged independent experts to review Jonatan's case and have supported their arguments with research – all to no avail. Karolinska Hospital's Anova clinic refuses to comment or conduct an inquiry into the case.

There are numerous studies showing that gender reassignment treatments can improve mental health and reduce suicidal ideation, particularly in the older generation of transsexuals. The problem with the more recent research is that it is conducted by researchers who work in the very services they are evaluating in their studies or receive funding from these services. In addition, the studies are based on surveys which do not follow up on participants long term.

One Dutch study from 2014, which is often cited because it found gender reassignment led to increased psychological well-being, sent surveys to patients one year after their surgery. The average age of the patients was 20.7 years.[190] This, as the Swedish long-term study demonstrates, may have been far too soon after surgery. The Dutch study is hampered by another typical problem: one out of five participants became untraceable and did not complete the final survey, resulting in incomplete data. In addition, one participant had died of necrosis during vaginoplasty.

Towards the end of 2019, however, a study was published which appeared to demonstrate that gender reassignment improved mental health. Conducted by Karolinska Institute and Yale, it showed that the longer the length of time since surgery, the less likely the individual was to

---

190 Annelou L. C. de Vries et al. (October 2014). 'Young adult psychological outcome after puberty suppression and gender reassignment'. *Pediatrics*, Vol. 134, No. 4.

seek treatment for psychological ill health.¹⁹¹ This finding is the opposite of that in the Swedish long-term study. Researchers Richard Bränström and John Pachankis had studied data from the entire Swedish population between 2005 and 2015, including 2600 trans people and had documented their hospital admissions. Since the study was based on verifiable data from hospital registers and not on surveys, it received recognition worldwide. Swedish daily *DN* carried a long article headlined "Trans people feel better after surgery" and stated "the mental health of trans people improves year on year following gender affirmation surgery."¹⁹² Magazines like *QX* and *Out*, with majority LGBTQ readerships, informed their readers that "Sweden's trans healthcare services improve trans people's mental health."

Yet when professor and physician Agnes Wold reviewed the data the study was based on, she found that, in fact, it showed the contrary. In a letter to the *American Journal of Psychiatry* and *Dagens Nyheter*, Wold wrote:

> Hence, among the individuals examined in the Bränström study, the risk of being hospitalized for a suicide attempt was 2.4 times higher if they had undergone gender corrective surgery than if they had not. Whether this is a causal relation, i.e. that surgery actually worsens the poor mental health in gender dysphoric individuals cannot be determined. Nevertheless, the data presented in the paper do not support the notion that surgery is beneficial to mental health in gender dysphoric individuals.¹⁹³

Thirteen of the 22 trans people admitted to hospital following suicide attempts in 2015 had undergone gender affirming surgery while nine had not. Risk of suicide was therefore higher for those who had had surgery. The study merely demonstrates that the risk decreases over time, Wold writes. Such a finding could just as well be presented as: "surgery not only leaves physical scars but also results in psychological scars, which to some extent fade over time."

---

191 Richard Bränström and John Pachankis. (2019). 'Reduction in mental health treatment utilization among transgender individuals after gender-affirming surgeries. A total population study'. *American Journal of Psychiatry*. <https://doi.org/10.1176/appi.ajp.2020.1778correction>.
192 Hans Arbman. (24 October 2019). 'Ny studie: Vuxna transpersoner sökte mindre psykiatrisk vård efter operation'. *Dagens Nyheter*.
193 Agnes Wold. (1 August 2020). 'Gender-corrective surgery promoting mental health in persons with gender dysphoria not supported by data presented in article'. *American Journal of Psychiatry*. p. 768. <https://doi.org/10.1176/appi.ajp.2020.19111170>.

Agnes Wold was not alone in writing to the journal to highlight the error; 12 other researchers did the same. Bränström and Pachankis were obliged to publish a correction in which they admitted that their conclusion stating that gender affirming surgery promoted mental health was not borne out by their data:

> Upon request, the authors reanalyzed the data to compare outcomes between individuals diagnosed with gender incongruence who had received gender-affirming surgical treatments and those diagnosed with gender incongruence who had not. While this comparison was performed retrospectively and was not part of the original research question given that several other factors may differ between the groups, the results demonstrated no advantage of surgery in relation to subsequent mood or anxiety disorder-related health care visits or prescriptions or hospitalizations following suicide attempts in that comparison.[194]

However, few laypersons read *The American Journal of Psychiatry* and neither *Dagens Nyheter*, *QX* nor *Out* published the correction – the readers of these publications still believe the incorrect information that research shows surgery improves mood and mental health. Agnes Wold is one of Sweden's most cited professors – not a day goes by without her being interviewed about everything from the pandemic to pregnancy. This time, though, her words went unheard.

Clearly, there are people whose mental health improves following surgery and who feel they have been granted a new life in their new body. As mentioned, several studies exist, particularly of the earlier patient group which mainly comprised older men. Few in this 'core group' of transsexuals regret their choice – in fact, one study showed that membership of the core group diminishes the risk of regretting one's decision to have surgery. However, another crucial factor in preventing regret is Real Life Experience prior to surgery.[195] People in this core group were likely to go through with surgery regardless of what is reported in the media and, if the procedures were all done in private clinics, they would be

---

194 Richard Bränström and John Pachankis. (2020). 'Correction to Bränström and Pachankis'. *American Journal of Psychiatry*, Vol. 177, No. 8, p. 734. <https://doi.org/10.1176/appi.ajp.2020.1778correction>.

195 Friedemann Pfäfflin. (2008). 'Regrets after sex reassignment surgery'. *Journal of Psychology and Human Sexuality*, Vol. 5, No. 4, pp. 69–85. And M. Landén, J. Wålinder, G Hambert and B. Lundström. (1998). 'Factors predictive of regret in sex reassignment'. *Acta Psychiatrica Scandinavica*, Vol. 97, No. 4, pp. 284–289.

a private matter – those who want breasts are free to purchase them and it is no one's concern should they choose to do so.

The problem arises when myths are spread about 'sex change' being the only way to happiness, and publicly funded health care provides treatment and surgery as a solution to psychological problems. Such myths can lead to a number of hesitant people deciding to undergo hormone tratement and surgery. This in itself risks exacerbating poor mental health and leaving physical scars which will never heal. Patrick, a British man who was placed on hormone treatment after only one 45-minute consultation, tells his story in an anthology:

> Transitioning made me suicidal. There have been several suicide attempts in the process of trying to transition. […] Once I started transitioning, I grew suicidal because I started to develop a sense of self which bore no connection with my physical reality […] Undergoing medical transition rendered me stuck in some kind of dead-end identity with a medicalized body that might look like a woman's body but without me being an actual woman […] After several suicide attempts and a fortune spent on surgeries, I managed to react, not just on an intellectual level but also emotionally.[196]

Gina from Sweden recounts similar emotions. Having initially felt euphoric immediately after her mastectomy, she soon began feeling unwell with a new kind of dysphoria surfacing. She had transitioned due to not fitting in as a woman, yet now she did not fit in as a man either. Gina subsequently decided to detransition and started the website detransinfo.se with another young woman who had also detransitioned. On their website, they write that hormones were unhelpful for their gender dysphoria, that they have several effects which healthcare services do not inform patients of, and that, "even if you have a strong feeling of belonging to a different sex, it is not a given that you will feel better in that other gender role."[197] The number of detransitioners has grown exponentially: membership of the international online forum r/detrans has gone from 300 to 37,500 in just two years. Many of the testimonies posted there are from minors who already had extensive surgery done to them, such as that of user "Clyde Fallon":

---

196 Patrick. (2019). 'Detransition was a beautiful process' in Michele Moore and Heather Brunskell-Evans (ed). *Inventing Transgender Children and Young People*, pp. 176–177. Newcastle upon Tyne: Cambridge Scholars Publishing.
197 <https://www.detransinfo.se/orsaker-till-detransition/>.

> I realised that I should have done more about my mental health as a girl and that my problem wasn't needing to transition but it was rather me needing to accept myself. I was never gonna be happy in my body without counselling. But with counselling I could have been happy in my female body. I want my old life back so badly. I feel like a girl and wanting to be a boy was just me wanting to be accepted. I didn't want people to make fun of me anymore. Now I'm 17 and I've thrown away my whole life. I'm turning 18 in Theo [sic][198] months but I can't go out and enjoy my life. I'm not even able to go to school as I'm mentally completely destroyed. I grieve my old voice and breasts! I want them back! I can't listen to my sisters as I'm jealous of them not having done this mistake.[199]

The 17-year-old speaks as if the burden lay on her: she has thrown away her life, she should have gone to therapy, she should have accepted herself. But what teenager does not make dramatic decisions? Should the choice to remove one's breasts really be available to a minor in the first place? Another participant replies: "You were manipulated by a system that wasn't interested in your well being."

A Swedish case which was reported to HSAN (a body similar to the UK Professional Standards Authority in Health and Social Care) concerned a 35-year-old, HIV-positive bi-polar man. Following only a phone call to health care services, he was prescribed hormones, without any further queries or assessment. The man later reported the service "partly due to side effects from the hormones but mainly because he had begun to doubt his transsexuality." The physician maintained that "the purpose had been to provide the best possible assistance to this patient" but was nonetheless cautioned by HSAN.

A clinic in the Swedish town Alingsås has begun offering a new type of treatment: trauma counselling for those who regret their gender corrective surgery.[200] In what must be a wholly unique phenomenon, the same clinic which carries out the treatment and surgery also provides care to patients traumatised by that very treatment.

As can be seen from the letter below, detransitioners tend to be extremely critical of the care they have received. The letter was written by

---

198 Theo = three.
199 <https://www.reddit.com/r/detrans/comments/wt41ya/my_life_was_destroyed_with_15_years_old_im_17_now/>.
200 <https://www.svt.se/nyheter/granskning/ug/har-behandlas-flera-som-angrar-sin-konskorrigering-fem-till-tio-personer>.

three young women who had been treated at Anova and regretted it. They wanted to read it out at a meeting for family members:

> Belief in the capacity of medicine to lessen gender dysphoria and make life easier is overrated. It works for some but, generally speaking, psychological ill health is not uncommon following transition. Even suicides occur – despite the fact we don't like talking about it. We also think it is not easy to understand the difficulties that come with 'integrating as a man' and being viewed as a man by society. We each looked forward to this before our transitions but realised during the process and in the years that followed that it was hard and unfamiliar and we never truly felt like 'men'. Instead, we often felt incredibly lonely.[201]

However, management felt that the meeting was not the "right forum" for their story and they did not receive permission to read their letter.

A mother of a girl who has begun having doubts about her gender reassignment wrote to me to say she was angry that no attempts were made to assess her daughter's psychological problems. She had grown up suffering from numerous mental health issues but no one within health care services was interested in hearing about them – all they could offer were hormones and surgery. She is now stuck in a half-way state between a girl and man, having never had the chance to become a woman. Her mother wrote this in a distraught letter:

> Throughout the whole process of gender reassignment, I was never invited to or offered one single meeting. I haven't met those who treated her and I don't believe staff were told about our family situation. As far as I'm aware, no exploratory conversations are offered to the individual seeking treatment for gender dysphoria either. One and only one treatment option is offered: hormones and surgery. I am so angry. I want to kick and scream and fight my way out of this cage. I want to shout from all the rooftops in the country in defense of mothers and our right and duty to think for ourselves when it comes to our children and to rely on facts![202]

In the Board of Health and Welfare's recommendations, parents who do not accept gender reassignment treatments for their children are instead viewed as problematic and obstructive. The child knows best and should

---

[201] 'S' and 'R'. (16 December 2018). 'Hälsning till Anovas anhörigmöte från tre detransitionerare'. *EnAnnanTypAvKvinna*. Published on <https://vettigt.blog/>.
[202] Letter from Martina. April 2020.

the parents have a different opinion, they require assistance to change it. The Board, in fact, recommends that parents be referred for psychosocial support to "help them support their child" and "grow accustomed to the child's or youth's gender dysphoria."[203] In the recommendations, it is explained that "efforts ought to focus on supporting guardians and other family members in cultivating an accepting and supportive attitude" and on being "compliant with puberty blockers and cross-sex hormone treatment."[204]

Anova clinic's Kid-Team even has a template for safeguarding alerts to social services which have, on a number of occasions, placed children whose parents were critical of medical interventions, into care. One example is that of a 14-year-old girl who phoned Bris (the equivalent of the UK charity NSPCC, the National Society for the Prevention of Cruelty to Children) and informed them her mother had questioned her selection of 'boy' on an online IQ test she had completed. The helpline advised the girl to report her mother to social services.[205] In another case, a girl complained her parents refused to use the pronoun 'he' when referring to her, at which point her school raised a safeguarding alert. When it transpired that her parents had been against puberty blockers too, the girl was placed in foster care by social services. Her father told me:

> She was placed in a family we didn't know. We weren't allowed contact with her for the first weeks. After three months, an investigation showed that we hadn't done anything wrong and she was returned home to us. By then, she had relapsed into anorexia. For nearly two years, we were visited by a family social worker whose task it was to check on our suitability as parents. Initially, they came twice a week. Even though she was so ill due to anorexia, the clinic wanted to prescribe puberty blockers, which we didn't agree to. Then in May of the following year, our daughter regretted everything and changed her mind. She came home one day and told us she didn't want to continue the process and abandoned it. The clinic tried to get her to continue the treatment but she never went back there again.[206]

---

203 'God vård av barn och ungdomar med könsdysfori. Metodbeskrivning och kunskapsunderlag'. (2015). Socialstyrelsen (Board of Health and Welfare), pp. 19–20.
204 Ibid.
205 Author's interview with 'V', mother of girl. March 2019.
206 Author's interview with 'R', father of girl. 21 March 2020.

Another parent, a mother who also wishes to remain anonymous, told me:

> My son started all this just before he turned seventeen. If I had known how it was going to turn out, I would've approached matters completely differently when he came to me and said he wasn't sure whether he really felt like a boy or not. I thought Ungdomsmottagningen [a drop-in clinic for young people] was a good place where young people could talk to someone and discuss exploring their identity but after only the first meeting, they wrote a referral to the gender clinic. My son took it as a diagnosis and went from doubting his gender identity to fully embracing a different gender identity and ordering hormones online. He'd never displayed feelings like this previously, had never felt ill at ease in his gender. I tried to talk to the trans health care services about my fear that he may have schizophrenia, which runs in our family. It wasn't just that he wanted to become a woman, he had also taken to barricading himself in his room, stacking stuff in front of the door and sleeping with a knife under his pillow. But they didn't want to listen to me and when he turned eighteen, the Anova clinic began prescribing hormones even though not everyone on the staff team agreed. A year later, I found a suicide note in his computer. The whole thing has been a nightmare – he's dumped his friends and doesn't speak to us parents anymore.[207]

This mother reported feeling that she had no say in anything and that trans services "tore" her son away from her. She emphasised that she never tried to forbid him from having treatment, but simply wanted to discuss it with him. I asked her whether it seemed to her that trans services are experimenting with young people. If only it were so, she replied – experiments are serious attempts to research something, which involve keeping records and drawing conclusions. In this case, she said, no one within health care services appeared interested in the consequences of their actions.

Yet criticism is beginning to surface from the inside, from doctors who have worked at clinics providing gender affirming treatments. Angela Sämfjord is a specialist physician with several years' experience in child and adolescent psychiatry at BUP (Sweden's child and adolescent mental health services – CAMHS). She had been appointed physician-in-chief when trans healthcare services in the region of Västra Götland were being established. To begin with, she assumed she would be seeing patients who

---

207 Author's interview with 'M', mother of boy. 27 April 2020.

fit the traditional pattern of presentation for trans people: "early and clear," i.e. presenting a gender identity different to that 'assigned' at birth early on and very evidently. Instead, she was faced with an avalanche of young people, mainly girls, with mental health problems:

> The youngsters who accessed trans services presented a much higher degree of psychiatric diagnoses and psychosocial problems than is encountered in the general child and adolescent mental health services demographic. They were like CAMHS deluxe! Some screening we did revealed alarming statistics. Around half of them had autism – compared to one per cent in the general population. It was also clear that their psychological ill health had begun a few years before or concomitantly with thoughts about sex change. We presented our findings to RFSL and hoped in our naivety that they would take them seriously. Instead, the RFSL representative threw their arms up in the air and proclaimed: Trans revolution![208]

That is when Sämfjord decided that she could not continue working for the service. She says it was a matter of conscience, since trans care had reached a point where it was impossible to turn patients down. Lobbyists make vociferous demands and doctors who do not supply the anticipated diagnosis are hung out to dry online. Rather than providing health care services, it got to a point where it was more about satisfying patients' demands. Sämfjord provides the following analogy by way of example:

> If a patient is told by her doctor that she doesn't have cancer, she's happy. But if a patient is informed by her doctor that she isn't trans, she becomes furious. It is a common occurrence for patients to travel to other clinics around the country in search of a different diagnosis.

There were also cases in which parents were more convinced than the patient her/himself and pushed for a particular outcome.

In March 2019, newspaper *SvD* published an article by seven physicians from Sahlgrenska Hospital in Sweden titled 'Sex changes on children are akin to medical experiments':

> In Sweden, as in several other countries, a rapidly growing experimental undertaking has been going on for a few years now. Each year in our country, hundreds of children are subjected to 'treatment' with hormones and later to genital mutilation in the absence of anything that even comes

---

208 Conversation with Angela Sämfjord. 4 April 2020.

close to a reasonable basis in terms of science and proven experience. Generally, these children are not participants in ethically sound clinical research. It is not uncommon that the treatment is carried out in the absence of parental consent. This is all occurring with the blessing of the National Board of Health and Welfare.[209]

The industry often points to statistics demonstrating that few people regret their transition. Firstly, however, few people have the courage to disclose publicly that they regret major decisions in life – having a child, joining a cult or going into exile – no matter how much one has had to suffer for this decision. Regretting a decision entails admitting that one has made the wrong one, which can be unbearable to live with when it cannot be undone. For those who transition, it may be difficult to see it as a decision at all, since this flies in the face of the established narrative.

Secondly, many studies only count those who have changed their legal sex and then changed it back again, which does not include everyone who has undergone treatment. Thirdly, almost all statistics are based on adults who transitioned at a time very different to now, when assessments were lengthy and comprehensive processes. It is not difficult to understand that if you think long and hard about the decision and it is not merely one hastily made in your teenage years and which is actually rooted in different problems, it is far more likely that you will be satisfied.

Of course issues also did exist with the old approach. One individual I talked to who transitioned at that time tells me that the long assessments could be experienced as a kind of resistance to be overcome at all costs. For her, this meant that she became determined to go through with the procedure. The challenge became a goal in itself, and she forgot to think about whether it was actually something she wanted. Still, there are a multitude of factors which indicate that those who transition following long periods of deliberation are satisfied to a larger extent than those who make a quick decision.

Yet medical transition is still mostly promoted as the path to well-being for one and all, despite there being indications that it can result in the exacerbation of mental health issues. Young people are being sold a promise of authenticity and normality, in the achieving of which no

---

209 Christopher Gillberg, Eva Billstedt, Jovanna Dahlgren, Elisabeth Fernell, Carolina Gillberg, Nouchine Hadjikhani and Darko Sarovic. (13 March 2019). 'Könsbytena på barn är ett stort experiment'. *SvD*.

particular care seems to be taken. Uttering the words 'gender affirming care' is easier than undergoing it and many young people with unrealistic expectations – not least those on the autistic spectrum with their often literal interpretation of reality – may be under the impression that it is really possible to wake up transformed into a complete woman or man. The industry disseminates this idea through slogans like "One Pill Makes You a Boy, One Pill Makes You a Girl" and markets the treatments as a way of fully changing sex.[210] As one patient told me, "They didn't explain that as a 185 cm tall seventeen-year-old with broad shoulders, it may be impossible for me to pass as a woman." Not everyone is going to look like YouTuber Blaire White. The fact that gender identity theory has become hegemonic within the state, school, sport and public documents does not mean that it is easy to be accepted in reality. The person who believes she will fully pass as a member of her new sex is often repeatedly reminded that others see her as something else. Men who have transitioned have to endure harassment and risk being victims of hate crimes. Homosexual men who have transitioned can feel excluded from the gay scene but also not accepted by the heterosexual world. Trans men often have an easier time of it provided they've developed facial hair, but the difficulty of manufacturing a functioning penis can make dating a nightmare since both heterosexual women and homosexual men are often looking for a person with a penis. Excluded from the male community, many trans men remain in the lesbian community, where they are frequently not welcome either since they are viewed as men. If the aim was to get rid of gender dysphoria, the result can often be the onset of a completely different gender dysphoria – one that cannot be banished through treatment.

Vanessa López, Miss Trans Star International and reality show star, writes in her autobiography *Jag har ångrat mig* (I regret it) that she no longer wants to use the term gender reassignment. Instead, she calls it "gender conforming." As a child, Lopez loved playing with dolls and didn't think for a minute that this would have something to do with her genitals. Dolls were dolls and they were fun to play with, period. "The fact I had a willy, unlike mum, didn't affect my identifying with the feminine."[211]

---

210 Diane Ehrensaft. (January 2009). 'One pill makes you a boy, one pill makes you a girl'. *International Journal of Applied Psychoanalytic Studies*.
211 Vanessa Lopez. (2014). *Jag har ångrat mig*, p. 191. Sweden: Two-Spirit Publisher.

But something happened when she grew older and came into contact with the outside world:

> It was when I went to nursery school that I began to realise there was something that wasn't quite right about me. Today, I would rephrase that and say there was probably something about the outside world that wasn't quite right.[212]

She could no longer be a boy and play with dolls. López was beaten up nearly every day, called a faggot and there

> was no one back then who explained to me that I could behave like a girl as much as I wanted and that boys were allowed to behave like girls without it necessarily meaning that they had to go all the way and surgically remake their genitals.[213]

López goes on to write: "I knew I was never going to be a successful man in a world in which femininity in men is viewed as something shameful."[214] Today, she feels a deep sorrow over not being able to have children and says: "If I were to advise young people today, I'd tell them that it's not you or your sex that there's anything wrong with. It's the imbalance in humanity that's the problem."[215]

'Allies' often like to portray themselves as trans people's knights in shining armour. They regard themselves as open and tolerant and are thus incapable of criticising what they see as a vulnerable person's own choice. Yet the encouragement a newly transitioned individual may receive from allies online, does not always translate into concrete support and she risks being left alone with her body. A symbol in the media, but marginalised in the real world, alone with her medicines and her doubts. On the one hand maligned by the far-right, on the other praised by left allies as a symbol of the avant garde – yet it is up to the trans person herself to hold her own and administer her injections year in year out. Should she regret her transition or express the slightest doubt, she risks being ostracised from the trans community and singled out as a traitor.

Interestingly enough, when doctors, detransitioners and parents started raising the alarm, healthcare services kept silent while the

---

212 Ibid.
213 Ibid. p. 192.
214 Ibid. p. 193.
215 Ibid. p. 194.

retaliation came from academics and thinkers. Most of these individuals seemed to – deliberately or not – have misunderstood the criticism; they were under the impression that trans people, and not *trans healthcare*, were being criticised. Essentially, they conflated the two.

Anna Dahlqvist dismissed criticism as "anti trans" in the magazine *Ottar* and claimed she could prove that the trans children's parents who had been critical of the care offered in fact had "connections to conservative Christian groups and radical feminists with trans-critical agendas."[216] She made the claim based on the fact that a Norwegian member of the Christian Democrat Party and a feminist commentator had expressed their belief in the existence of two sexes.

Art critic Ulrika Stahre's piece in *Aftonbladet* was a dismissive shrugging of the shoulders: "The fact that some people do not feel at home in their bodies and receive assistance to either take things further or find other solutions is definitely not the biggest problem around." The main problems, according to Stahre, are "the widening gap between social classes, unemployment and climate anxiety," and ended her article by inviting a "happy and content trans person" to contribute to the debate.[217]

In *Expressen*, commentator Myra Åhbeck Öhman wrote that the critique of puberty blockers was a "caricature of moral panic" which was "out of step with the times, narrow minded and one dimensional."[218] She claimed puberty blockers were effective and cited three studies, among them a "large meta analysis which shows that 52 out of 56 studies demonstrate that transitioning has a positive effect on mental health." Unbelievably, she appears not to have read any of the studies herself, as not one of them concerns puberty blockers. Furthermore, none of the studies is of the new group of teenage girls, with the majority consisting of surveys of older males who transitioned as adults a long time ago. It is also not true that 52 of the 56 studies show a positive effect on mental health from transitioning. It is clear that Åhbeck Öhman is less interested in finding out the real effects of puberty blockers, as she signs off by encouraging readers to choose "which side of history they want to be on."

---

216 Anna Dahlqvist. (20 June 2020). 'Antitrans-allians'. *Ottar*.
217 Ulrika Stahre. (2 September 2019). 'Nej det finns ingen transmaffia'. *Aftonbladet Kultur*.
218 Myra Åhbeck Öhman. (29 July 2020). 'Anna Björklunds försvar av J.K. Rowling är moralpanik'. *Expressen*.

The same nonchalance can be found in nearly all the articles on the topic by cultural commentators. Their stance is one of principle only, they display little interest in investigating matters themselves and are more concerned about being on the right side of history – whatever this means. Yet the most serious problem is that they make use of a hodgepodge of sloppily googled articles in order to defend treatments whose serious adverse effects they do not know. Why is it that individuals who purport to be on the side of trans people advocate treatments which risk being directly harmful for their health? And the silence from the actual health care providers was conspicuous in its absence.

CHAPTER 24

The Industry Under Pressure

It might be said, in retrospect, that it was the case of Keira Bell which turned the tide.

Briton Keira Bell was 15 when she first accessed trans healthcare services. After only three hour-long conversations, she was prescribed puberty blockers and a year later, was put on testosterone. At 20, she had surgery to remove her breasts.

Three years on, Bell regretted having had the treatment and surgery. She sued the clinic on the grounds that a minor does not have the capacity to consent to puberty blockers, accused the clinic of providing misleading information and argued that the process contravened Article 8 of the European Convention on Human Rights, which forbids state interference in private and family life.[219]

In December 2020, the High Court found in her favour. Following the judgment, the Tavistock Gender Identity Development Service, a publically funded and state-run unit, can no longer prescribe puberty blockers to children.[220] The historic judgment states that puberty blockers are to be considered an experimental treatment whose results are as yet unclear, that the purpose of the treatment has not been clarified and that it has life-changing consequences. The treatment cannot be considered 'time for the patient to reflect', as it is more similar to a fast-track to hormone therapy,

---

219 In the High Court of Justice: Case No: CO/60/2020, Between Quincy Bell (2) Mrs A and the Tavistock and Portman NHS Foundation Trust.
220 Ibid.

which in turn can lead to infertility. For these reasons, this treatment cannot be equated to normal medical treatment, which aims to prevent, alleviate or cure disease. A child under 16 cannot be presumed capable of consenting to such treatment.

The day after the judgment, the National Health Service ceased treating children under 16 with puberty blockers.[221] Although in 2021, the Appeals Court did not uphold the High Court judgment, in July 2022, the NHS announced that Tavistock would be closing for good.[222] Following a report from the NHS by paediatrician Hilary Cass, it was concluded that the clinic had adopted a series of unscientific practices, such as overlooking health issues other than gender dysphoria. It also stated that "health staff feel under pressure to adopt an 'unquestioning affirmative approach'."[223]

Sweden's Karolinska Hospital announced in May 2021 that it would cease to apply the Dutch Protocol, and not treat minors at all except within clinical studies.[224] The decision was presented worldwide as though Sweden had outlawed puberty blockers, which was not the case. The decision only concerned one hospital, which also later softened its decision to announce it would still continue to treat those who had begun treatment.

In 2022, the Swedish Board of Health and Welfare announced new national guidelines, which recommend "caution" when treating minors with hormones. Risks of hormone treatment are now said to outweigh benefits. Hormone treatment is now principally to be prescribed within a clinical study. If outside of a clinical study, this has to be a decision taken by both a multidisciplinary conference and the parents of the child. Regarding GnRH analogues, these should be used for gender dysphoria only as an exception or in a clinical study. No youth in Tanner stage 2 should be given puberty blockers, as it is considered unethical not to let the youth first be exposed to their natural puberty. Furthermore, puberty blockers for Tanner stages 3 and 4 are only to be given if the minor has a

---

221 Amendments to Service Specification for Gender Identity Development Service for Children and Adolescents (E13/S(HSS)/e).
222 Andrew Gregory. (29 July2022). 'NHS to close Tavistock gender identity clinic for children'. <https://www.theguardian.com/society/2022/jul/28/nhs-closing-down-london-gender-identity-clinic-for-children>.
223 Ibid.
224 <https://lakartidningen.se/aktuellt/nyheter/2021/05/karolinska-satter-stopp-for-hormonbehandling-vid-konsdysfori/>.

stable "psychosocial" situation and does not have any other psychological issue such as trauma, substance abuse or is at risk of suicide.[225] This, in many ways, is a return to the type of cautionary policies of 2007. The report states furthermore that very little is still known about the safety and efficiency of treatments, and that very little new research has been added to the body of knowledge since 2015.

After the decision to close the Tavistock, the gender identity industry has started to come under pressure worldwide, and voices are now being heard in Australia and Scotland to close down treatment of minors as well. Of all aspects of gender identity ideology, the hormone treatment of children has become by far the most controversial in society at large.

---

[225] Socialstryrelsen. (February 2022). 'Stöd, utredning och hormonbehandling vid könsinkongruens hos barn och ungdomar'. Update of national guidelines on care of children and adolescents with gender dysphoria.

PART 3

THE ONE SEX THEORY

CHAPTER 25

A Tale of Trans People?

Gender Identity theory often purports to be a story for and about trans people, laws are reformed for the sake of trans people and anyone questioning the theory is told to 'listen to trans people'. All of a sudden, everybody from corporations to presidents to church leaders seems concerned with the plight of this one group.

As the preceding analysis has demonstrated, gender identity theory rather victimises trans people. From the moment a person is classified 'trans', she is considered to be deviant. Despite the stubborn insistence that being trans is a positive characteristic, her body is viewed as faulty and in need of fixing. Her life and fertility are sacrificed along the way and she is offered no help or apology if her body is damaged in the process. Should she be suicidal prior to the interventions, this is used as a reason to prescribe hormones, while if she suffers from suicidal thoughts *after* treatment, professionals look the other way. If she commits suicide or dies, the services that treated her accept no responsibility – she has become a symbol, not a human being like others. She is not considered worthy of a future and her suffering is only of interest when it can be employed as ammunition in political arguments which are often entirely unrelated to her circumstances.

Despite many insistences, she is not the protagonist of this story, but a prop to be used at will in a narrative with implications and consequences reaching far beyond her life. This narrative seeks to radically redefine sex in its entirety and concerns a much larger group of people. Gender identity theory does not just create the story of the trans person but invents a whole new identity as well: the 'cis-person'.

CHAPTER 26

Woman: A Dangerous Word

The word woman has become problematic. Increasingly, it is being replaced with terms like 'uterus bearer', 'menstruator' and 'chest feeder'. In England, the term 'non-trans women' is sometimes used.[1] A group established to discuss women's genital problems was described by the magazine *ETC* as "a group for all vagina bearers."[2] Second-hand shop Emmaus advertised a discount for "all those who identify as non-men" on International Women's Day in 2017.[3] Sanitary pad manufacturer Always decided in October 2019 to remove the female symbol from their packaging, following complaints from customers that it caused distress and was not inclusive enough.[4] Tampon brand Tampax was not to be outdone by this move and, a year later, ceased using the word woman and began addressing their advertising campaigns to "people who bleed." In an effort to celebrate diversity, they declare, "Fact: Not all women have periods. Also a fact: Not all people with periods are women. Let's celebrate the diversity of all people who bleed!"[5] Tampax's advertising regularly includes statements about breaking down taboos around menstruation

---

1 <https://www.versobooks.com/blogs/4090-i-m-not-transphobic-but-a-feminist-case-against-the-feminist-case-against-trans-inclusivity>.
2 Karin Holmberg. (20 November 2018). 'Ha ett underbart fittliv'. *Dagens ETC*.
3 'Feministisk rabatt 8 mars 2017'. <http://emmausbjorka.se/2017/02/21/feministisk-komensationsrabatt-8-mars/>.
4 Heather Murphy. (22 October 2019). 'Always removes female symbol from sanitary pads'. *New York Times*.
5 Instagram post by Tampax. (15 September 2020).

yet the company has merely replaced one taboo with another: the word woman. "People with periods can do everything men can do, but do it better – AND while bleeding" reads one of their Instagram posts, demonstrating in the same sentence that the word *man* is not taboo and that it continues to be used as the opposite of woman. However, that word, 'woman', must no longer be uttered. Man is ok, woman is not. The whole approach is full of mixed messages: one is to celebrate, the company demands, as if there was a party going on, yet it is not clear for whom we are celebrating. Who are the people with periods who are not women? One guess is that Tampax refers to trans men, i.e. a small group of biological women who would be offended by being called women. Yet this group, as demonstrated, would hardly celebrate getting their period and most do anything to get rid of it, the period being seen as – precisely – a sign of being female. Most trans men who take hormones would not even have their period. The group of people who celebrate menstruation but still abhor the thought of being called women must be a rather minuscule group within an already minuscule group; the number of women who celebrate their period already being quite small to begin with. Added to that, members of this group would probably be insulted anyway by Tampax's notion that people with periods are, by definition, not men and that men do things worse.

How to make sense of this confusion? There is one common denominator: woman is erased. We find it everywhere so-called inclusive language is being used. Inclusive language is itself a misnomer since in reality it means to exclude the word woman.

This is especially so in the reproductive rights debate. Planned Parenthood, the largest sexual and reproductive health organisation in the US, celebrates the removal of taxes on sanitary products for all "menstruators in New York."[6] When US States legislate to prohibit abortion, those who speak out about an attack on women's rights are promptly reprimanded: abortion is *not* a women's issue, claim hundreds of articles in *Forbes*, *Rewire* and *Amnesty International*, since "people of all

---

6 Meghan Murphy. (7 September 2016). 'Are we women or are we menstruators'. *Feminist Current*. <https://www.feministcurrent.com/2016/09/07/are-we-women-or-are-we-menstruators/>.

genders have abortions."⁷ And when Roe vs Wade was overturned in the US supreme court, many opponents did not even mention women as the ones who would be affected. As the Center for Reproductive Rights put it, the affected would be "especially Black, Indigenous, and other people of color, members of the LGBTQ community, people with disabilities, young people, and people living on low incomes." What all these groups, who could need abortions, would have in common is omitted.⁸

In December 2020, Denmark's Kvindemuseet, one of the world's first women's museums, announced they were changing their name to KØN-Gender Museum Denmark. By way of explanation, management stated that the word woman excludes while the word gender "includes all people."⁹

Several British and American companies have taken to writing 'womxn', explaining that the substitution of the letter *a* for *x* is for the purpose of "including black and trans women." They do not elaborate on what it is about the letter *a* but not the letter *x* which excludes black women specifically, though one thing is clear: something about the word woman has suddenly begun to stick in people's throats. The magazine *Ottar* asks the question: "Can we talk about women?" and interviews the trans author Maria Ramnehill, who says:

> All women do not have a vagina and all those with a vagina are not women. It's as simple as that. [...] An example could be radio station P3's programme *Musikhjälpen 2013*, whose theme was 'All girls have the right to survive their pregnancy'. To be more inclusive, this slogan could have been rephrased as 'Everyone has the right to survive their pregnancy'.

Ramnehill further suggests we should refer to 'non-men', a term which encompasses all those who do not benefit from a patriarchal social structure. Thus, according to Ramnehill, instead of saying 'there should be more women on executive boards', we could say 'there should be more non-men on boards'.¹⁰

---

7   S. E. Smith. (1 March 2019). 'Women are not the only ones who get abortions'. *Rewire News*.
8   <https://reproductiverights.org/supreme-court-case-mississippi-abortion-ban-disproportionate-harm/>.
9   'Kvindemuseet skifter navn til KØN'. (5 December 2020). Kvindemuseet. <https://kvindemuseet.dk/nyhed/nyt-navn-til-kvindemuseet/>.
10 Hugo Ewald. (7 December 2014). 'Kan vi prata om kvinnor?' *Ottar*.

Ramnehill wants us to do away with the words girl and woman but says nothing about the word man. This word, in contrast, is not seen as problematic or exclusionary; it is a point of reference that all others must relate to, like the sun at the centre of the solar system. The suggested term 'non-men', implies the existence of two groups: men and everyone else. The first of these, man, is a fixed category and is not carved up into 'sperm producer', 'scrotum bearer', 'penis haver' but remains whole and functions as its own reference point (the term 'non-woman' is not applied to him). In the other group, which used to be called 'woman', we now find 'everyone else'. The independent status of this group has been dissolved and they can now only be referred to by their organs and what they are *not*.

Similarly, Bobby Noble, professor of sexuality studies, claims the word woman should be abolished:

> Critical trans perspectives should be making it much harder to make truth claims about the universalizability of 'women'– experientially or otherwise – without at least using it with much more precision to identify a relation to 'woman' no longer reducible to the female body or the nefarious 'women's experiences'.[11]

Like Ramnehill, Noble argues that it is the word woman which is problematic, not the word man. Further, he claims that neither the body nor lived experience ought any longer to provide a basis for solidarity and political action – even the act of raising one's hand and asking a history lecturer to name female historical figures is problematic, according to Noble:

> Doesn't the gender-panicked imperative to 'remember the women', mark an unequivocal gender fundamentalism, where such fundamentalisms themselves – not unlike those of nationalism, military-state, white-supremacist or Christian, to name only a few – function to ground a feminist imaginary and its methodology of social, moral and biological coercive normalization?[12]

The message here is: don't rock the boat of male dominance, girls – doing so brings you dangerously close to creating a fundamentalist, white-supremacist military regime! Yet lecturing solely about men in history

---

11 Bobby Noble. (2012). 'Trans. Panic. Some thoughts toward a theory of feminist fundamentalism'. In Anne Enke (ed). *Transfeminist Perspectives in and beyond Transgender and Gender Studies*, p. 50. Philadelphia: Temple University Press.
12 Ibid.

is not considered exclusionary by Noble. The above text is part of an anthology which calls itself feminist, but which tears to shreds all attempts at female solidarity using a battery of threatening analogies. In itself, this is nothing new – the history of the women's movement being one of backlashes – but contrary to the reaction of the extreme right, which does not masquerade as something it is not, the liberal backlash is clad in the language of the women's movement and feminism. Thus, the reader interested in feminism feels 'at home' and lets down her guard despite the fact the message is a classically patriarchal one of guilt and shame: don't try and think for yourself woman! You are problematic!

"Avoid: woman!" is emblazoned in large red lettering on Sweden's national health service website. As far as possible, the word woman is to be avoided when discussing bodies. For instance, one should avoid statements like "many (women) feel worried prior to giving birth" and should instead use language about body parts: "There is often a smallest common denominator, for example body parts or hormones."[13]

It is becoming increasingly common to reduce women's experiences of sexuality and reproduction to being solely about organs. This creates big challenges for the feminist movement, which is having to reformulate oppression as if it was body parts being oppressed instead of women. When sexuality educator Sandra Dahlén's book about vaginas, *Hallongrottan* (The Raspberry Cave), was published, the word woman did not feature in discussions. The vagina was portrayed as a separate entity that had sex independently of the woman it was part of. It even possessed a personality: "Does your vagina think you should change jobs? Does it think you should send the kids away more often?"

In an interview, Dahlén is asked, "What is the vagina's status in today's society?" She responds: "The vagina is a very charged space, one subjected to an extraordinary amount of violence, both in war- and peacetime."[14] Discussing the vagina without ever mentioning women lends a cryptic air to Dahlén's statements: it is as though we are all walking around harbouring an illogical hatred toward this thing, a hatred that has no context or history, as if "the vagina" would be a charged space even if it was lying around in a fridge, as if there was no connection between that hatred and

---

13 <https://www.1177.se/riktlinjer-och-material/sprakliga-riktlinjer/diverse-ord-och-uttryck-a-o/k2/kvinna---undvik/>.
14 <https://www.etc.se/kultur-noje/slidan-ar-missforstadd>.

the historical oppression of women. The vagina would thus be in need of a political struggle of its own, as well as the uterus, the period and the cervix – naturally, all separated!

Sweden's Left Party launched one of its healthcare reforms in July 2019 in a similar fashion: "An intervention that saves lives. Free cervical screening for all people with wombs."[15] When they received criticism for their phrasing, the reply was the predictable "not all people with wombs are women." Putting aside the strategically incomprehensible issue of selecting the smallest target group imaginable – few, if any, would identify as 'womb bearers' – the main question is: what is the Left Party's definition of sex? If it is not what is between your legs, what is it? A stereotype? A feeling? An essence? And if the word sex is not to exist anymore, the question of how to formulate a critique of patriarchy arises.

American author Naomi Wolf claims use of the word woman can no longer be justified:

> But when there is now a trend of female-to-male transgender Smith undergraduates raising questions about 'what is a Smithie?' – and even what is a woman, or a man – how do we justify women-only events, training or ideologies?[16]

Who, then, was Wolf's book *The Beauty Myth* – with its subtitle *How Images of Beauty Are Used Against Women*, and use of the word woman ten times on the first page alone – directed at? Wolf responds: "So many men and trans people have read *The Beauty Myth* and thanked me for it. I didn't write it only for readers born with uteri." On the question of what a woman is, she has this to say: "Woman is whoever wants to be a woman. Why police other people's gender choices? Who cares? What does it matter? Honestly. Being a good person matters."[17] Sex is now, according to Wolf, a *personal* choice and not a structural form of oppression. Yet if sex is now so unimportant as to be superfluous, does this not render the arguments in Wolf's earlier work impossible? In 1991, she wrote:

> The beauty myth tells a story: The quality called 'beauty' objectively and universally exists. Women must want to embody it and men must want

---

15 <https://www.facebook.com/vansterpartiet/photos>.
16 Naomi Wolf. (15 February 2013). 'Do we still need women-only spaces?' *The Guardian*.
17 <https://twitter.com/naomirwolf/status/1288919444131991552>. (July 20 2020.) Account since suspended.

to possess women who embody it. This embodiment is an imperative for women and not for men [...][18]

If we cannot speak of men and women any longer, can the above analysis even be made? How are we to understand that beauty myths affect one half of the population in an entirely different way to the other half? If being a woman is a matter of personal choice, does it not follow that being affected by beauty myths is a personal choice as well? Yet again, we are confronted by the same asymmetry, which sets aside the word man as unproblematic – Wolf comments without hesitation that several men have read her book – while women are reduced to "readers with wombs," a term far less inclusive than the term woman, since even women born without a womb and those who have had a hysterectomy are affected by beauty myths. After all, it is not the uterus that must comply with the idea of beauty, but the woman.

These calls for the abolition of the word woman are usually met with an uncomprehending shrug of the shoulders – what's the big deal? It's just about being inclusive! If everyone doesn't feel represented by certain terms, why continue to use them? Framing it as a question of inclusion makes the choice appear an uncontroversial no-brainer, akin to inviting the whole class to a child's birthday party. Who would be against this? Surely only bitter individuals who want to ruin things for everyone else! Inclusive language comes, as a consulting company says, without a cost, but "not using it in a business context has economic costs."[19]

Let us assume for a moment that this happens: that we abolish the use of the word woman due to discovering that 0.25% of the population with XX-chromosomes does not want to be referred to with this word; that a further 0.25% with XY-chromosomes want to be called women and that another 0.5% do not want to be called anything at all. Let us thus assume the word woman, when used in conjunction with menstruation and pregnancy, is deeply distressing to this 1% of the population. Why, in such a situation, would abolishing the word man not also be required? It is exclusionary in precisely the same way. According to this logic, all words should be abolished. No word is 100% comprehensive in what it refers to, covering every member of the category it denotes – the word

---

18   Naomi Wolf. (1991/2002). *The Beauty Myth: How Images of Beauty Are Used Against Women*, p. 12. New York: Harper Collins.
19   <https://www.witty.works/en/blog/post/what-is-inclusive-language>.

'black' does not include individuals who have albinism, 'working class' does not include pensioners, not to even mention the word 'elderly', which is forced upon people who do not feel old but are so in years. How would any words for anything exist if we were to take this argument to its logical conclusion?

When musician Salif Keita, who has albinism, sings "I am black / My skin is white …" we understand what he means, without it being necessary for him to start campaigns to abolish the term 'black'. All words are by definition generalisations which create exceptions. For many years, we have known of the existence of transgender people without discontinuing the use of the word woman. Yet gender identity theory argues that, rather than the exception proving the rule, the exception is now meant to overthrow the rule. The exception, now, *is* the rule.

Several far more serious consequences arise from abolishing the word woman. If we cannot say 'woman' anymore, we also cannot discuss women's health, discrimination of women in medical research or women's bodies in the first place. Genitals are compartmentalised into one topic, menstruation into another, pregnancy into a third and so forth. We thus lose the ability to consider women's oppression as a whole, seeing only our body parts as separate from one another, with their own independent existences. Rather than our body parts being part of us, we become appendages to them: we walk around as bearers of our vaginas and wombs but do not exist beyond them as a group. None of these neologisms contain a liberating potential: no one is happy referring to themselves as a 'womb bearer' and it is hard to picture 'menstruators' uniting in rebellion. What we are witnessing with the proposal to abolish the word woman is in fact an incredibly far-reaching alienation of women – an alienation that is not being imposed on men to the slightest degree. This alienation is aided by a linguistic violence that carves up women in our consciousness, producing a collage of body parts that can be dismembered and rearranged any old way. It is not only the possibility of seeing structural sex discrimination vanish with this outlook, but also the opportunity to understand oneself as a *self*, a person. Woman is no longer permitted to be, as Simone de Beauvoir wrote, a *situation*.

The name of our sex is not a minor detail. Without the word 'woman', women disappear as political subjects, and so does any meaningful kind of feminism. A common name is the foundation of all groups. Any political organising starts with naming the subject in question: who are we?

Certainly, women will continue to exist even if we are no longer referred to as women – we will continue to be born, give birth, die and breathe. Yet in the absence of an awareness of the situation of our sex, we cannot understand our circumstances and will remain unable to organise for our betterment. This is why all oppressed groups must have a name. All – workers, the colonised, homosexuals, black people – have named themselves, sending the message: this is who we are. Those white people who insist on being colour-blind do not comprehend that it is precisely through the erasure of the possibility to mention skin colour that the opportunity to fight for better conditions is also erased. Similarly, erasing the word woman is a full frontal attack on the women's movement.

Yet something remains disturbing about the word, as Karolina Ramqvist's words in the novel *Alltings början* (The Beginning of Everything) remind us:

> I do not know what is wrong with the word woman, but something is. It is difficult to read it, write it, utter it. On the other hand, it is very easy to use the word man. […] It's normal and not messy or sticky at all. It's nothing![20]

At the level of biology, this is of course utter nonsense. Men's bodies produce a significant amount of mess and statistically they are not more common or normal than women's bodies. Rather, the illusion of man as the standard is one brought about as a result of the culturally created gender hierarchy. It is the very same illusion which surfaces in the current discourse regarding the word woman. At this stage, we are still permitted to talk about women's genitals – in fact, as we have seen in this chapter, references to breasts, vaginas and wombs are very much welcome – so long as one doesn't mention they are in any way connected to women. In the next stage, however, even sex organs are banished from the discourse.

---

20 Karolina Ramqvist. (2013). *Alltings början*, p. 115. Stockholm: Norstedts.

CHAPTER 27

Vagina: A Dangerous Word

In 2014, two private US women's colleges, Mills College and Mount Holyoke, decided to change their definition of woman. From then on, the definition would be decoupled from biology, allowing all those who self-identified as women to apply to the institutions. Mount Holyoke's president Lynn Pasquarella explained: "We recognize that what it means to be a woman is not static [...] we acknowledge that gender identity is not reducible to the body."[21] A year later, Mount Holyoke cancelled their annual performance of Eve Ensler's *The Vagina Monologues*, saying the play "is problematic because it is not inclusive of trans women." The theatre board's spokeswoman Erin Murphy explained the decision in an interview:

> Gender is a wide and varied experience [...] one that cannot simply be reduced to biological or anatomical distinctions, and many of us who have participated in the show have grown increasingly uncomfortable presenting material that is inherently reductionist and exclusive.[22]

Eve Ensler countered that her play had not mentioned women, only vaginas, but the decision was not reversed. It appears vaginas are now also taboo. At Washington University, the play continues to be staged, though the word vagina has been removed and it is now called *The (Blank)*

---

21 Dominique Mosbergen. (3 September 2014). 'All-women's Mount Holyoke College changes policy to welcome transgender students'. *Huffington Post*.
22 Tyler Kinkade. (16 January 2015). 'Mount Holyoke cancels 'Vagina Monologues' for not being inclusive enough'. *Huffington Post*.

Monologues. Where the word vagina would have appeared, there is now an empty, unnameable void, bookended by brackets.[23]

We are now very far indeed from gender identity theory's introductory talk of openness and acceptance of everyone as they are. We are also a long way off from the next layer, which believes everyone ought to find their own gender identity and which views men and women as opposites. In this third camp, women are a problematic category that must be renamed, questioned and whose sex must be replaced by an empty space. Women's bodies are considered threatening and exclusionary while men's bodies continue to exist freely and are not subjected to similar treatment. Worth noting is that it is *women's* speech about women's bodies which is labelled problematic. Men are still permitted to name women's sex – the gender police do not rush in to porn sites and demand that 'pussy' and 'cunt' be replaced by *(blank)* on the grounds that they exclude people. (Just imagine human traffickers forced to change their script to: Let me fuck your [blank], show me your [blank]). Yet when women speak of their own sexuality, it is considered inappropriate for them to name their own sex organs. The women's movement is apparently not meant to be liberating – it is meant to be *inclusive*!

Nor is it the word vagina itself that is made taboo – it is only taboo when it can be associated with women. Listen to this definition, from a manual about safer sex from the Human Rights Campaign Foundation:

> Dick: We use the word dick to describe external genitals. Dicks come in all shapes and sizes and can belong to people of all genders.
>
> Front hole: We use this word to talk about internal genitals, sometimes referred to as a vagina. (…)
>
> Vagina: We use this word to talk about the genitals of trans women who have had bottom surgery.

Thus, women may no longer call their vagina a vagina, as this word is now reserved for men, or "trans women who have had bottom surgery." We will have to be content with the word, "front hole", in a very symbolic reversal, as gender reassignment surgery for men *does* create a hole which does not

---

23 Katherine Timpf. (20 February 2019), 'Students drop "Vagina" from The Vagina Monologues to be more "inclusive"'. *National Review*.

lead anywhere, whereas the female vagina is a channel through which we create and give life to humanity.²⁴

When Donald Trump's words "grab them by the pussy" hit headlines in the midst of the 2016 election campaign, there was an explosion of anger. Large marches called 'Women's Marches' were organised all over the USA, also spreading to Europe. Feminist Krista Suh designed a pink hat in the shape of a vulva in a move to symbolically reclaim the organ from Trump. The hat was crocheted by thousands of women all over the world and was the marchers' response to the red caps worn by Trump's supporters, yet it eventually came to be seen as controversial by the very leaders of the marches. Organisers advised against wearing the hats in several cities, saying the vulva could be considered an exclusive symbol. The magazine *Bustle* attempted to talk sense into women and get them to leave the hats at home:

> With the renewed vulnerability of trans kids making headlines and the targeting of trans women of color continuing its bloody rampage into 2017, now is not the time for the vagina-centricness of the women's march. […] There's no doubt that the 'pussy'-centric signs and chants of the Jan. 21 women's marches privileged cis women over trans people, and that feminist circles as a whole privilege cis women.²⁵

These warnings appear to have gone unheeded. One paper reported that the organisers' admonitions "didn't stop thousands of women knitting pussy hats and excitedly posting photos of Fallopian tube-themed march placards to Instagram."²⁶

Interestingly enough, few of those who tried to prohibit the vulva hats were trans people themselves. The proportion of trans people who care about something as irrelevant as other people's choice of headwear is likely to be insignificant if not altogether non-existent. Either the trans person in question has a vagina or has had one (and in both cases they can relate) or the trans person has a penis and would presumably be able to fathom the existence of other genitals – or why not make their own hat?

---

24 <https://assets2.hrc.org/files/assets/resources/Trans_Safer_Sex_Guide_FINAL.pdf>.
25 Noor Al-Sibai. (6 March 2017). 'How to acknowledge your privilege at The Women's Strike'. *Bustle*.
26 Chloe Sargeant. (22 January 2018). 'Until the Women's March is inclusive of all women, I can't identify with it'. *SBS News*.

The whole point of the marches was that Trump, who by this time had become President, thought that vulvas *in particular* were a body part that could be grabbed without asking. Thus, the raison d'être of the marches was that people who have vulvas are *not* privileged. Still, it was demanded that those with vulvas retreat into the background – at their own march – in case the penises felt distressed and excluded.

All these struggles might seem trivial to some – why fight about a hat? Again, this is not about a hat. Nor is it about trans people per se. Trans people are just the most efficient argument used at this time in history to tell women what we can or cannot do in our own movement, how we must and must not conduct our struggle, how we are allowed and not allowed to speak about our own bodies, our opinions and our own experiences. It is a way of disrupting women's energy and guilt-tripping us for speaking our minds and being creative. It could thus be interesting to remember the origin of the word trivial, as Professor Mary Daly pointed out: it comes from the Latin tri via, three roads, which is a place where three roads met during the Roman Empire and where common people, especially women, from different villages would meet and naturally, talk would arise.[27] Their talk was seen as irrelevant by the higher classes, and ever since, women's talk has been referred to as trivial.

---

27 Mary Daly. (1979). *Gyn/Ecology, The Metaethics of Radical Feminism*, p. 78. London: The Women's Press.

CHAPTER 28

The Creation of the Cis-Person – or How We Fell In Love with Gender Roles

Gender identity theory supposedly seeks to abolish the binary pair man/woman, yet in the process it institutes a different binary: the trans person/cis-person.

The prefix cis means 'on this side' and gained traction in the 1990s as a term referring to people who were not trans. It is most commonly used in reference to women: since the term woman has been broadened to include people born as men, women born as women have been rechristened cis-women. The word was added to the Oxford English Dictionary in 2015[28] and is defined below by the Swedish Secretariat for Gender Research:

> The word cis-person is often used to show the relationship between an individual's legal and biological sex and their gender identity. An example of a cis-person would be someone born with a vagina (biological sex), being registered as 'female' (legal sex) and who sees and has always considered herself a woman (gender identity). This individual expresses herself as a woman (gender expression) (see also binary/linear gender) through her choice of clothing, body language, hair style and behaviour. These individuals can be called cis and a central feature of the position of a cis-person is that it is often associated with cultural conceptions

---

28   <https://public.oed.com/blog/december-2015-update-new-words-notes/>.

of normal, natural and healthy and is a position which entails many privileges.[29]

This is a particularly interesting definition in that it raises more questions than it answers. For instance, what does it mean to always have "considered" yourself to be a woman? Is it sufficient to have discovered your genitals or is a wider awareness required and if so what? What is meant by expressing one's gender identity through "clothing, body language, hair style and behaviour"? What constitutes female behaviour and who decides this? The phrase "is associated with" establishes a fact, yet the authors do not take responsibility for the statement, instead gesturing toward vague cultural norms.

At first glance, it may seem a definition that is accessible to everyone: we are all aware of the existence of women's clothing and men's hair styles. Applied to individuals, however, the statement reveals an unworkable analytical category. A woman can have long hair (feminine, according to many) but work as the CEO of a bank (a position previously only held by men). Does this make her a cis-person? Is Pippi Longstocking a cis-person? How does someone express his manhood "through behaviour"? Does attending a football match once a year qualify you? And where to place male body-builders in this binary, with their huge muscles and oiled bodies posing in front of audiences wearing only miniscule, glittery swimsuits?

These are precisely the kinds of questions which the field of gender studies normally sets out to ask. But the appearance of the term cis seems to have resulted in this academic field ceasing to carry out its primary task, namely questioning gender roles. What is actually being communicated with the word cis, is that the majority of people *fit into their gender role*. Both Margaret Mead and Judith Butler have been done away with in one fell swoop. Gender is no longer a conflict, a power structure, nor something which is continuously being renegotiated. Suddenly, gender roles have become static, natural and eternal. As the publically funded Youth Centre writes:

> If you are happy in your gender and do not want to change it, this is called being cisgender. If you feel that something is not right or that

---

29 'Kunskap om genus'. Nationella sekretariatet för genusforskning (Swedish Secretariat for Gender Research). <https://www.genus.se/ord/cis/>.

you're not happy in the gender others say you are, this is known as being transgender.³⁰

Not only are most people said to fit into their gender role, they are also said to be happy in it! Based on this definition, one might well wonder whether any cis-people exist at all. Logically, most people must fall outside these criteria and the Youth Centre goes on to advise that if "something" does not feel right, then "gender affirming care exists, which involves changing the body through for example surgery or hormone treatment." So there are two options: be happy and feel comfortable in your gender or have surgery. Freeing oneself from gender roles, creating one's own self, or finding feminism are not included as alternatives. The message to young people is that those who do not fit into these restrictive norms should alter their body as soon as "something" does not feel right.

Most definitions of cis-persons include the words "happy/content" and "comfortable with." Matilda Åkerlund of Umeå University writes that a cis-person is "content with the sex they were born into."³¹ Thus, if most people are cis-gender and if being cis-gender means being content in one's gender role, the implication is that gender roles are not contentious for 99% of people.

From Wollstonecraft to de Beauvoir, feminist thinkers' main task has been to highlight the exact opposite of this contention, demonstrating how gender roles are *not* a neat fit for people. As Gerda and Åsa Christenson argue in their essay "Cis är inte feministisk analys" (Cis is not a feminist analysis):

> Being feminist is to question established gender norms and restrictive expressions of gender. It is *not* experiencing gender expression as linear nor believing that one's gender identity has 'always' been linked to or must be linked to gender norms. Most feminists view gender primarily as a social construct. The idea of cis – of the gender linear person – is one which feminism has been fighting against since time immemorial. A feminist analysis would therefore also never conflate cis with a privilege:

---

30 <https://www.umo.se/jag/sexuell-laggning-och-konsidentitet/trans-och-cis/>.
31 Mathilda Åkerlund. (28 August 2018). 'Representations of trans people in Swedish newspapers'. *Journalism Studies*. <https://www.tandfonline.com/doi/full/10.1080/1461670X.2018.1513816>.

feminism views the gender linear as a construct and form of confinement which it strives to destroy.[32]

Responding to Christenson and Christenson's article, trans activist Lukas Romson writes that "their lack of awareness of their privileged position as cis women is in very poor taste" and they should not be opining on the matter in the first place: "Let's make this clear once and for all, how individual trans people, the trans movement and trans feminism defines terms is not something cis people should comment on. Period."[33] In another response, trans author Maria Ramnehill writes that Christenson and Christenson are "unknowledgeable," "have never had to give particular thought to what it's like being a trans person and yet they write articles about it" and that "they do not have a patent on feminism."[34]

Yet Christenson and Christenson were not analysing trans people and their experiences, but the term cis – a term that purports to define women like them. Both Romson and Ramnehill's comments imply that 'cis-women' should not be allowed to discuss the word cis. Thus, women are to be defined by others, should not have an opinion on this definition and, although they are women born as women, they have no right to comment on the matter. We have reached a stage in which merely holding an opinion about oneself is seen as an unwarranted incursion into the territory of the trans issue. The term cis is primarily used as the opposite of trans – those who are not trans are cis. As noted by Elizabeth Hungerford, the pair is even more binary than the man/woman pair:

> Occasionally, a person might describe themselves as neither cisgender nor transgender, but you absolutely cannot be both. That wouldn't make any sense. Cis and trans are opposites, mutually exclusive categories. Like man and woman, cis and trans constitute a binary. Cis/trans is the new gender binary.[35]

---

32 Gerda Christenson and Åsa Christenson. (17 June 2014). 'Cis är inte feministisk analys'. *Feministiskt Perspektiv*.
33 Lukas Romson. (25 June 2014). 'Cispersoner kan inte definiera transkamp'. *Feministiskt Perspektiv*.
34 Maria Ramnehill. (20 June 2014). 'För nyanslöst för en progressiv feministisk rörelse'. *Feministiskt Perspektiv*.
35 Elizabeth Hungerford. (2016). 'Female erasure, reverse sexism, and the cisgender theory of privilege'. In Ruth Barrett. (ed). *Female Erasure: What You Need to Know About Gender Politics' War on Women, the Female Sex and Human Rights*, p. 39. California: Tidal Time Publishing.

The word also has an additional characteristic: it is first and foremost used to refer to women: 'cis-gender woman' results in 268,000 listings on Google, while 'cis-gender man' results in 189,000. The term further implies that a woman must be referred to as what she is *not*, i.e. born a man. Cis thus entails a new definition of woman in which she is once again defined in relation to man. The word woman already comes from old English "wife of man" meaning an exception to the rule; now, in addition, she is *the type of woman who was not born a man*. She is relegated to a subcategory of her own category.

The cis-woman, we are told, is a woman who is satisfied with her gender role. She is content and has never given the matter much thought. Above all, she is privileged, for if there is any word that crops up most often in connection with cis-woman, it is the word privilege. She is lucky because she was born a woman and continues to be one. And since she is so lucky, she ought to be permanently apologetic about it and learn that both she and her sex must stay out of the limelight.

Woman – the oppressed sex with a right to say no – has swiftly been argued away from public discourse and replaced with the cis-woman – an individual said to be in a position of privilege who must grovel and apologise. And man, are people apologising! Successful women are standing in line to humbly explain how privileged they are to have been born women. US politician Alexandria Ocasio-Cortez says in an interview: "I'm a cisgender woman. You know, I will never know the trauma of feeling like I'm not born in the right body, and that is a privilege that I have."[36] In the fashion magazine *Elle*, women are informed that it is privileged and spoilt to fight for women's rights since a group exists which is much more oppressed:

> Where cis women can choose to push and challenge gender stereotypes, transgender women, men and non-binary people have to oppose them in order to live as their true selves. Trans people, and especially trans women, routinely die for exercising the freedoms cis feminists are working to attain.[37]

---

36   *The Intercept* Podcast. (29 January 2019). 'Alexandria Ocasio-Cortez on her first weeks in congress'.
37   Sady Doyle. (20 January 2018). 'It's trans remembrance day, and it's way past time cis women show up for trans rights'. *Elle*.

Being a woman has suddenly become akin to being a billionaire, and standing up for women's rights has become equated with siding with the powerful. One gets the impression women never suffer from domestic violence, never get discriminated against in the workplace, never die from men's violence or childbirth, whereas men who transition "routinely" die all the time, and that this is somehow women's fault for daring to challenge gender stereotypes. Articles like these are drenched in guilt-tripping which is absent from articles directed at men. Men's magazines do not carry reports of what life is like for trans men, nor are their readers admonished to put their own needs to the side for the sake of their brothers who happened to be born women. Nor do they contain pieces on how men ought to support trans women. Yet the essence of texts aimed at women is that it is selfish to fight for their rights and especially selfish to 'challenge gender stereotypes'.

US trans activist Sam Dylan Finch lists 130+ "unearned advantages" that cis-people benefit from.[38] These include being spared questions on how one has intercourse, being able to move around freely without being stared at, receiving competent health care, not being discriminated against in the workplace, not being bombarded with articles about how people of their gender are murdered, being allowed to wear clothes and uniforms which align with one's gender, not being sexually objectified and potential partners knowing what their genitals look like and what to call them.

Sound familiar? Finch has just described what most women go through on a daily basis. Receiving poorer health care due to one's sex, being groped, subjected to sexual violence and inappropriate, probing questions, reading articles about how women are killed by their partners because they are women – this is unfortunately well-known territory for us women. The text thus turns the very harassment and injustices the women's movement fought against into *undeserved privileges*. We should feel pleased that we are allowed to dress in alignment with our gender, despite us having done nothing to deserve it. We should be thankful that we are permitted to wear high heels and veils, since these 'align' with our gender. If we follow this analysis to its logical conclusion, even a girl who is genitally mutilated at nine and married off at 12 is a cis-person and

---

38 Sam Dylan Finch. (29 February 2016). '130+ examples of cis privilege in all areas of life for you to reflect on and address'. <https://everydayfeminism.com/2016/02/130-examples-cis-privilege/>.

thereby privileged – her sexual partners know what they are to call her genitalia: cunt! Similarly, a homosexual man in Saudi Arabia or Uganda would, according to this interpretation, be considered 'normal, natural and healthy' – and privileged:

> [...] cissexual privilege is the idea that cissexuals inherit the right to call themselves female or male by virtue of being born into that particular sex. In other words, cissexuals view their gender entitlement as a birthright.[39]

The new political figure known as the cis-woman really only has one task: to come in second place. This is a task that all cis-women must approach with the utmost seriousness and they must understand that not even feminism is for them. In an article in the magazine *Brand*, the literary critic Anna Remnets refers to trans women as "the most vulnerable women." Women who do not understand this, she goes on to say, harbour an "intolerant and exclusionary view of the most vulnerable in patriarchy: trans women." They peddle "conspiracy theories claiming that trans women are men" and if they cannot see this then "feminism is not going to liberate anyone but white ciswomen."[40]

The epithet 'white' is routinely bandied about when cis-women are being defined. Its purpose is to justify the idea that women belong to an elite. Yet what it is actually saying is that women, by definition, are white and that no other women exist. In response to this kind of justification, the user Fleshphobe writes on Tumblr:

> Black women aren't your prop for arguing that males are a part of the lesbian community. We're just as female as any other ethnicity of woman and having dark skin is in no way comparable to having a fucking dick ...[41]

Attempts to narrow the referents of the term woman – which refers to half the world's population – to a politically obsolete elite consisting only of privileged, ignorant, upper-class white women are often made by those who belong to this group themselves, so-called 'white cis-women'. This can seem odd – are they not pulling the rug out from under their own feet? On the other hand, it may be a smart move, in that a seemingly self-critical

---

39 Julia Serano. (2007). *Whipping Girl: A Transsexual Woman on Sexism and the Scapegoating of Femininity*, p. 168. New York: Seal Press.
40 Anna Remnets. (2018). 'Hur radikal är radikalfeminismen?'. *Brand*, No 1.
41 <tumblr.com/fleshphobe> (post deleted).

attitude allows them to secure their position, symbolically distancing themselves from their identity. Striking first, they anticipate the critique that could be directed toward them, by being the harshest critics of their own circumstances. Thus they are no longer 'the white cis-woman' but 'the critic of white cis-women'.

That the subject of feminism is women has until recently been as irrefutable as it is that the subject of socialism is the worker. Both are movements which arose to address the specific situation of a particular group. This fact does not exclude other groups from being able to support the cause, nor that the group's interests have not overlapped with those of other groups. It also does not mean that feminist-minded transitioned men would not have a great deal to contribute when their goals and those of feminism are shared. What is being argued now is that women ought to realise that they are not the protagonists of their own movement. Since "trans women are often economically the most vulnerable" and "merely insinuating that ciswomen are worse off and that they somehow own the position of being subjected to patriarchy's violence and oppression is prejudiced and divorced from reality," writes author and former spokesperson of the Swedish Green Party's youth group Alexander Alvina Chamberland.[42]

It is interesting to note that to be subjected to oppression is here referred to as some kind of knighting ceremony. To be oppressed is to "own a position of being subjected to violence" as if the impact of violence itself was secondary to the political legitimacy arising from claiming a position of oppressed. It is also striking how many of the terms – cis-privilege, cis-normativity, cis-sexism – are lifted straight out of feminism's terminology, and now aimed at feminism itself. Instead of sexism, we we are now supposed to say cis-sexism. This neologism, explains literary critic Sam Holmqvist, means that "normative genders are seen as more legitimate than non-normative ones."[43] Yet if 'cis' is the norm, is 'trans' not then a way of adapting to this norm? Isn't 'trans' an attempt to become 'cis'? Is it not precisely the gender linearity – the alignment of body and soul – which gender reassignment surgery and hormones strives toward? Does this not mean that it is, in reality, the person who remains in their

---

42 <https://www.facebook.com/alexalvinachamberland/>.
43 Sam Holmqvist. (2016). 'Att skriva transhistoria. Cisnormativitet och historiens könsöverskridare'. *Tidskrift för genusvetenskap*, Vol. 37, No. 4.

biological sex but refuses to conform to the gender role assigned to that sex who is the true gender bender? Isn't he who refuses to be gender congruent and doesn't care about matching sex with gender the real champion of diversity? These questions present a significant conundrum for advocates of gender identity theory: how to simultaneously conform *and* retain the position of outsider? Iwo Nord, Signe Bremer and Erika Alm build on Susan Stryker's texts and argue:

> Stryker anchors her theory in the bodily experience of trans sexuality yet her point is not that the trans sexual body which undergoes surgery and/or hormone treatment should in itself be an expression of cisnormativity. What she claims is that, despite the medical profession's normalising aims, the body that is reshaped through medical interventions is "something more, and something other than the creatures our makers intended us to be." In other words, Stryker emphasises the constitutional instability of the subject while simultaneously writing out the bodily inscription as intersubjective, an act which enables subversion.[44]

These nonsensical linguistic acrobatics are designed to ensure that the adjective 'subversive' must not be applied to cis-women, since they can never become "something more." Thus, trans women are women, but they are also "more" than that. To actually perform acts of subversion is secondary to inhabiting a position of "the subversive" which implies discursive power in academia and online debates, enabling one to start a sentence with the words "As a … (insert oppressed group) I believe …"

Moreover, the cis/trans axis has come to replace the sex-based power hierarchy of man/woman as an analytical tool in several contexts. A clear example of this can be seen in an interview with actor and director Andrea Edwards, who produced a play based on Valerie Solanas' *SCUM Manifesto*, which she staged in 2011 with Erik Holmström. The play divided the audience into sections based on sex – men had to sit on one side of the theatre, women on the other. When the men entered, the women were already seated, applauding ironically to demonstrate how men are used to being praised. Women sat on golden cushions and were offered sweets and grapes. Men were addressed in condescending tones, told they had "monkey brains" and that their sex constituted an error of evolution. The ensuing debate was harsh. Several male critics felt the play incited violence

---

44 Iwo Nord, Signe Bremer and Erika Alm. (2016). 'Cisnormativitet och feminism'. *Tidskrift för genusvetenskap*, Vol. 37, No. 4.

and were particularly critical of the division of the audience by sex. Police officers in civilian clothing had to be present since the actors had received death threats.[45] There was a clear gender gap in the play's reception: male reviewers criticised it, females appreciated it. In *Brand* magazine, Andrea Edwards said:

> I really want to emphasise that the hatred and threats were directed exclusively at the women involved in the project. If the hatred had been about the staging of *SCUM Manifesto* as such, then Erik would have been subjected to the same, if not more aggressive, attacks. This isn't about hatred of feminism but about hatred of women.[46]

The hatred was thus not directed at feminism as a concept but at women as a sex. The ensuing reactions also proved the play's point that sex matters. Seven years later, Edwards is asked if she would stage the play again. She says she would, but adds:

> But if I'm honest, I'm also a bit frightened, because the performance is problematic in that it's very cisnormative: there's seating for men on one side and women on the other. In the end, we managed to solve this when we staged it by collaborating with a trans organisation that helped us modify the ticket purchasing system – but the annoying fact remains that there are only two galleries in the theatre.[47]

Edwards is here assuming that the existence of trans people precludes a feminist analysis of patriarchy. Now let's reflect on this: does the presence of a few individuals who have transitioned, overthrow patriarchy's central tenet, the oppression of women by men? Exceptions to rules have always existed and a practical solution can be found. The division of the audience could be done according to sex or gender – a point could be made whichever one is chosen – but one would still be able to retain the original separation between men and women. What gender identity theory increasingly demands, however, is use of the exception as a lever to

---

45 Sabinah Gustavsson. (2014). 'En scum affär. En grundläggande retorisk analys av recensioner som behandlar Turteaterns uppsättning av SCUM manifestet'. Unpublished essay. Litteraturvetenskapliga institutionen. Uppsala universitet.

46 Eva-Maria Benavente Dahlin. (2012). 'Det handlar om kvinnohat, inte om feministhat'. *Brand*, No. 2.

47 Rebecka Bohlin. (10 December 2018). 'Jag är sugen på att sätta upp Scum-manifestet igen'. *Dagens ETC*.

overthrow the entire rule, making it impossible to separate men and women. And in the end, the play was never put on again.

The trans issue is repeatedly used as a pretext to stop discussing sex and power. Suddenly, it is "sensitive" to speak about men and women. But is it a new thing, or is it the same old misogynist sentiment returning in a new guise? Disagreement about the division of the audience into men and women is exactly the same complaint that incensed male viewers seven years earlier when the same play was performed, but what was then considered *reactionary* is now seen as *progressive*. The content of the criticism is almost identical: exposing the relationship between sex and power is controversial and dangerous.

On the face of it, it may seem that the problem lies in discussing biology, since "we must not be limited by our biology." Such assertions appear appealing: we are more than just our bodies, biology is not destiny and so forth. Yet if we cannot talk of biology, we cannot mention the word trans either, since what is seldom mentioned is that the category 'biological sex' is in fact a prerequisite for the terms trans and cis. Any mention of the words 'trans' and 'cis' is referring to biological sex. The basis of the dichotomy is precisely the relationship to one's own biological sex. Those who remain in the sex they were born in are now known as 'cis', while those who want to 'cross over' to the other sex are known as 'trans'. When defining cis, the Swedish Secretariat for Gender Research writes without hesitation that those born with a vagina are women, just as Mathilda Åkerlund writes unambiguously about being "born in a specific sex." Thus, the proverbial bathwater is brought flooding back just as quickly as it was washed down the drain and what is now considered 'problematic' is not talk of biology but an analysis of power based on sex.

This is an example of the asymmetry of gender identity theory. As long as one employs the dichotomy cis/trans, one is permitted to use biological sex as a common denominator. Yet if exactly the same dichotomy is used to advance an analysis of men and women in patriarchy, the thought police are summoned. Trans author Julia Serano, who coined the term cis-person with others, writes in the book *Whipping Girl* that it is time to cleanse language of words like "biological woman," since Serano claims there is no difference between biological women and trans women: "as someone who has had estrogen in her system for five years now, shouldn't I be considered a 'biological' woman?"[48] Yet at the same time, the book is filled with references to "cis-women" and the privileges they enjoy, cis-women who don't understand how lucky they are to not have to apply layer upon layer of foundation to cover their stubble,[49] cis-women who laugh disparagingly at men's fear of wearing pink,[50] and ungrateful cis-women who try to play the victim:

> When I look into trans women's eyes, I see a profound appreciation for how fucking empowering it can be to be female, an appreciation that seems lost on many cissexual women who sadly take their female identities and anatomies for granted, or who perpetually seek to cast themselves as victims rather than instigators. [51]

Serano applies a double standard which has become one of the key features of gender identity theory: on the one hand, biological women do not exist as an oppressed group; on the other, when speaking of a privileged group, they suddenly do exist. Yet if one is being consistent, the word woman is not more exclusive than the words trans, cis or man, as they are all based on exactly the same biological division. 'Women' and 'cis-women' are one and the same, namely those born with XX-chromosomes. Gender identity theory is lifted straight from feminism, it is just that the concepts have swapped places: woman/man is substituted with trans/cis. Trans woman are, according to this theory, in the position previously occupied by women, while women now inhabit the position of men and are thereby redefined as perpetrators.

Banning of the concept of biological sex has turned out only to apply to the category 'woman'. When 'trans' and 'cis' are to be defined, the biological dichotomy between sexes resurfaces and reigns unfettered – *now* it must no longer be questioned. It is no longer fluid and shifting but fixed. A biological woman cannot decide to call herself a trans woman: to be one, she must have been born a man. She is dispatched to the category cis-woman and becomes privileged as a consequence. Unless of course she decides to change sex and become a trans man – in which case she will be considered privileged because she is a man. In this new gender structure,

---

48   Serano. (2007). p. 173.
49   Ibid. p. 302.
50   Ibid. p. 287.
51   Ibid. p. 380.

no platform exists from which women can speak without being labelled privileged.

In 2018, the Scottish parliament decided to replace the term 'biological woman' with 'cis-woman,'[52] thus keeping the same division but in a different form. The category *woman* is expanded to include men and the word woman in the sense of the *political subject of feminism* now also comprises men and women. It has become taboo to say 'woman' if one means only biological women, yet there is now a different word to refer to this group, one with the obligatory prefix 'cis', which equals privilege. Thus, according to gender identity theory, it is only possible to speak of the group biological women as a *privileged group*. At the drop of a hat, women as an oppressed group have been reinvented as privileged and the definition of the most oppressed has become … those born with a penis!

---

52 <https://www.heraldscotland.com/news/17438641.iain-macwhirter-get-over-it-cis-women-are-just-on-the-wrong-side-of-history/>.

CHAPTER 29

Gender Self-Identification

Most Swedish readers will not have heard of memo 2018:17. But Spaniards will not have been able to avoid hearing about 'Ley Trans', and all Canadians know what Bill C-16 is. These are all law proposals which seek to decouple medical gender reassignment from legal sex, enabling individuals to change the sex in their passport and other ID documents through an online application. Argentina, Norway and some states in Australia have already implemented similar laws. The Swedish proposal states that anyone who is 16 years or older should be able to change their legal sex without having to provide a reason (in an earlier proposal the age limit was 12).[53] Changing sex will thus become as easy as changing your address – all you have to do is inform the state which sex – or rather which gender – you feel you belong to.

The purpose of the new laws is allegedly to facilitate procedures for trans people. In Spain, the proposal was accompanied by the slogan 'Despatologización Ya!' – stop medicalisation now. The Spanish government's view is that it should not be necessary to alter one's body in any way in order to live as a member of a different gender; treatment and medical certificates would no longer be necessary steps in changing the sex on your passport. Passports in particular are often named as an obstacle for trans people who are trying to pass as their new gender, since these can lead to questions and stares at airports. The Swedish law proposal

---

53 Socialdepartementet. Regeringskansliet (Government Offices of Sweden). (29 July 2022). 'Förbättrade möjligheter att ändra kön', p. 95.

concerns "an individual's right to define their gender," but it is specifically directed at trans people, a fact made clear when its authors state the law is for "people who feel their gender identity is not in alignment with the gender recorded in the national register."

Yet the outcome of these laws in reality is the exact opposite of their stated purpose – they open the door for everyone who is *not* a trans person to change their legal sex. Presumably, few if any trans people would want no contact whatsoever with health care services while still wanting to change the gender on their ID documents. What would be the point? What man would want a passport that says 'woman' when he does not resemble a woman in the slightest? Would this not merely lead to even greater problems at airports? Legal sex is usually the last thing a trans person changes, only after undergoing social and medical transition. There may be individuals who are satisfied taking hormones without undergoing genital surgery, but this is already possible today since laws in Sweden, Spain and other countries allow change of legal sex for those who have only just begun hormone treatment.

What we are witnessing now is something much more wide-ranging, namely the *codification of gender identity theory into law*. These are proposals of historic magnitude, much more so than their authors seem to comprehend. Gender will become an identity in its own right, completely unconnected to the body. No longer a material, biological fact, nor an innate identity or a social construct dependent on how others view a person, gender would become entirely a personal matter: everyone is free to choose which gender they belong to.

Yet in reality, gender is *not* a matter of personal choice. It is primarily a social structure affecting others as well as the individual. Statistics, sports, changing rooms, prisons, strip search regulations, refuges, anti-discrimination measures, quotas and medical research are all examples of areas with sex-based divisions. If any man is allowed to change his sex merely because he feels like it, it is not difficult to see how this would lead to problems for women. A man who changes his legal sex to female in the absence of any contact with health care services is still a man physically and in terms of appearance.

The consequences of these laws have received no recognition in Sweden. Scarcely any debate has taken place regarding the proposal; even feminist groups and leftist political organisations seem to view the matter as a non-issue and nothing to quibble about. During work on the proposal, which has been carried out in collaboration with the police and several trans-rights organisations, not a single women's rights organisation was consulted. The impact assessment merely briefly states:

> The proposal is not deemed to have any consequences on local authorities' decision-making powers, public services, the ability to reach integration policy targets nor on equality between women and men.[54]

The situation is different in Great Britain, Canada and Spain, where the feminist movement has mobilised. In Great Britain, a number of feminist organisations have been set up expressly to combat the legal changes. These include Woman's Place UK, Declaration on Women's Sex-Based Rights and Fair Play for Women. Due to this massive resistance, gender-self ID was not introduced in the reform of the Gender Recognition Act in 2020.[55] In Canada, Meghan Murphy from the feminist magazine *Feminist Current* held public meetings and wrote articles opposing Bill C-16, yet the bill was approved. In Spain, the organisation Contra el Borrado de las Mujeres (Against the Erasure of Women) was set up by the country's most eminent feminists, lawyer Paula Fraga and philosopher Alicia Miyares. In their manifesto, they write:

> Sex is the basis for the discrimination and violence which we women are subjected to. Eliminating the category of sex and replacing it with gender self-identification is a misogynistic act. Abolishing sex as a legal category nullifies all actions against structural inequality.[56]

One may be in favour of women-only spaces including trans women, but these laws and proposals go far beyond such inclusion and are about something altogether different. They allow entry to all women-only spaces to men who are *not* trans women. It thereby becomes every man's right to decide whether he wants to be a woman. Every Tom, Dick and Harry can register himself as a woman and gain entry to women's prisons, refuges, all-female shortlists, and changing rooms.

One could argue that nobody would do this – that it is an exaggeration worthy of conspiracy theorists to think that men's interest in gaining access to women-only spaces would stretch to such drastic actions and that, if it did occur, it would be limited to a very small number of individuals.

---

54 Ibid. p. 140.
55 <https://commonslibrary.parliament.uk/research-briefings/cbp-9079/>.
56 <https://contraelborradodelasmujeres.org/contexto/>.

CHAPTER 30

A Room of One's Own

The law on gender self-identification in Norway came into force on 1 July 2016. That month, a student, Birgitte, entered the changing room at Sis Sports Centre in the city of Stavanger and saw a naked man with a penis in the showers. She asked whether he had got the wrong changing room and received the reply that he was a woman and had a female ID number. Birgitte went to the front desk to inquire and was informed that men were indeed not allowed entry to the women's changing room.

Six months later, in February 2017, Birgitte saw the same penis in the women's changing room. When she asked the person what he was doing there, she received the following reply: "What the hell is your problem? It's none of your fucking business!"[57] By this time, the sports centre had changed its policy to allow everyone legally registered as female to use the women's changing room. The fact that the man had a fully intact male body made no difference. Following this episode, Birgitte began getting changed in the toilets. She told me that several other women started showering at home.

This was not the end of the story. The man reported Birgitte to the Equality and Anti-Discrimination Ombudsman, claiming that her questioning his right to be in the women's changing room amounted to harassment. He stated he "felt deeply offended at her insinuation that he was not a woman." He further claimed that he was significantly more likely

---

57 Diskrimineringsnemnda (Anti-Discrsimination Tribunal). Sak (Case No.) 68/2018.

than women to be subjected to male violence and therefore had a greater right to protection in the form of using the women's changing room.

The fact that the man had changed his legal sex to female also meant he received free legal assistance from JURK (legal counselling for women) in his case against Birgitte. The organisation was established in 1972 by the women's movement to provide support for women who experienced for instance male sexual violence, but its new policy extends support to "anyone who defines themselves as a woman." The man, who was now called Sandra, therefore qualified.

The Norwegian law on gender identity discrimination specifies trans people as a particularly vulnerable group, since they challenge traditional notions of gender. The law states: "harassment based on gender identity and gender expression encompasses an individual's sense of their own gender, i.e. that which is not immediately visible to others."[58] Thus, a person can be harassed due to an invisible characteristic, without the harasser being aware of this characteristic. Returning to Birgitte's experience, her objection to the individual's presence in the changing room would not, according to the new Norwegian law, be an objection based on his very visible sex. It would be discrimination based on gender identity because the man sees himself as a woman, a fact that was not visible. Thus the difference between him breaking the law and her breaking the law, lies in how he perceives himself – a fact she can neither see nor change.

The case was followed closely by the media. The Students' Union at the University of Stavanger declared they supported Sandra "fully, due to her raising an important debate of principle" and hoped for a finding against Birgitte.[59] The penis bearer also received support from trans activists who celebrated him as a role model and "one of many who have recently begun claiming their place in public spaces," according to an article in *Stavanger Aftenblad*, which concluded with the words: "Where should Sandra shower? Wherever she wants to."[60]

The Equality and Anti-Discrimination Ombudsman found that Birgitte had discriminated against the penis bearer on grounds of gender

---

58 Ibid.
59 Facebook post. (4 March 2017). Studentorganisasjonen StOr at University of Stavanger.
60 Karoline Skarstein. (29 March 2017). 'Sandra er mitt forbilde, og jeg ble rørt da Studentorganisasjonen gikk ut og støttet henne'. *Stavanger Aftenblad*.

identity/gender expression. Given that she was aware from their first meeting that he identified as a woman, she ought to have understood that questioning this could "upset" him. The Equality and Anti-Discrimination Tribunal reached a different decision, with a three to two majority in Birgitte's favour, citing an "unclear legal situation" and the fact that Birgitte had reason to believe individuals with a penis were not to use the women's changing room due to her initial conversation with front desk staff.

Another case which has become famous world wide is the Brazilian wax affair. In Canada, 16 women who work doing Brazilian waxes on women were sued in the Human Rights Tribunal when they refused to wax a scrotum. The women were all small business owners with immigrant backgrounds, mainly from East Asia, and several of them worked from home. The scrotum in question was that of Jonathan Yaniv, who had recently changed his name to Jessica Yaniv and who had previously been reported to the police for asking 14-year-olds to send him photos of their used tampons.[61] Yaniv sued the salons one after the other for significant amounts for gender identity discrimination. Since his legal sex is female, he argued, the beauty therapists were obliged to wax his scrotum. In vain, the women countered that they were not trained in the techniques required to wax a scrotum and that Yaniv could approach salons which did offer the so-called manzilian wax. Yaniv has thus far been unsuccessful in his request for damages but his lawsuits have led to several of the female business owners going bankrupt.[62]

When Canadian feminist Meghan Murphy tweeted about the case, writing "men are not women" and using the pronoun "he" to refer to Yaniv, she was permanently banned from Twitter. Twitter maintains that trans people are a protected category and that "misgendering or deadnaming of transgender individuals" is an infringement of their conduct policy. Paradoxically, anyone can call themselves trans, which entails membership of this protected category and leading to everything one has done using one's previous name becoming unmentionable.

Many assume that the above cases are exceptions and are not to be taken seriously. Granted, it is highly unlikely that women's changing

---

61 <https://thepostmillennial.com/exclusive-15-year-old-alleged-victim-of-jessica-yaniv-speaks-out>.
62 Helen Joyce. (25 July 2019). 'A Canadian human rights spectacle exposes the risks of unfettered gender self-ID'. *Quillette.com*.

rooms will be filled with hordes of men who have changed their legal sex just to mess with others. However, creating concrete opportunities for people to take action and then claim that no one will take this action is odd to say the least. Laws must take into account the fact that people's actions are unpredictable and assess risks. The second major issue is that finding ways to enter women's spaces is precisely what sex offenders and abusers do. If there is anyone who is going to take advantage of this possibility, it is them. Who else would want to register as a woman without wanting to be one? There is a reason we have created women-only spaces and if anyone regardless of their sex can claim entry to these simply by virtue of saying they are a woman, this makes a complete mockery of the protection such spaces offer.

Another argument that is often floated around says it is no big deal for a woman to see a naked man every once in a while and that sex-specific changing rooms are unnecessary. One may well subscribe to this opinion, yet there are enough women who, for cultural, personal and experiential reasons would under no circumstances want to be naked in a changing room with unfamiliar naked men (no matter how they identify), to make this argument irrelevant. The mere risk of this happening is sufficient for a significant number of women to cease feeling at liberty to use changing rooms, regardless of what others think about gender self-identification. Therefore, it is very clear that legal changes of this type will lead to women's access to public spaces being severely restricted. As British commentator Stephanie Davies-Arai puts it: "In the name of inclusion, girls are being excluded from their own facilities."[63]

In Canada, Bill C-16 has already resulted in problems at homeless shelters. One case involved a homeless woman fleeing sexual violence having to share a room with a "bearded, hairy man who talked about sex" and who did not seem to be a trans woman at all. When the resident relayed her concerns to staff, telling them she did not want to sleep in the same room with a person who she clearly felt was a man, she was informed "she was discriminating," since the person's legal sex was registered as female. The homeless woman had to move out and sleep on friends' sofas.[64]

---

63   Quoted on <https://twitter.com/Agnes_KB/status/1191270323649499136>.
64   Joseph Brean. (2 August 2018). 'Forced to share a room with transgender woman in Toronto shelter, sex abuse victim files human rights complaint'. *National Post*.

Cases like these are particularly serious because women in homeless shelters are often fleeing extremely violent men. In one Canadian case that ran for 25 years, the country's oldest rape crisis center, Vancouver Rape Relief and Women's Shelter, lost its public funding in 2019 for not hiring a biological man as a rape counsellor. The man, who identified as a woman, argued that he had the right to work at the service, while the shelter argued it was important for women who had been raped to receive counselling from someone *they* considered to be a woman.[65]

A growing number of women's shelters around the world have adopted policies which define the word woman as all those who identify as women. It is formulated as a matter of inclusion, openness and 'welcoming all sisters'. Often, these assertions are accompanied by deceptive questions like "Who's welcome in feminist spaces? Who's excluded?" followed by the explanation that trans people are the most likely to be victims of violence and therefore in most need of protection.

The fact that trans people are at risk of violence is well-documented. However, what is seldom mentioned is that the type of violence differs. When women are victims of violence, it is overwhelmingly in the context of a relationship, while trans people are significantly more likely to be victims of hate crimes by unknown perpetrators. The Swedish Public Health Agency's 2015 report on trans people's health states: "When it comes to violence, the perpetrator was in most cases unknown to the victim and the violence occurred in a public place."[66]

As a result, the type of support required often differs radically. Yet rather than investigating the specific type of support trans people need, the solution called for is for women's shelters to change their definition of sex. As Swedish women's shelter employee Lea Honorine notes, exclusionary policies have in practice never existed, since women's shelters operate on a principle of never asking for ID numbers or registering service users due to safety. Therefore, if a trans woman who passes as a woman requests a space at a shelter, no questions are asked. Cases even exist of homosexual men fleeing violence being supported by women's shelters.

---

65 Camille Baines. (21 March 2019). 'Trans woman hopes funding cut will send message to Vancouver rape crisis group'. *The Canadian Press*.
66 Folkhälsomyndigheten. (2015).'Hälsan och hälsans bestämningsfaktorer för transpersoner'.

Viewed from a practical perspective – there are both women and trans people who require protection from men – practical solutions exist which address both groups' needs without restricting either groups' rights. LGBTQ organisations could, for instance, invest in creating nation-wide shelters for trans people which are specialised in providing the specific type of support required. What is happening as a result of gender self-identification laws is something completely different and is circumscribing women's spaces.

The ideological battle regarding sex and gender is also being played out in women's prisons. Being incarcerated, the women concerned are by definition not offered a choice in the matter and are not asked their opinion. In December 2019, the Swedish murderer Kristoffer Johansson was moved to a women's prison (Hinseberg), following his change of legal sex to female. Johansson was sentenced to ten years' imprisonment for murdering and dismembering his Thai ex-girlfriend, 20-year-old Vatchareeya Bangsuan. The Prison and Probation Service's report contains no deliberation on the safety of female inmates, stating only that the applicant cited "special circumstances" and that Hinseberg prison "offers suitable activities and security."[67] This despite Hinseberg being a category-2 prison (equivalent to category C in the UK) with a significantly higher proportion of communal spaces, while the men's prison Johansson was previously held in was a maximum security category-1 institution (equivalent to category-A in the UK). No category-1 women's prisons exist in Sweden.

Media reports stated Johansson's sex-change treatment consisted only of an oestrogen plaster and testosterone blockers.[68] Scandal ensued after he was transferred to the women's prison, where his behaviour generally contravened the rules. He wrote pronographic novels about the staff, made threats of violence and of harming and killing the prison rabbits.[69] (Women's prisons in Sweden often host pets for the children of inmates to play with on visits.) Following his release, Johansson has dedicated himself

---

67   Kriminalvården (Swedish Prison and Probation Service). (4 November 2019). Beslut placering (Placement decision). No. 2018/457.
68   Kim Malmgren. (21 September 2018). 'Kim Johansson styckade sitt ex – korrigerar sitt kön i fängelset'. *Expressen*.
69   Johan Ronge. (1 January 2020). 'Raseri i kvinnofängelset: Hotade honom till livet'. *Expressen*.

to threatening feminists on the internet. On his Instagram account, he is seen posing with weapons, displaying drawings of sawn-off body parts and calling himself a Terf-hunter. He contacts feminists who have been critical of him or of trans activism, threatening them and their partners with statements like "it's not so smart of them considering what I was convicted of."[70]

In Sweden, there are currently three men who have murdered women or girls who have applied to change their sex to female. Ulf Olsson, who murdered ten-year old Helén Nilsson after abusing, raping and starving her over several days, claimed in 2005 that he felt he was a woman and was reported to have taken hormones.[71] Another man who stabbed his parents to death in January 2020 had changed sex from male to female one year prior to the crime. The headlines in all media read: "Woman convicted of double murder in Hjo."[72]

In the wake of Johansson's success, several other men convicted of abuse of women have begun applying for transfer to women's prisons. One such case is that of B, a 62-year-old man sentenced for violence toward his girlfriend.[73] With the help of his lawyer, Silas Aliki, an active participant in the trans debate, B has applied to be transferred to a women's prison despite not changing his legal sex nor undergoing any form of gender reassignment treatment whatsoever. The application states that B "has identified as female since childhood but was only able to and dared seek help for this years later" and that incarceration in a men's prison entailed "a risk that she be subjected to threats or violence." Moreover, B does not intend to undergo any treatment for male perpetrators of violence against women since he does not consider himself to be a man. B's current placement also "does not enable her to attend any intimate partner violence programs since the institution only offers programmes aimed at men who commit intimate partner violence." In the end, B's application was rejected because he had not changed his legal sex. He reported not having begun the process since it "can take several years." Should the

---

70 <https://kuriren.nu/bli-prenumerant/artikel/grm3gp1j>.
71 Per Lindelöw and Lars Palmborg. (31 March 2005). 'Helén-mannen på väg att bli kvinna'. *Expressen*.
72 <https://www.svt.se/nyheter/lokalt/vast/kvinna-begars-haktad-for-dubbelmord-i-hjo>.
73 Förvaltningsrätten (Administrative Court) in Göteborg. (2 May 2019). Dom (Sentence) 12186–18.

Swedish proposal mentioned earlier become law, B will be able to change legal sex and transfer to a women's prison without any difficulties.

Hundreds of similar scenarios have occurred over recent years in Great Britain, Ireland, the USA, Canada and Australia. With self-identification now being the only requirement for changing one's legal sex, and legal registration as female being the only requirement to gain entry to a women's prison as an inmate, applications have come flooding in. Among those who have been granted transfer are Canadian Adam Laboucan (convicted of assaulting infants), Matthew Harks (who has assaulted more than 60 girls), and British Karen White (who attacked female inmates following transfer to a women's prison and had to be relocated to a men's facility).[74] Meanwhile, 170 inmates in Colorado's men's prisons have submitted a joint application to women's prisons.[75]

In 2015, the British Association of Gender Identity Specialists authored a letter addressing the massive increase in male sex offenders applying for gender reassignment treatments with the express purpose of being transferred to women's prisons. Physicians who interviewed the prisoners were of the opinion that far from all had a genuine feeling of being born in the wrong gender and that it had become standard practice to accept these applications, a situation which "oblige[s] medical practitioners to advance a plan the basis of which is the facilitation of subsequent sexual assault."[76] It is becoming less common for an application to even be required: in October 2020, the state of California introduced a law allowing inmates to specify whether they wished to serve their sentence in a women's or men's prison, according to their self-identified gender.[77]

If the price for pretending to be a trans person was previously much too high for most people who lacked serious intentions – you had to pay with your penis – nowadays it is sufficient to see oneself as a woman. This could be considered a very low price to pay indeed for gaining access to

---

74 April Halley. (12 October 2019). 'Male-bodied rapists are being imprisoned with women. Why do so few people care?' *Quillette.com*.

75 Jamiyla Chisholm. (11 December 2019). '170 incarcerated transgender women sue Colorado corrections for discrimination'. *Colorlines*.

76 Dr James Barrett President, British Association of Gender Identity Specialists. (20 August 2015). Written evidence submitted by British Association of Gender Identity Specialists to the Transgender Equality Inquiry, p. 6.

77 Jonathan McDougle. (7 October 2020). 'California to house transgender inmates based on gender identity'. *CBS News*.

a setting of women who lack liberty to move around freely. Cases even exist of sex offenders being granted early release once they have changed gender, since their new, lower testosterone levels are presumed to decrease the risk of reoffending.[78] To date, there are no known cases of a trans man having applied for transfer to a men's prison.

---

78   Jimmy McCloskey. (17 January 2020). 'Pedophile who molested baby freed from jail after transitioning to become a woman'. *Metro UK*.

CHAPTER 31

Unspeakable Violence

In December 2018, several Swedish media outlets carried reports of a woman being prosecuted for grievous crimes related to child pornography. She is alleged to have had in her possession 13,656 indecent images and videos of children being raped: the crime was judged "grievous" due to the particularly young age of the children and the especially callous way in which they had been exploited, according to the summons. The prosecutor was interviewed commenting on how unusual it was for a woman to commit this type of crime.[79] Comments immediately began appearing on various internet fora, saying things like: that shows you women are no better than men etc. Some male commentators expressed excitement and curiosity about the woman and wanted to find her.

Now, the individual was in fact a man, and was even registered as a man at the time the crime was committed. He changed his legal sex to female in August 2017, according to national records, while the crime was committed on 10 July 2016.[80] What appeared to be a woman was in fact a man, a far-right sympathiser and with a career in the armed forces to boot.[81] Three months later, the man was placed on probation but was referred to as a woman throughout by the media. The fact he had been a man was only highlighted on one Russian sensationalist news site.

---

79 <https://www.norran.se/nyheter/blaljus/tusentals-barnpornografiska-bilder/>.
80 See Luleå tingsrätt (District Court). Case No. B 121–17.
81 <https://www.forsvarsmakten.se/sv/aktuellt/2016/06/stolt-soldat-i-lulea-pride/>.

When I decided to investigate the matter, the Tax Agency was initially unwilling to provide confirmation of the change in the person's ID number, declining to respond to my queries on the grounds that the matter was 'sensitive'. After three calls, I obtained confirmation that he had been assigned a female ID number one year earlier. Yet when I wanted to write a piece for the newspaper *Metro* on the story, I was told I could not refer to the prosecuted as a 'man' and had to use 'person' instead. I did not accept this and the piece was cancelled. 'Man' was thus the controversial word – not the crime or describing the person who had committed it but the act of calling him a man. Had this man been sentenced to prison, the number of women convicted of child pornography crimes would have increased by five per cent. Crime, and in particular sexual offences, are highly gendered phenomena: men commit 98 per cent of sexual offences according to Brå (The Swedish National Council for Crime Prevention),[82] making crimes of this nature very much a male domain. The same is true for violence in general: 90.4 per cent of murders and 79 per cent of assaults are committed by men.[83]

Our naming of the world around us matters. Being able to call men's violence against women *men's* violence against *women*, and not 'domestic violence', 'family violence', 'initimate partner violence' or the French 'crime passionel' has been a long, persistent battle for the women's movement. Revealing power relations and who does what to whom has not been easy. Without a doubt, the word man is the most controversial in this context. The same word which in general language is so neutral and universal, becomes incredibly charged in the context of criminal acts against women and children. As we well know, the classic headline reporting a rape does not read 'Man suspected of rape' but 'Alleged rape of woman'.

What is going on here is that as soon as a man decides he is a woman, our ability to name him vanishes into thin air. He undertakes a kind of linguistic exiting from patriarchal existence and becomes the victim rather than the perpetrator. Feminism's entire terminological apparatus is thus sidelined. Regardless of whether he has committed the archetypal male

---

82 <https://www.bra.se/statistik/statistik-utifran-brottstyper/valdtakt-och-sexualbrott.html>.
83 <https://sahlgrenska.gu.se/forskning/aktuellt/nyhet/stora-skillnader-mellan-kvinnor-och-man-som-begar-dodligt-vald.cid1377316 och https://www.bra.se/statistik/statistik-utifran-brottstyper/vald-och-misshandel>.

sexual offence – murder and dismemberment, indecent exposure, use of child pornography – we are not permitted to consider him a man.

With just one simple act, namely uttering the words "I am a woman," a sex offender can hit the switch and turn off the entire feminist analysis. Not only does he cease to be a man in discourse, he becomes the woman of all women, the most oppressed among the oppressed.

There are few other acts that allow a criminal to be completely acquitted and simultaneously to metamorphose from the accused to the accuser. Suddenly, the perpetrator becomes a victim who requires protection from both men, who will abuse him, and women, who will terf him – and liberal feminists fall over themselves rushing to his defence. The gender change even applies retroactively, meaning that the crimes a man committed when his legal sex was male will be referred to as crimes committed by a woman if he transitions in the future. Interestingly, his successes are not subject to corresponding treatment: the medals Caitlin Jenner won as Bruce have not been taken back with the explanation that it was 'actually' a woman who competed in the men's category.

Thus, male violence is gender washed and labelled as female. When an intellectual is permanently banned from Twitter because she referred to a male perpetrator as 'he', when articles are cancelled because they call a male perpetrator of crime 'he' and when public sector employees are fired for referring to perpetrators as 'he', what exactly is this about? It is about the establishment of a new hegemony in which we are *not permitted to talk about men's violence*.

The Spanish far-right and anti-feminist party Vox, whose roots lie in fascism, are among those who have realised this and applaud it. Following the launch of the Ley Trans bill by Spain's Minister for Equality Irene Montero, a proposal which would entail men's violence against women being redefined based on gender self-identification, Vox spokesperson Macarena Olona tweeted: "I would never have thought that Irene Montero's feminism would be our best ally. Violence knows no gender. We are now taking the first steps toward abolishing sexist laws!"[84]

---

84 <https://twitter.com/macarena_olona/status/1326098944888287233>.

CHAPTER 32

Every Man's Right

While we have been focusing on the foreground, something remarkable is taking place in the background: gender roles have suddenly lost their meaning. One of the premises of gender identity theory, as we have seen, is that gender identity is innate. Thus, a loving boy who likes playing with dolls is, according to this theory, definitely a girl. Now the same individuals who argued this, claim that a man who mutilates women, rapes them and ejaculates on them is without a doubt a woman if he says so. Suddenly, there is no longer anything male or female – suggesting otherwise is merely prejudice and both sexes are equally violent. As we saw in the previous chapter, the courts and media are now obliged to refer to a career soldier who downloads large amounts of brutal child pornography as a woman merely because he said he was.

Gender identity theory has undergone yet another metamorphosis. In its initial stages, it was all about gender spectra, tolerance and diversity. In the next stage, the words 'brain', 'genes', 'foetal stage' and 'innate' were the order of the day. A woman is a person who is empathetic, likes skirts and displays an interest in social issues, we were told. Yet when the theory begins its passage toward making legal changes, these fixed points vanish. The word 'woman' is now a free for all which men can lay claim to without having to care about any roles at all: a woman is what *he* says it is. His words, regardless of whether he is a convicted sex offender behind bars, now supplant all theories. At once, the previously rigid system reverts to plasticity. This constitutes the deep ideology of gender identity theory.

Gender identity theory can thus be described as consisting of three layers, where each new layer erases the previous one. The outermost layer is a veneer of tolerance, celebrating diversity and everyone's right to be themselves. This layer is peeled back to reveal a rigid thinking about gender norms in which only baby blue and baby pink exist and the only choice is to conform, if necessary through medical interventions. In this second layer, no tolerance exists for femininity in boys and a terrible end is said to befall those who fail to adapt to gender norms: death. It is said this is set in stone, has been so since time immemorial, and transcends history and culture. Yet no sooner have we resigned ourselves to this state of affairs, than another layer is uncovered overthrowing the diktats of the previous one. Now there is no sign of biology as far as the eye can see and every man who claims he is a woman is one, regardless of his appearance or behaviour. Thus, with one single utterance, he can turn the tables and claim to be the victim of gender discrimination all the while continuing to be a man physically. It is notable that this is the only category of discrimination which can be invisible and depend entirely on the individual's own feelings.

Thus, when the new laws are to be explained and justified, we are told gender identity is a biological fact, but when they are to be implemented and applied, gender identity has all but disappeared and in its place we find that a man's words are law.

The same duality is evident in the writing of many gender identity theory proponents – the work of author and trans activist Julia Serano is one example. Serano claims to have a "female soul" and has argued for the existence of a "female essence." One might thus reasonably assume Serano believes in the existence of something female. Yet when it comes to questions of female-only spaces, all talk of essence disappears:

> Indeed, some of the most common arguments used to deny trans women the right to participate in women-only spaces also happen to be the most antifeminist. For example, many argue that trans women should be barred from women's spaces because we supposedly still have "male energy." But by suggesting that trans women possess some mystical "male energy" as a result of having been born and raised male, these women are essentially making the case that men have abilities and aptitudes that women are not capable of. Another popular excuse for our exclusion is the fact that some trans women have male genitals (as many of us cannot afford or choose not to have sex reassignment surgery). This "penis" argument not only

objectifies trans women by reducing us to our genitals, but propagates the male myth that men's power and domination somehow arise from the phallus.[85]

Hence, the argument is that a penis does *not* a man make. Nor does "energy" make a person male or female. Now the claim is that men do not have any special characteristics and essence no longer exists. (Here, however, Serano mistakenly assumes that when women speak of "male energy" they are referring to positive attributes like talents and capabilities and not, for instance, to arrogance.) Serano thus deconstructs the very same gender previously constructed and demonstrates in the process how gender identity theorists jump at will between different layers of their theory. Sometimes there is an essence to femaleness – a soul, a set level of oestrogen – yet when women are to define what a woman is, this argument no longer applies. Is there something female, or isn't there? It seems, only when it can be used to define trans women as women, but when women want their separate spaces, then "female" does not exist. The exact same arguments Serano uses to argue the existence of a female essence are not valid when women want to use them to exclude men.

All gender identities are not for the taking, however. The woman who wants to call herself trans woman soon realises this is not allowed: men can be women, but women cannot be trans women. The various women who have tried to do this online, have met with replies such as "calling yourself a trans woman is appropriating an experience you do not have" and "inaccurate and frankly rude."[86] Woman is apparently for everyone – trans woman only for men. Men who, just a second ago, denied being men at all and claimed to be women the exact same way a woman was.

And so we hit a wall: man's sovereign right. Sex has become his possession: it is what he says it is.

---

85 Julia Serano. (2007). p. 239.
86 <https://forum.emptyclosets.com/index.php?threads/does-anyone-identify-as-an-afab-transwoman.420822/>

CHAPTER 33

Invisible Trans Men

Does every woman, then, have the same right? Can she become a man if she so wishes? Can she choose to sit out her sentence in a men's prison, use men's changing rooms, receive men's salaries and in practice be accepted as a man? Interestingly, the entire debate has centred around men's right to enter women's spaces, while few women have shown interest in gaining access to spaces reserved for men. Hardly any literature exists on the situation of trans men and nobody is demonstrating for their right of access to anywhere. Studies of trans people in prisons abound – each and every one of them concern trans women. I have found one article about trans men in prison in an academic journal and it is about why there are no studies of trans men in prisons.[87]

In the US, where the debate around gender segregated bathrooms rages, trans men have hardly been mentioned. It is generally assumed that, if trans women are to use female toilets, then trans men should use male toilets. The lack of coverage may be something to do with the fact that, as trans man Jackson Bird writes in a rare article on the subject, it is difficult for a person with a vagina to pee in a urinal.[88] Devices do exist for the purpose but, as Bird writes, those that are realistic enough to be used in public do not always function properly and result in a pair of

---

87 Elias Lawliet. (2016). 'Criminal erasure. Interactions between transgender men and the American criminal justice system'. *Aleph, UCLA Undergraduate Research Journal for the Humanities and Social Sciences*, Vol. 13.
88 Jackson Bird. (24 September 2019). 'A trans guy on adjusting to men's bathroom culture'.

wet trousers. Thus the trans man is left with the lone booth in the men's bathroom, about which Bird writes, "I spend so much of my time outside occupied restroom stalls that I've considered penning an essay series entitled, 'Waiting for the Cis Men to Stop Pooping: The Life and Times of a Trans Man'."

And yet, the considerable dilemma that trans men experience in the men's toilets has not resulted in any demands for the removal of urinals. The same is true for trans men in men's changing rooms: I have not succeeded in finding anyone who has lodged a complaint nor found any anecdotal evidence from upset males who have suddenly come across a naked person with a vagina parading around a men's changing room. Accounts about these spaces relate exclusively to trans men's fear of being outed as women and thereby risk being subjected to sexual harassment. A trans man often passes with her upper body but her lower body still retains female genitalia and therefore "undresses under a towel, so as not to expose his genitalia to other users of the changing room," as performance artist Jason Barker has described.[89]

Almost all the headlines regarding 'the first trans person' are about a trans woman. During the 2010s, trans people were selected for political office in several US states: Kansas, Vermont, Arkansas, Delaware, as well as in other countries including the Philippines, France, New Zealand, Australia, Romania, Belgium, Brazil, Venezuela, Uruguay, Peru, Portugal, Poland and Italy. They were all trans women.

As a rule, trans women's entry into politics is described as a milestone in the battle for justice. From a women's rights perspective however, it is difficult to see it as anything other than the same deck with the cards shuffled around, since trans men are conspicuous by their absence in the world's parliaments. It appears to be even harder for a woman to enter politics as a man than it is as a woman.

While trans women reap success after success in the world of sport, there are few examples of trans men succeeding in men's sport. Occasionally, one reads about a female athlete who has changed sex, but since she is no longer permitted to compete in the female category having taken testosterone, she usually disappears from the world of sport as soon

---

89 Catherine McNamara. (2010). 'Using men's changing rooms when you haven't got a penis. The constitutive potential of performing transgendered masculinities'. Central School of Speech and Drama.

as she becomes a he. Occasionally, she might make an attempt to compete in the male category but seldom reaches the podium. As a female athlete, she was already overshadowed by men's sport, as a trans man she loses even this place in the shadows.

While trans women often achieve greater success in the public arena as women than they enjoyed as men, the opposite seems to be true for trans men. For a man, gender reassignment can mean he goes from being a mediocre athlete to breaking world records in the women's category; from playing a minor part in a reality TV show to being Woman of the Year, from a regular teen to the constituency women's officer for the Labour Party as happened in the UK.[90] For women on the other hand, gender reassignment rarely leads to career advancement. A trans man may get headlines if 'he' becomes pregnant, if 'he's' the face of a tampon advertisement or stars in a porn film – the three most common headlines containing the word transman. If he becomes a trans activist, he must settle for playing second fiddle to trans women's cause, just as lesbians had to stand aside for gay men. Sometimes, it is even the very same individuals we are talking about, having been lesbians in the '90s gay movement and trans men in the 2010s trans movement – still in second place.

Trans men also find it significantly more difficult to participate in dating on the gay scene: a mere 12 per cent of homosexual men report being open to dating a trans man, while 29 per cent of lesbian women state they are open to dating a trans woman, according to one US study.[91]

Overall, silence persists when it comes to trans men. It is almost as though they do not exist. They are still treated as women – that is, belittled and rendered invisible – yet they do not officially belong to the group 'women' anymore and are therefore excluded from the category of woman as a political subject, along with the movement for her liberation, namely feminism.

For all that is said about male privilege, trans men do not seem to get any of it. The only thing conceded to them are the pronouns; other than that, males do not share power, spaces, brotherhood, prizes or political offices with them. They are not allowed to really be men, which leaves us

---

90   Lucy Bannerman. (20 November 2017). 'Trans teenager Lily Madigan voted in as a Labour women's officer'. *The Times*.
91   M. J. Murphy. (5 February 2020). 'Why (some) gay men won't date transmen', *Medium.com*.

with the following equation: men can be women, but women cannot be men, men can be men, but women cannot be women (only cis women), men can be trans women, but women cannot be trans women. Men can be everything, women nothing.

CHAPTER 34

Open Female Spaces, Closed Male Spaces

In an essay on the UK left-wing publisher Verso's blog, philosophers Lorna Finlayson, Katharine Jenkins and Rosie Worsdale write about gender self-identification laws in Great Britain. They begin by stating that several feminists have opposed the proposals, on the grounds that they risk exposing women to men's violence in prisons, for example. They go on to question this concern:

> Although we do have overwhelming evidence that men commit violence against women at much higher rates than women commit violence against either women or men, this evidence does not establish that the basis of this heightened risk is, as critics of self-ID claim, male biology and/or male socialisation.[92]

The writers hypothesise that identity itself could be the deciding factor, that is, the feeling of being a man could be the reason behind men's violence. Thus, perhaps if a man no longer identifies as a man, he is not as dangerous as he would otherwise be? Yet in the next breath, they observe, "We don't pretend to know for sure, though. We don't think that this is something that anybody knows." And therefore, they conclude, it is not possible to claim that women need separate spaces either, for example in prisons.

---

92 Lorna Finlayson, Katharine Jenkins and Rosie Worsdale. (17 October 2018). "'I'm not transphobic, but …'". A feminist case against the feminist case against trans inclusivity'. *Verso Books* blog.

As it happens, it is incorrect to say that this is something that nobody knows. On the contrary, the largest statistical review ever compiled on the topic (the Swedish 2011 long-term study) shows that men who transitioned committed crime at significantly higher rates than women, a finding which led the study's authors to conclude that trans women "retain a male blue-print when it comes to offending. The same was true for violent crime."[93] It is therefore *not* the case that men who transition automatically stop being violent. Moreover, this fact is likely to be true to an even higher degree for men who undergo no treatment whatsoever but merely self-identify as women. Yet these philosophers appear to adopt 'we do not know' as a stance of principle, seeming to argue that we should not be interested in knowing, since this is a matter which we ought to know nothing about.

Predictably, this intellectual shrugging of the shoulders is superseded by a sudden clarity when the authors discuss whether trans women and men who identify as women ought to be allowed entry to men's spaces. Now, these people's safety is without a doubt in danger:

> The well-established vulnerability of trans women to violence at the hands of cis men means that requiring trans women to have to use spaces designated for men jeopardises not only their comfort but also their safety. As we have seen, the proposal to instigate 'third spaces' is less of a proposal than a way of washing one's hands of the issue. Even if such spaces could be created, their use would 'out' people as trans, which is still a highly stigmatised identity.[94]

Suddenly, the philosophical discussion about what makes men dangerous is absent: now they are without question extremely dangerous and no trans woman should have to be in the same room as a man. The authors imply that a perpetrator of violent crime who is a biological man can, by identifying as a woman, renounce his violent tendencies. Yet, if it were this easy to do so, why is it not possible for all men to just do it?

The model these philosophers are advocating is in fact a two-room model: a closed male space and an open female space. This model is just as binary as the previous one, however more asymmetrical. The male space

---

93 Cecilia Dhejne et al. (22 February 2011). 'Long-term follow-up of transsexual persons undergoing sex reassignment surgery. Cohort study in Sweden'. <https://doi.org/10.1371/journal.pone.0016885 2011>.
94 Lorna Finlayson, et al. Ibid.

is constructed as homogenous, monolithic, exclusionary and violent. The women's space is for the leftovers – women, trans people, non-binary people – and is required to be inclusive yet not in need of protection. This model also neatly summarises gender identity theory: the male name, male sport, male spaces, all are retained intact while female spaces are opened up.

At least the previous model, based on biological sex, was symmetric: no one could gain access to the other's space. Moreover, it did not take account of stereotypes: regardless of dress, appearance or how people identified, biological sex was what counted. The new model allows male space to be preserved intact and even strengthens the surrounding walls, since *no men who dress like women, no feminine men and no men who deviate from gender stereotypes belong there.*

An example of this model is the Catalonian parliament building, where the toilet signs have been changed. One is for women, trans people, wheelchair users, children and, astonishingly, menstrual cups. The other is for men.[95] The room that used to belong to women is now an open category, an assembly point for all the leftover non-men and otherwise deviant minorities. The men's room remains exclusively male, for the ruling elite only – no others are allowed entry to it, not even wheelchair users.

How are the borders of this male space policed? The answer is implicit in Finlayson, Jenkins and Worsdale's article: with threats of violence. Trans women should not be in men's spaces as this could prove dangerous. Why do the authors not question this (presumed) violence?

The shocking answer is that no one in this debate does so. No contributors problematise this intact male space for the simple reason that its threats of violence are naturalised. Men fight and rape anything feminine – that is just how things are and there is no need to challenge the status quo. Yet the fact that women, for the same reason, might find it unpleasant to be naked in a room with people they consider to be men – well, *that* is just prejudiced and must be challenged vociferously! Tolerance is not required of men, only of women, since women's spaces cannot threaten violence. The staggering truth is that what implicitly dictates the boundaries of men's spaces is the law of violence. Violence is used to create and maintain

---

95 Photo taken by Catalan member of parliament Ángeles Álvarez. <https://twitter.com/AAlvarezAlvarez/status/1335483900236353536>.

this boundary, calling out: do not enter! The room's towel-clad occupants need not even do the threatening themselves – philosophers, lawmakers and authorities are more than happy to oblige. And thus, the new gender model's structure is created: closed male spaces, open female spaces.

It is not the term 'man' which is being fragmented, questioned, substituted with non-woman, mxn or m*n. Gender identity theory only entails questioning the category 'woman', along with an implicit affirmation of man as a category. Since women gained formal equality in the west, male territory is policed through violence and informal structures while that of women is policed through rules. It is not possible to access male power structures or be accepted as a man by men in their changing rooms by appealing to any *rule*: it is men themselves who must accept outsiders into their space. A woman cannot say: I am a man now, let me be prime minister! Or: I may have a vagina but I am nevertheless a man so don't rape me! Neither of these are definitions of man which men are expected to adhere to.

Where does this leave women? In the mentioned philosophers' text, three categories emerge: the perpetrator of violence (man), the one requiring protection (trans woman), and the one who does not perpetrate violence but does not require protection either (woman). The trans man is not mentioned at all. What, then, does the opening up of the category 'woman' mean for women's status? It means that a woman remains a woman no matter what she is called: *her* being and room for manoeuvre is not expanded. In the trans economy, she will be ignored and trampled upon whatever gender she identifies with.

The issue of nudity in changing rooms illustrates this point. The arch patriarchal and highly illogical rule regarding nudity tells us: men want to see naked women, women do not want to see naked men; men want to show their naked body to women, women do not want to be naked in front of men. The age-old male practice of indecent exposure has been revived on the internet where millions of men shamelessly send images of their genitals to women they have never met and enjoy the idea that women are looking at their penis. When she sees his penis, patriarchal logic dictates, he has power over her. Yet this power also manifests when *he* sees *her* naked, for a man who sees a woman naked is able to ruin her life. He can, in certain cultures, wreck her chances of marriage and he can publicly ridicule her so that she is beset by a horrific shame. He can spread her images at school, to her colleagues and parents and bring her to the verge of suicide. A woman, on the other hand, has no power over a man she sees naked: the only meagre vengeance she could possibly mete out is to spread the rumour that he has a micropenis.

Opening women's changing rooms to anyone who wishes to call themselves a woman changes absolutely nothing in this power dynamic. In the meeting between the post-postmodern patriarchy and traditional patriarchy, women are left in the firing line with only themselves to rely on to resolve their predicament.

This is deep patriarchy returning, right through the three layers of gender identity theory, carrying the same basic contradictions as any patriarchy. All patriarchal systems subscribe to a set of moral norms. These can be: men should be breadwinners, women should be stay-at-home mums; men should behave like gentlemen, women should not put out; men should be strong and not cry and so forth. Many mistakenly believe that these rules *are* patriarchal, but the moral rules themselves do not necessarily constitute oppression – had they really been applied. Differing roles are not in and of themselves a sign of oppression. What actually characterises patriarchal systems is the fact that men are free to break the rules, while women are punished both when they comply and when they resist. For instance, a rule might state that extra-marital sex is wrong, and then only punish women who have sex outside marriage. Another might stipulate that adultery is against the will of God, only for the betrayed wife to be told forgiveness is the highest virtue. A moral rule might require a man to provide for his family, but the same community looks on in tacit approval when he impregnates women and flees the scene without any consequences. An oft-cited so-called gender role is that men should supposedly be strong and not cry, and yet the man who "dares to show his feelings" goes viral and receives applause. The core of patriarchal ideology, as with all exercise of power, is not the rules but the double standard.

This is precisely the structure we see returning in gender identity theory. On the surface, it creates new norms for men and women, yet in reality, only men are granted freedom to truly act. The end result is that both sexes become the sole property of man.

CHAPTER 35

"The End of Women's Sport as We Know It"

Even if we do believe in male and female souls, and a soul independent from the body, there is one sector in which bodies matter: sport. In this arena, biological sex plays a decisive role. Participation in all sports, with the exception of horseriding and chess, is divided according to sex. Certain sports are even segregated by age, height (fitness competitions) and weight (boxing, rowing).

Yet the new definition of woman has reached the world of sport as well, leading to fundamental changes in the rules of women's sports. Before the Rio Olympics, the IOC (International Olympic Committee) released new guidelines stating that, to be eligible to compete in the female category, a man had only to identify as female and show that his hormone levels had been ten nanomoles/litre for at least one year, regardless of the sport. Previously, genital surgery had also been required, but this is no longer the case. After the Tokyo Olympics in 2021, the IOC rules were changed once again. Now there is no longer a hormone level limit for participating in the female category – "until evidence determines otherwise, athletes should not be deemed to have an unfair or disproportionate competitive advantage due to their sex variations, physical appearance and/or transgender status."[96]

---

96 International Olympic Committee. (16 November 2021). 'IOC Framework on Fairness, Inclusion and Non-Discrimination on the Basis of Gender Identity and Sex Variations'.

The Swedish Gymnastics Federation now allows all athletes to self-select their category up to the junior level (13 to 18-year olds) of the Swedish championships.[97] Seventeen US states allow adult males to compete in the female category as long as they identify as women.[98] The rules vary for other sports associations: the American NCAA (National Collegiate Athletic Association) requires only that hormone treatment to lower blood testosterone has continued for one year, without stipulating a maximum amount of testosterone allowed at the time of competing. The same is true for the marathon association WSER (Western States Endurance Race). This organisation allows all athletes to compete in the female category with the caveat that, should a person born male achieve tenth place or higher, proof of hormone treatment for the period of one year is required.[99]

What was remarkable about the IOC's previous rules was that they appeared to be completely arbitrary and not based on any research. Permitted levels of testosterone were set at ten nanomoles/litre for all sports, without consideration of the fact that men have greater advantages in some sports compared to others. Moreover, the level itself was very high: men's testosterone levels are normally around 30 nanomoles/litre while women's are around two nanomoles/litre.[100] Genetics professor Eric Vilain, who assisted in the writing of these rules, explained that the level was set high because it would otherwise have been impossible for males to compete in the female category:

> It is not about making everybody biologically equal, and I think that is a common misconception when we start talking about transgender athletes [...] People want transgender [females] to be physiologically identical to [born] females, and if they're not, it's unfair. That is not possible. [...]

---

97 Ellen Hellmark. (30 November 2020). 'Gymnaster får välja tävlingsklass oavsett juridiskt kön'. *SVT (Sveriges Television)*. <https://www.svt.se/sport/gymnastik/gymnaster-far-valja-tavlingsklass-oavsett-juridiskt-kon>.
98 Martina Navratilova. (26 June 2019). 'The trans women athletic dispute with Martina Navratilova'. *BBC* Documentary.
99 Stephanie Case. (9 May 2019). 'Western States Has New Rules for Transgender Athletes', *Outside Online*.
100 Stephane Bermon, David J. Handelsman, and Angelica L. Hirschberg. (October 2018). 'Circulating testosterone as the hormonal basis of sex differences in athletic performance', *Endocrine Reviews*, Vol. 39. No. 5, pp. 803–829.

> The goal is to create a pathway to include the transgender athlete, not create total equality.[101]

During the Tokyo Olympics, transgender inclusion in women's sports was a big debate, as a New Zealand weightlifter Laurel Hubbard participated in the +87kg woman's weightlifting competition. Hubbard competed in the male category under the name Gavin Hubbard ten years earlier, and had not been particularly successful, but in 2017 he set a new world record in women's weightlifting (in the clean and jerk category), lifting a whole 19 kilos more than the silver medalist. Despite Hubbard failing all three lifts in Tokyo, many voiced concern about the future of female sport. Belgian weightlifter Anna Vanbellinghen, also in the +87 category, protested that "the whole thing feels like a bad joke" and that it was unfair to females.[102]

The IOC admitted the need for revision, yet when the new rules came, any formal barrier to males competing in female sports had been removed. Instead of stricter rules, the IOC issued ten principles aimed at promoting inclusion. From now on, the main aim is to protect the "vulnerabilities of transgender people and people with sex variations." Gender identity is not a reason for exclusion from any sports category. This means that, athletes do not have to undergo any medical transition, nor are gynaecological examinations or any other type of "invasive physical examinations" allowed.[103] Should an athlete have unfair advantages, this argument must be brought and proven after the event rather than before competition. The IOC does not state that sex, specifically and in and of itself, is an unfair advantage, which could lead to females being excluded from competing in their own category, but not males. The new framework was developed "following an extensive consultation with athletes and stakeholders concerned" – yet when i emailed the IOC Press Office to ask for a list of those consulted, i receive the reply that "We cannot disclose names as the consultation was done on the basis of confidentiality of those who took

---

101 Fred Dreier. (18 October 2018). 'Commentary: The complicated case of transgender cyclist Dr. Rachel McKinnon'. *VeloNews*.
102 Brian Oliver. (30 May 2021). 'Exclusive: Rival weightlifter speaks out on transgender Hubbard's presence at Tokyo 2020'. *Inside the Games*.
103 International Olympic Committee. (16 November 2021). 'IOC Framework on Fairness, Inclusion and Non-Discrimination on the Basis of Gender Identity and Sex Variations'.

part."[104] We thus do not know what the criteria were for being on the IOC's list of stakeholders, nor what expertise the framework is relying on. What we do know is that 250 anonymous individuals have decided that being female is no longer a criteria for competing in female sports.

The new era has, predictably, meant that several men are achieving success in women's sport. A new world record in women's track cycling was set at the 2018 World Championships by gender studies professor Rachel McKinnon, who was born male. The erstwhile record holder Sarah Caravella-Fader withdrew before the race to protest the inequality of McKinnon being permitted to compete in the female category, while the bronze medalist Jennifer Wagner-Assali complained after the competition.[105] American swimmer William Thomas competed for three years on the men's team and was ranked 462 as a male swimmer, but after being allowed to join the women's team under the name Lia, shot up to number one in the NCAA (National Collegiate Athletic Association) 500-yard freestyle race.[106] Commenting on the female swimmers' parents' protests, Thomas says that "trans people don't transition for athletics. We transition to be happy and authentic and our true selves." Somewhat contradictory, Thomas also states in the same breath that his ultimate goal is reaching the Olympics.

In May 2019, construction worker Mary Gregory, who had come out as trans two years earlier, broke four world records in women's weightlifting in one day. When it was noticed during drug tests that Gregory had a penis, the athlete responded that this was of secondary importance since he is

---

104 "Dear Kajsa, Thanks for getting in touch. We cannot disclose names as the consultation was done on the basis of confidentiality of those who took part. Some even signed a confidentiality document. Only the persons involved can disclose. This is done to protect the athletes who took part. Best, The Media Relations Team International Olympic Committee." Email from IOC Press Office, 9 September 2022.
105 Fred Dreier. (18 October 2018). 'Commentary: The complicated case of transgender cyclist Dr. Rachel McKinnon'. *VeloNews* and Leah Simpson. (20 October 2018). 'It's definitely NOT fair: American cyclist lashes out after losing world championship to a trans woman.' *Mail Online.* <https://www.dailymail.co.uk/news/article-6296975/American-cyclist-lashes-losing-world-championship-trans-woman-wont-accept-apology.html>.
106 Katie Barnes. (18 March 2022). "Amid protests, Penn swimmer Lia Thomas becomes first known transgender athlete to win Division I national championship". *ESPN.*

"like any other woman. 100 per cent female. I get my hair styled female. Ears pierced, nails painted."[107] Following massive protests, Gregory was later stripped of the records.

In strength sports, what is mainly at stake is world records, but when it comes to aggressive contact sports, the risks are a great deal more serious. When MMA (Mixed Martial Arts) fighter Tammika Brents competed against ex-marine Fallon Fox who had changed gender eight years earlier, Brents not only lost the match – she also sustained concussion and a broken skull bone before the referee called time.[108] In an interview afterwards, Brents said:

> I've fought a lot of women and have never felt the strength that I felt in a fight as I did that night. I can't answer whether it's because she was born a man or not, because I'm not a doctor. I can only say, I've never felt so overpowered ever in my life and I am an abnormally strong female in my own right. Her grip was different, I could usually move around in the clinch against other females but couldn't move at all in Fox's clinch.[109]

Upon discovering McKinnon's world record in track cycling, tennis player Martina Navratilova spontaneously tweeted: "You can't just proclaim yourself a female and be able to compete against women!" As a result, she was hit with a barrage of hate. Navratilova says she reacted to this by considering whether there was something wrong with her, whether she could have phrased her remarks differently, and tweeted: "I am sorry if I said anything anywhere near transphobic – certainly I meant no harm – I will educate myself better on this issue but meantime I will be quiet about it. Thank you."[110] This is Martina Navratilova talking, winner of 18 Grand Slams, world number one for 332 consecutive weeks, openly lesbian since 1981 and campaigner for homosexual rights for 30 years. However, having studied the matter and reflected on it, she wrote an article for the *Sunday*

---

107 Dawn Ennis. (7 June 2019). 'Trans powerlifter smashes records and draws backlash'. *Outsports*.
108 *BJJ World*. (21 October 2018). 'Transgender MMA fighter breaks skull of her female opponent. Are we becoming too careful not to offend any group of people?' <https://bjj-world.com/transgender-mma-fighter-fallon-fox-breaks-skull-of-her-female-opponent/>.
109 Alan Murphy. (17 September 2014). 'Exclusive: Fallon Fox' latest opponent opens up to #WhoaTV'. whoatv.com.
110 <https://twitter.com/Martina/status/1075921080991256581>.

Times in which she stated that "If anything, my views have strengthened." She writes that decreasing hormone levels is insufficient:

> A man builds up muscle and bone density, as well as a greater number of oxygen-carrying red blood cells, from childhood. Training increases the discrepancy. Indeed, if a male were to change gender in such a way as to eliminate any accumulated advantage, he would have to begin hormone treatment before puberty. [111]

Navratilova was widely supported, but in certain circles her name has been dragged through the mud. From one day to the next, she was thrown out of the LGBTQ group she helped found, Athlete Ally, which made the following statement: "trans women are women, period. They did not decide their gender identity any more than someone decides to be gay, or to have blue eyes. There is no evidence at all that the average trans woman is any bigger, stronger, or faster than the average cisgender woman."[112] A swathe of articles condemned Navratilova, and the contempt and condescension that oozes from these articles towards one of our era's greatest tennis stars makes one wonder whether women's sport is still just a charity case. In an article typifying this tone, Isabelle Bartter, web designer and socialist who was known as Allan Bartter a few years earlier, writes in the *Socialist Worker*:

> I play Ultimate Frisbee. I fell in love with this sport in 2003 when I was a freshman in high school. I left all other sports for it. I didn't apply to a single college or university that didn't have an Ultimate team. [...] I've left my blood on the field. I've left my tears on the field. I've left everything I had left in me on the field. I have been injured, and I have been healed by Ultimate. I have always tried to live up to the spirit of the game, but I'll be the first to admit that I haven't always been a gracious winner or a humble loser. I hope I have been both more often than not, but I have certainly grown up in Ultimate. It is my home. It's my community. My history is

---

[111] Martina Navratilova. (17 February 2019). 'The rules on trans athletes reward cheats and punish the innocent'. *The Sunday Times*.

[112] Joanna Hoffman. (19 February 2019). 'Athlete Ally: Navratilova's Statements Transphobic and Counter to our Work, Vision and Values'. *Athlete Ally*. < https://www.athleteally.org/navratilovas-statements-transphobic-counter-to-our-work-vision/>.

why reading comments like those made by Martina Navratilova are so hurtful to me as a trans woman athlete.[113]

The article is certainly clear on two points: Bartter is extremely keen on frisbee and on the word 'I'. What is unclear however, is why this implies that female athletes do not have the right to compete on an equal footing, nor how all this relates to socialist workers.

The same double standard is applied here as in the discussions concerning male and female spaces: if proponents of gender identity are quick to argue the differences between 'male' and 'female' in the brain when it comes to a passion for the colour pink, this conviction is turned on its head when sport is concerned. Suddenly, there are no differences between men and women. England's FA (Football Association) considers it a myth that men are taller and stronger than women, since "women come in all shapes and sizes."[114]

RFSL (The Swedish Federation for Lesbian, Gay, Bisexual, Transgender, Queer and Intersex Rights) employs the same argument to advocate for abolishing sex-segregation in sports, saying it is a myth that men are better at sports than women:

> The underlying assumption that those who were assigned the sex 'male' have an unfair advantage compared to those assigned the sex 'female' has been dismissed by several researchers. Despite evidence of overlaps between women's and men's sporting achievements, and knowledge that differences within the male group are often greater than differences between the sexes, it seems the idea that men are better at sports dies hard. One explanation for this is that assumptions regarding binary gender and male superiority are rarely challenged – in fact they are sooner reinforced – in the highly gender segregated business that is sport.[115]

The 2017 public inquiry 'Transpersoner i Sverige' (Trans people in Sweden) addresses the issue of sport and is in favour of abolishing sex-based categories in sports, at least for young people because "no research exists which supports the view that trans women or trans men benefit from

---

113 Isabelle Bartter. (12 March 2019). 'Trans athletes won't be sidelined by bigotry'. *Socialist Worker*.
114 The Football Association. (March 2016). 'A guide to including trans people in football', p. 28.
115 Mathilda Piehl, Aleksa Lundberg, Jonah Nylund, Eva Linghede, Moa Hansson and Dorna Behdadi. (October 2020). 'Trans och idrott. Ingen ska lämnas utanför'. *RFSL*.

advantages in athletics *at any stage of transition*" (my italics).[116] "At any stage of transition" means prior to beginning treatment, when gender identity is merely an idea. This would mean that there are no physical differences between men and women at all – an astonishing discovery considering world records in almost all sports. The authors of the inquiry state they have based their findings on a 2016 research review which includes eight articles and 31 competition rules from sports associations. They maintain that the research reviews "state" there is no evidence for imposing separate categories for the biological sexes in sports.

What the inquiry does not mention is that seven out of the eight articles consist of interviews with various groups about their experiences of sport.[117] Not a single one of the studies which the inquiry is based on measures concrete *results*. Just one of the studies measures physical capacity by comparing trans women's and trans men's muscle mass before and after hormone treatment, but it does not reach the conclusion the Swedish inquiry reaches. It *does* state that women undergoing testosterone boosting treatment can acquire muscle mass comparable to that of some men after one year – but this does not mean that men's levels decrease to those of women: "After one year of androgen deprivation, mean muscle area in M–F had decreased significantly but remained significantly greater than in F–M before testosterone treatment."[118]

The study concludes there is insufficient evidence to provide a definitive answer to the question of whether sports ought to be sex segregated and that small differences can make a big difference when it comes to sport. They note that presumably, trans men (women who have transitioned) could compete with men, while there is no certainty that the same is possible for trans women.

Nor do the other studies cited reach the conclusions the inquiry attributes to them. One is a philosophical discussion concluding that it

---

116 Remiss SOU (Statens Offentliga Utredningar, Official State Enquiries). (2017). 'Transpersoner i Sverige – Förslag för stärkt ställning och bättre levnadsvillkor', No. 92, p. 363.
117 Jon Arcelus, Walter Pierre Bouman, Emma Haycraft and Alice Bethany Jones. (2017). 'Sport and transgender people. A systematic review of the literature relating to sport participation and competitive sport policies'. *Sports Med*, Vol. 47, No. 4, pp. 701–716.
118 M. C. Bunck and L. J. Gooren. (2004). 'Transsexuals and competitive sports'. *European Journal of Endocrinology*, Vol. 151, No. 4.

is not easy to decide on the matter, partly due to female athletes growing in height and partly due to the limited number of people concerned: "the incidence of gender dysphoria syndrome is low, and consequently the frequency with which transsexual athletes might be expected to have a significant impact on a given sport should be similarly low."[119] Several of the studies are qualitative studies in which trans people speak of their experiences of sport and competitive sports.[120] In fact, one is an interview with just a single individual, a trans woman, about experiences of playing ice hockey.[121]

Is this really the basis on which the future of women's sport in Sweden is to be decided? Why are research findings distorted like this in a public inquiry? The main question, however, is whether this topic falls within the remit of the inquiry in the first place. One of its tasks is to "propose concrete interventions to improve conditions for trans people." The inquiry should therefore address practical solutions which might make life easier for 0.5 per cent of the population. The chapter on sports is introduced by the observation that trans people lead a more sedentary life than the wider population and have unhealthier habits.[122] From this point, which is about the need for daily exercise and general health, the authors suddenly leap to the demand that *professional athletes* ought to be allowed to choose whether to compete in male or female categories. What follows are proposals which would apply to society as a whole by radically redefining sex. Removing the female category in professional sports is unlikely to help the sedentary individuals for whom concern was feigned at the beginning of the chapter, as they presumably simply need to get out and move around.

---

119 J. C. Reeser. (2005.) 'Gender identity and sport: is the playing field level?'. *British Journal of Sports Medicine*, Vol. 39, No. 10.
120 See, for example, Owen D. W. Hargie, David H. Mitchell and Ian J. A. Somerville. (22 April 2015). 'People have a knack of making you feel excluded if they catch on to your difference. Transgender experiences of exclusion in sport'. *International Review for the Sociology of Sport*.
121 Jodi H. Cohen and Tamar Z. Semerjian. (2008). 'The collision of trans-experience and the politics of women's ice hockey'. *International Journal of Transgenderism*, Vol. 10.
122 Remiss SOU (Statens Offentliga Utredningar, Official State Enquiries). (2017). No. 92. 'Transpersoner i Sverige – Förslag för stärkt ställning och bättre levnadsvillkor', p. 349.

This constant sliding from problems for a few, to solutions for everyone, ending in limitations for women is typical of almost all areas into which gender identity theory has entered. Another example are the difficulties which a few individuals experienced with sex-specific ID numbers in Sweden leading to the solution that these should be abolished for *everyone*. The proposed solutions are allegedly to provide support for and facilitate things for trans people but their actual result is to curtail women's rights.

Lobby groups, sports associations and lawmakers repeat the mantra that women's sports must be inclusive and welcome everyone, but what this implies in practice, is that female sports cannot remain female. 'Inclusivity', 'human rights' and 'everyone being allowed to participate' are the buzzwords. Martina Navratilova's documentary *The Trans Women Athlete Dispute* includes footage of several male professional athletes who wish to compete in the female category – some having done no more than apply lipstick and had their hair cut in a bob. A professional golfer tells viewers that he has no interest in taking hormones but definitely wants to compete against women because he would feel anxious at having to go out there amongst all those men. A Formula One driver who has competed for years as a man reports that he feels he is a better driver as a woman and reckons he can become a role model for women drivers. A football player who has not had any treatment whatsoever feels it is obvious he should be allowed onto a female team since, according to him, he identifies as a woman and men would thus think it strange to see him on the pitch."[123] He does not appear to have considered what the women would think. Martina Navratilova is visibly touched by this and concludes that perhaps she is the one who needs to reconsider and says she did not set out to hurt anyone. She concludes that the questions around trans people's daily exercise raise a number of challenges regarding changing rooms, sex segregation and in particular attitudes.

Yet we are not talking about little league football or beach yoga here, but professional sports. The latter is about competition, not about inclusion. Most of us will never come anywhere near competing in the Olympics, nor is it a human right to be able to do so. Professional sports is about records, money and prestige. What is to stop states taking advantage

---

123 Martina Navratilova. (26 June 2019). 'The trans women athlete dispute with Martina Navratilova'. *BBC Documentary*.

of the new rules and entering biological men in female categories in order to win more medals? For those who think this is unrealistic, we only have to study the case of the Iranian women's football team. In 2015, eight of the players were men awaiting sex change.[124]

Some commentators go so far as to argue that female sports ought to be abolished altogether in favour of one mixed category. Sociology professor Elle Cashmore maintains this is the "end of female sports as we know it"[125] and that, inevitably:

> ... it's a question of time before we will have to remove the distinction between male and female sports. This is the 21st century, and we are entering a new era. Self-ID is already valid in prisons and politics, so why not sports? The landscape of women's sport will not look the same in ten years.[126]

All this is occurring precisely at the moment that female sports is finally beginning to gain ground. Not until 1928 were women permitted to compete in the Olympics since, for the French aristocrat founder of the modern Olympic games, Pierre de Coubertin, the Olympics were "the solemn and periodic exaltation of male athleticism" with "female applause as reward."[127] And not until the year 1990 were all Olympic categories opened to women, while still today there are five Olympic sports which only males compete in, such as Greco-Roman wrestling and decathlon.

Until relatively recently, women's participation in sport was a controversial topic. Women have long been prohibited from taking part by notions about sports decreasing their fertility and female athletes being unfeminine. Afghan women were not permitted to take part in the Olympics until 2004 and their participation is again threatened after the Taliban takeover. The IFBB (International Federation of Bodybuilding and Fitness) abolished its female category Ms Olympia in 2014, saying that

---

124 <https://womenintheworld.com/2015/10/01/eight-players-in-irans-womens-soccer-team-are-men/>.
125 Ellis Cashmore. (29 June 2021). 'Will transgender athletes bring the end of women's sport as we know it?' *Fair Observer*. < https://www.fairobserver.com/culture/ellis-cashmore-transgender-athletes-womens-sport-gender-inequality-news-53621/>.
126 Martina Navratilova. (26 June 2019.). 'The trans women athlete dispute with Martina Navratilova'. *BBC Documentary*.
127 <https://www.smithsonianmag.com/science-nature/rise-modern-sportswoman-180960174/#Fukt0kXYIrjhYWFg.99>.

overly muscular women gave the sport a bad name. (In 2020, Ms Olympia was relaunched.) In Iran, female sports cannot be broadcast on TV or played in front of a male audience. Yet the number of women in sports and competitive sports is higher than ever. For many girls from poor backgrounds, sports can even be a way to escape poverty and avoid forced marriage.

We need only to study world records to understand why sex segregation in sports is necessary. The male world record in marathon running is, at the time of writing, two hours one minute, while the female record is two hours 14 minutes. The male record in 100 metres sprint is 9.58 seconds, the female one is 10.49. For high jump, the figures are 2.45 metres and 2.09 metres respectively and for pole vault 6.20 metres for men and 5.06 for women. These results do not mean that men are better people or that they train harder, but that our bodies are different. Prior to puberty, these differences are small, but after puberty, which entails an increase in testosterone levels for men, males achieve on average ten to 12 per cent better results in running and swimming and 20 per cent better in high jump and long jump. Testosterone levels in themselves are not the sole reason – it is the body which testosterone creates during puberty. As researchers David J. Handelsman, Angelica L. Hirschberg and Stephane Bermon write in the *Journal of Endocrinology*, women have on average 50 to 60 per cent of upper arm muscle mass compared to men, 65 to 70 per cent thigh muscle mass and 60 to 80 per cent leg strength compared to men. Young men also have on average 12 kilos more skeletal mass than young women.[128] In the absence of a female category, few women would have the opportunity to become professional athletes.

What is the situation when it comes to male sports? This is where things get interesting. Trans men have been, according to the IOC and other sports bodies, eligible to compete in men's sports without restrictions – but they are not permitted to undergo testosterone boosting treatment due to WADA (World Anti-Doping Agency) regulations. To do so, they must apply for special dispensation, and the rules and procedures for this are far more complex and time-consuming than for the male who wishes to compete with females. Several female athletes who have transitioned

---

[128] Stephane Bermon, David J. Handelsman and Angelica L. Hirschberg. (October 2018). 'Circulating testosterone as the hormonal basis of sex differences in athletic performance'. *Endocrine Reviews*, Vol. 39, No. 5.

have had to cease competing following the notification that they are excluded from the female category as they are no longer women and cannot compete in the male category due to taking testosterone.[129]

Few trans men have achieved success in male sports. While the permitted testosterone levels for women's categories have been adapted for *the express purpose of including men,* no proposals exist for how male categories can include women. Solutions could include implementing a handicap system similar to that in golf, changing the points system, forced quotas or special relief for the team that includes a trans man — but the matter is not even being discussed. No documentaries are being produced concerning trans men in sport and the public inquiry does not so much as mention it. The only issue being debated is opening up the women's category.

Yet again, we are faced with open female spaces, closed men's spaces. This change entails woman being left without a category of her own: she cannot compete in the male category, while in her own category she risks losing to a man. She is not even allowed to be the second sex, she is relegated to the second sex of the second sex. Meanwhile, for the man, things are looking bright: he retains his dominance in the male category and should he not succeed there, he can hop over to the female category where success is guaranteed. Yet again, we see the female category being expanded through imposition of rules, while the male category is defended by means of physical strength.

---

129 SVT. (23 January 2019). 'Noel Filén Hammarström, "Var som en spik i hjärtat'. <https://www.svt.se/sport/basket/noel-soker-dispens-att-spela-med-damlag>.

CHAPTER 36

"It Started with the Realisation that Women Do Not Exist" – A Fatal Blow to Equality Policies

Now that the term woman is questioned and there are calls for its abolition – what are the implications of this for equality politics? As is well-known, the terms 'woman' and 'man' are at the very heart of equal opportunities policy. The overarching aim of, for example, Swedish equal opportunities policy is to create the same opportunities for women and men, including rights and duties in all areas of life.[130] In 1994, Sweden adopted the term 'equality integration', meaning all governmental and official decisions must include an equality perspective in the decision-making process at all levels and at all stages of the process. The government body Statistics Sweden therefore keeps separate statistics according to sex, the purpose of which is expressed very clearly in their report: "Statistics which are presented by sex mean that girls and boys, women and men are visible."[131] All data, texts, tables and diagrams must show results for women and men separately. A prerequisite for this is the country's system of ID numbers, which are sex specific, and which make Sweden a world leader in the collection of statistics concerning women's and men's living conditions. In addition, surveys and inquiries of all kinds gather data on biological sex.

---

130 Statistiska Centralbyrån (Statistics Sweden). (2004). 'Könsuppdelad statistik. Ett nödvändigt medel för jämställdhetsanalys' (Statistics by sex: A necessary tool for gender analysis), p. 6.
131 Ibid. p. 9.

Every other year, Statistics Sweden issues the publication *Women and Men in Sweden: Facts and Figures*, which summarises the state of equality in the country. It provides data on the numbers of women and men in the country, their age, higher education qualifications, earnings, unpaid work, health, political office holders and crime. This publication is used by companies, local authorities, researchers, journalists and activists – it states in black and white what inequality looks like. Those who claim we 'have already achieved equality' or that 'we have no problems here with inequality' can be countered by using the facts in this publication, as can those who claim there have been no developments.

Now, even this is being questioned. The 2017 inquiry regarding trans people in Sweden suggests that "the possibility of introducing completely sex-neutral ID numbers" be explored, that "we presuppose that self-identification should be the basis of individuals' selection of sex category" and that, rather than asking questions about sex, surveys ought to ask, "What sex are you? By sex, we mean gender identity, that is, the gender you yourself feel you are."[132]

Several political parties in Sweden are submitting proposals to abolish legal sex. The Liberal Party's Robert Hannah has petitioned Parliament to remove sex-specific ID numbers: "The purpose of introducing gender-neutral ID numbers is that individuals, many of whom are trans people, will not be 'gender identified' when identity documentation is shown."[133] In the petition, Hannah does not address how sex-based statistics are to be gathered if ID numbers become gender-neutral. Several politicians in the Left Party, among them Nooshi Dadgostar, Linda Snecker and Rossana Dinamarca, are in favour of investigating the possibility of "implementing gender-neutral ID numbers."[134] Even the Feminist Party is in favour of abolishing legal sex completely.[135]

---

132 Remiss SOU (Statens Offentliga Utredningar, Official State Enquiries). (2017). No. 92. 'Transpersoner i Sverige – Förslag för stärkt ställning och bättre levnadsvillkor', p. 489 and p. 463.
133 Robert Hannah. (21 September 2016). 'Ett tredje juridiskt kön och könsneutrala personnummer'. Motion to parliament. Motion No. 2016/17:58.
134 Lotta Johnsson Fornarve et al. (V-Left Party). (5 October 2017). 'Förstärkta rättigheter för transpersoner'. Motion No. 2017/18:3596.
135 <https://feministisktinitiativ.se/politik/sexualpolitik/konsidentitet-och-konsuttryck/>.

Why would feminist parties want to do away with the most important tool in battling inequality? Both the Left Party and the Feminist Party emphasise the continued importance of being able to gather sex-based data, however neither party explains how this would be possible if the tool for doing so is scrapped. Both parties insist that "the individual's self-identification must be the deciding factor" but do not seem to have considered whether it is sexist stereotypes that should be the basis of statistics or the material reality of biological sex. These discussions also raise the question: does a man stop enjoying male privileges the day he identifies as a woman?

Similar proposals are now streaming in from several directions. Sweden's most prominent philosopher Torbjörn Tännsjö was initially sceptical of the trans movement's demands. He expressed apprehension regarding "the deviation from sexual norms" and maintained that "robust biological differences" still exist between the sexes.[136] Ten years later, Tännsjö has not only jumped on the bandwagon but seems to be aspiring to take the driver's seat. Now he says that biological sex is a "private matter" and demands that all divisions based on sex in healthcare, sport and statistics be abolished.[137] "Sex-segregated sport is wrong," he writes in a column in the major daily *DN*, and argues this is because sex is a complicated issue which it is not possible to define and we should instead consider separation based on alternative categories, such as better and worse.[138] Women should not be allowed separate changing rooms either, he writes in another article, so as not to "provoke trans people" at sports facilities.[139]

Biological sex, according to Tännsjö, should no longer be considered a political issue: "I'm increasingly leaning towards the conviction that we should stop talking about [biological] sex."[140] He goes on to say that it is

---

136 Torbjörn Tännsjö. (24 September 2009). 'Transplanterad livmoder ett steg mot fullt könsbyte'. *DN Debatt*.
137 Torbjörn Tännsjö. (3 January 2020). 'Avskaffa all särbehandling på grund av kön'. *DN Debatt*.
138 Torbjörn Tännsjö. (7 May 2019). 'Fallet Semenya visar att könsuppdelad idrott är fel'. *DN Debatt*.
139 Torbjörn Tännsjö. (8 January 2020). 'Kön bör vara en privatsak'. *DN Debatt*.
140 Pi-samtal:"Vad skiljer egentligen kvinnor och män?" (Torbjörn Tännsjö, Angelica Linden Hirschberg and Markus Heilig in conversation.) (5 December 2019). *Fri Tanke*. <https://fritanke.se/video/pi-samtal-vad-skiljer-egentligen-kvinnor-och-man/>.

time to stop gender discrimination, but he is not referring to discrimination of women in the work place, the gender pay gap or medical research bias. Tännsjö only wants to abolish the formal rules which *benefit* women in sport, statistics and changing rooms. Participating in a philosophical panel discussion, he explains how he arrived at this conclusion: "It started with the realisation that women do not exist."[141] To snickering from the audience, Tännsjö explains on the all-male panel that the term woman is unnecessary:

> Should she be eligible to compete with women who have lower testosterone levels than her? Is this not unfair? Well, then it is the testosterone level that's important. If one wants to have vaginal intercourse with her, then it is important that she has a vagina. If she is at risk of haemophilia, then it is the chromosomes that are important.

By reducing women to fragmented body parts, Tännsjö renders all of culture and sexuality incomprehensible – sexuality is hardly only about 'having a vagina'. Above all, however, he renders the women's movement utterly impossible. We cannot address women's situation if we cannot say that women exist. Note that Tännsjö is not arguing that men do not exist. It is true that women's rights have long been a thorn in the side for Tännsjö, but until now he has restricted his opinions to being in favour of legalising the buying of sex and surrogacy. He has never dared go as far as to demand the abolition of woman herself, and thereby the foundation of equal opportunities policy. By utilising gender identity theory, he is able to attack all demands of the women's movement while simultaneously appearing progressive.

It is often claimed that the reason for abolishing legal sex is to facilitate dealings for trans people and allow for collecting data on them as a specific group. It is clear that there is a point to investigating trans people's situation. One must of course study that too at times. Yet when we ask questions about sex we are looking to find out about something different, namely how living conditions differ between those born with a vagina and those born with a penis. If we ask instead what gender people feel they are, we will receive different answers. Equal opportunities policy is based on biological sex *precisely because evidence exists that biological sex matters.*

---

141 Klubb Apollo. (1 October 2019). 'Finns individen? Kollektiva drömmar och den fria viljans dilemma'.

It is not equality between young and old, blue-collar and white-collar workers or trans people and cis people that is the subject of the question – other measures and surveys exist to gather data on these differences. Equal opportunities policy and the tools that make it possible are about remedying the injustices that exist between biological women and men.

What Tännsjö, Hannah and others are proposing is not an additional perspective. They are suggesting that we remove a perspective, namely the foundation which equal opportunities policies are based on. Without legal sex and sex-specific ID numbers, we will no longer be able to conduct sex-based analyses of income, pensions, crime, patient data, wealth and family benefits. In addition, legal sex is the basis for equality integration in the workplace and in education. When universities set targets of 50 per cent women for all newly recruited teachers and researchers, it is legal sex which allows them to measure success in reaching this target.[142] It is a simple procedure and can be carried out even when applications are anonymised. Using first names to decide is not nearly as efficient – in a multicultural society it is not always easy for recruiters to know an applicant's sex judging only by their name and many names are unisex.

The journey of the women's struggle from subversive movement to official politics has been long and hard. It faces constant resistance at all levels of society and there are many who dislike the work countries do on equality. Yet it would be political suicide to argue in favour of abolishing legal sex by saying one is against equality. When the demand comes from a more progressive place – in the name of facilitating things for a minority – suddenly liberals, feminists and philosophers are onboard and it is suspiciously easy to pull the rug out from under the whole of equal opportunities policy. It is telling that the far-right Swedish Democrats also want to abolish legal sex. They, however, do not need to beat around the bush by appealing to trans and non-binary people.

---

142 Karin Thorsell. (18 September 2018). 'Chalmers mål: 40 procent kvinnliga professorer om tio år'. *Tidningen Ingenjören*.

CHAPTER 37

"She Deserves a Kick in the Ovaries"

At this point one may wonder how proposals to abolish female sports, hamper equal opportunities endeavours, sterilise young homosexuals, place male sex offenders in women's prisons and forbid us from referring to women can be considered progressive. One might also ask what these proposals even have to do with trans people and where the debate around it all is. After all, the changes concerned will have far-reaching consequences, each of which merits thorough debate and review within academia, politics and society at large.

One quickly realises however, that questioning gender identity theory and protesting against changes implemented on the basis of it is no mean feat. In just ten years, a culture of backlash and reprisals has emerged against women who attempt to argue and take action against these changes. They have found themselves barred from Twitter, losing their jobs, being subjected to or threatened with violence and ending up as persona non grata.

When British researcher Maya Forstater (an expert on tax policy) expressed her views regarding legal proposals which redefined sex, her employer decided not to extend her contract beyond her probation period. Believing that sex was a biological and material category rather than a feeling was an unacceptable opinion to hold according to her employer, the organisation Centre for Global Development. In December 2019, an employment tribunal ruled against Forstater, and found that her views did "not have the protected characteristic of philosophical belief" and were therefore not covered by freedom of expression but were "absolutist," "offensive and exclusionary."[143] Forstater appealed to the Employment Appeal Tribunal, which on the contrary ruled that gender-critical views should be seen as a protected philosophical belief, and that "only views akin to Nazism or totalitarianism were unworthy of protections for rights of freedom of expression and thought."[144] The case was then sent back to the employment tribunal which ruled in July 2022 that Forstater had been discriminated against and suffered victimisation as a result.[145]

No woman speaking out on the subject of gender identity theory is exempt from severe consequences, no matter how powerful or rich she is. Ever since author J. K. Rowling began voicing her criticism of gender identity theory, she has been subjected to an organised boycott campaign. Bookshops have removed Harry Potter books from their shelves, she has had to return a human rights award and newspapers have encouraged fans to boycott Harry Potter products.[146] Even the quidditch league, which owes its existence to Rowling inventing the sport in her Harry Potter books, has decided to rename itself quadball to distance itself from Rowling, due to her views on gender.[147] The many articles which have been written about Rowling on the topic hardly ever seek to address her comments in a factual manner. A typical headline reads "Rowling criticised for transphobic remarks" without the article explaining what is transphobic about her remarks.

Academics such as professor of philosophy Kathleen Stock are harassed at work, with students and colleagues putting up posters with the text "Stock Out" to the point that she has to resign.[148] I myself have been fired from a position as editor-in-chief at the magazine *Arbetaren*, before I had the chance to start, due to letters and online claims that I am transphobic, after this very book was published in Sweden. Indian

---

143 Owen Bowcott. (18 December 2019). 'Judge rules against researcher who lost job over transgender tweets'. *The Guardian*.
144 Haroon Siddique. (10 June 2021). "Gender-critical views are a protected belief, appeal tribunal rules". *The Guardian*.
145 Haroon Siddique. (6 July 2022). "Maya Forstater was discriminated against over gender-critical beliefs, tribunal rules". *The Guardian*.
146 <https://www.independent.co.uk/arts-entertainment/games/feature/>. hogwarts-legacy-jk-rowling-harry-potter-boycott-transphobia-b485188.html>.
147 Manish Pandey. (21/7/2022). "Harry Potter: Quidditch renamed to Quadball over JK Rowling link". *BBC News*.
148 Nadeem Badshah. (7/10/2021) "University defends 'academic freedoms' after calls to sack professor". *The Guardian*.

feminist Vaishnavi Sundar had a similar experience. She had made a film about workplace sexual harassment, the first of its kind in India. The film was titled *But What Was She Wearing?* and was ready for release for 8 March 2020; it was set to be a milestone of the Indian #metoo movement. But it was never screened. Following Sundar speaking out against men who had undergone no gender reassignment treatment being allowed access to women's prisons, screening after screening was cancelled. A US group known as The Polis Project was found to be behind the boycott.[149]

When Nigerian author Chimamanda Ngozi Adichie said in an interview that "When people talk about, 'Are trans women women?' my feeling is trans women are trans women," all hell broke loose. Adichie was blasted with threats of boycott and, shaken and shocked, she had to wriggle out of her own opinion:

> From the very beginning, I think it's been quite clear that there's no way I could possibly say that trans women are not women. It's the sort of thing to me that's obvious, so I start from that obvious premise. Of course they are women but in talking about feminism and gender and all of that, it's important for us to acknowledge the differences in experience of gender. That's really what my point is.[150]

Adichie may have got away with just a scare but has been careful not to express her opinion on the matter this clearly again. Things panned out worse for the founder of *Feminist Current* and one of Canada's most renowned feminists, Meghan Murphy, who has been permanently barred from Twitter having tweeted "Men are not women."[151] Her lectures about gender identity theory and consequences for women of changes in the law have often been cancelled following pressure and threats.[152] Even the event 'An Evening with Canceled Women' at New York Public Library – a conversation with female intellectuals who had all been silenced or

---

149 Vaishnavi Sundar. (4 March 2020). 'I was cancelled for my tweets on transgenderism'. *Spiked Online*.
150 Damola Durosomo. "Chimamanda Ngozi Adichie Continues to Defend Her Comments on Trans Women During D.C. Appearance". *OkayAfrica*. (n.d.).
151 *BBC*. (22 May 2019). 'Twitter-ban feminist defends transgender views ahead of Holyrood meeting'.
152 <https://dailyhive.com/vancouver/gender-identity-meghan-murphy-sfu-cancelled>.

cancelled due to their texts about the consequences for women of gender identity theory – was cancelled.[153]

In these times of heated public debate, it sometimes appears that the number of victims of online hatred has gone through the roof, turning it into a genre of its own: testifying publicly about receiving public hatred and garnering sympathy for it. Being hated does not necessarily mean that one is right and claiming that one has been silenced by the elite has also become something of a rhetorical trick, since the same people who claim to have been censured often crop up the following day with even more followers and a bigger platform. That which is truly censured is, naturally, what we never hear about.

Yet the exclusion of those who try to discuss aspects of gender identity theory follows a unique systematic approach. Firstly, all women who express themselves on the matter are subjected to exclusion and silenced but barely any men are. Male commentators who express their views receive few if any retorts and are not cancelled or physically attacked. Secondly, it makes no difference what these women say or how carefully or humbly they express themselves – they are subjected to the same harsh treatment regardless. Those who attempt to address the topic from an intellectual standpoint are, as a rule, not engaged with on an intellectual level and are instead labelled 'transphobic' without any further discussion, with demands that they be barred from expressing their opinion on any subject in future, hold any job or be seen in public places. The gender identity question has become a valley of death. This is where you go to die, no matter how famous or popular you have been, even if you are the most best-selling author in the entire world. The same double standard is apparent when it comes to social media: male-dominated fora such as the Swedish Flashback or Spanish Foro Coches are rife with racism, sexism, trans- and homophobia and even Nazism – no one intervenes and the content is passed off as freedom of expression – while female dominated fora such as British Mumsnet are shut down or heavily moderated for including discussions about what a woman is. Thirdly, women are shut out of their own movement, from the platforms they themselves were involved in establishing and developing, and thus have nowhere left to

---

153 Richard Bernstein. (21 December 2020). 'On the left, a new clash between feminists and transgender activists'. *The Daily Signal*.

turn. When I meet Meghan Murphy in Stockholm, she tells me what being critical of gender identity theory led to for her:

> I can never find work again. I've lost the jobs I did have in journalism. I used to work with editors at rabble.ca, a progressive magazine, but after writing a criticism of the idea that the word 'menstruators' ought to replace the word 'women', my articles were removed, I was labelled 'transphobic' and forced to quit. My name has been dragged through the mud […] I can't show my face in 'progressive' circles. I used to have an active social life, I know most people in our part of Vancouver. Nowadays, I no longer go out without my boyfriend. I'm not famous enough to be recognised on the street, but I'm afraid nonetheless that someone will come up to me and punch me in the face. I'm frightened my house will be broken into. People are sometimes polite and kind when they meet me but then I see that they've spread shit about me online. It makes you very paranoid. [154]

Murphy has since had to go into exile in Mexico, a fate which has been common for intellectual dissidents from all over the world – however, gender-critical feminists who have to go into exile are not labelled dissidents or awarded prizes the way their male counterparts debating religion or geopolitics are.

In 2016, an exhibition by trans activist group Degenderettes ran at a San Francisco public library. The items on display included a blood-stained tank top with the writing "I punch terfs," a banner with the text "Die Cis Scum"[155] and a painting bearing the text, "May Terfs Wither Cold and Alone." There was also a collection of axes, sledgehammers and pride-coloured baseball bats, the reason being that "the Degenderettes twirl the classic American symbol of home defense (sic) baseball bats, because this is not a war between nations, it is a fight that has come to their door." These baseball bats and sledgehammers are also sold as merchandise by the Degenderettes.[156]

The exhibition generated heated debate. Was it, as the artists and organisers claimed, an anti-fascist, grassroots protest highlighting trans people's vulnerability, or was it violence against women legitimised by

---

154 Kajsa Ekis Ekman. (January 2018). 'Feministen som kom ut i kylan'. *Kvinnotryck*.
155 <https://fourelementsfitness.com/2016/12/10/color-guard-an-exhibition-of-baseball-bats-as-lgbtiq-flags-by-the-degenderettes/> Seen Jan 4, 2019, link defunct. Also on <https://www.facebook.com/events/1822265287988883/>.
156 <https://degenderettes.com/order#baseball>.

means of an ostensibly progressive aura? Conservative commentators argued that both sides of the debate were proof that 'gender ideology' had hijacked the public sphere, that art had degenerated and that public libraries should be defunded, while some socialists considered debates about these matters "culture wars" devoid of meaning which should best be ignored in favour of a focus on class struggle.

What, then, is a 'terf', why has it replaced 'feminazi' as the most common slur by far against feminists, and why should they be assaulted and attacked? Terf is an acronym which stands for 'trans exclusive radical feminist'. Few feminists – if any – have referred to themselves as 'terfs' and it is only recently that there has been an attempt to de-weaponise the slur by reclaiming it in an ironic way. It is used about women who believe in women-only spaces, who focus too much on women in their feminist struggle or, as in the case of Liv Strömqvist, who have written a comic about women's genitalia. The internet abounds with statements such as "TERFs like Germaine Greer are committing acts of genocide" and "if you are a terf i literally want to take a knife and stab it directly to your throat and twist it around."[157] The hatred is often aimed directly at the female body: "that terf deserves a punch right in the ovaries" and "I'd pay to watch someone violently rip her ovaries from her abdomen", as two trans activists discuss on Twitter. "Terfs can choke on my girldick" is one of the most common threats, displayed with the following wording on a banner at Dresden Pride 2022: "Terfs can suck my huge trans cock."[158]

There are few well-known feminists who have not been labelled a 'terf' at one point or another. In fact, the term has been normalised to such a degree that calling a woman a 'terf' is now sufficient to immediately discount and oust her from a conversation. *Kontext Press* publishes lists of Sweden's "top five anti-trans women" (with me in first place) and claims that these feminists believe that "it is TRANS PEOPLE and not capital, racism and sexism which are the root of women's oppression."[159] None of the feminists on the list have said anything of the sort but are, in the view

---

157 <https://twitter.com/RobbieTravers/status/662683596336062464/>. <https://speakupforwomen.nz/dont-call-women-terfs/>. Latter link now defunct.
158 Quoted on <terfisaslur.com> and <https://twitter.com/andrewdoyle_com/status/1566461347617193984>.
159 Silas Aliki. (15 March 2020). 'Lista: Topp fem transfientliga feminister'. *Kontext Press.*

of *Kontext Press*, guilty all the same due to having praised sisterhood, written books with titles like *Haggan* (The Hag) about old women's sexuality and for being "extremely heterosexual." Others, like a young representative of the Left Party's youth wing Ung Vänster, take things further and print tote bags with an image of a chair and the text "Throw this in your local transphobe's face," along with lists of who should receive this treatment. While such incitement to violence may appear rather silly, the problem is that this kind of language is usually part of a wider context in which some spread hatred, others point out targets and still others take action with the latter often being psychologically-ill individuals and violent criminals. Thus, while a young leftist publishes exhortations to assault women, the newly freed murderer Kristoffer – now Kim – Johansson sets up an Instagram account on which he poses with weapons, calls himself a *Terfhunter* and posts death threats to the women on the lists published by the young leftist.

No male counterpart exists for the term 'terf'. Despite the fact that it is overwhelmingly men who carry out violence against trans people, there is no word for them. Neither is there a movement identifying or accusing men who murder trans people. The artist group Degenderettes write in their exhibition catalogue that their aim is to raise awareness about trans people being murdered and name Brandi Seals, "a black trans woman murdered in December 2017" including all those who died of AIDS as a result of President Reagan's politics.[160] Yet it is feminists, not Seals' murderer and not Reagan, who are the subject of their hatred and deserving of assault with baseball bats. It is precisely this pattern: *male violence – women as scapegoats,* which returns time and again. Swathes of articles begin with descriptions of how trans people are subjected to violence, to then leap to the accusation that *feminists* are responsible for this violence. In an article in the *Huffington Post*, trans activist Kelsie Bryn Jones writes:

> When a cisgender woman is murdered, the violence against the murdered woman is eclipsed by the way that trans women are more often than not mutilated, dismembered, or set on fire in an orgy of hate.[161]

---

160 <https://sfpl.org/uploads/files/pdfs/Degenderettes-Labels.pdf>.
161 Kelsie Brynn Jones. (2 August 2014). 'Trans-exclusionary radical feminism. What exactly is it, and why does it hurt?' *Huffington Post*.

Jones claims that murders of trans women overshadow murders of cis women in their brutality. The message is that women who are murdered are privileged compared to those who were born male. Who perpetrates this violence and why? The text remains silent on these points and does not name the murderers, preferring to place blame on terfs, which it defines as "a loosely-organized collective with a message of hate and exclusion against transgender women." The entire text is centred around this blaming of women who use the wrong pronouns and concludes with self-victimisation: for his brave struggle against terfs, Brynn Jones has "been bombarded with spam, pornography, and signed up to various mailing lists" – though it is unclear how this relates to the matter at hand.

Thus, dead trans people are used as hostages in a political campaign which stands little chance of putting an end to the murders. Statistics regarding murders of trans people in the US in the first half of the 2010s show the following: trans people's risk of being murdered is, relatively, lower than that of 'cis' people. However, this is not the case when it comes to Black and Latin American trans people, for whom the risk is *considerably* greater.[162] Of the 28 trans people killed in the US in 2017, 24 were black and of the 20 trans people killed in the US in 2018, 14 were black.[163] Structural racism appears to be a key component in the majority of these murders. Several of the murders have an unknown motive; some are clear hate crimes, others are linked to drugs and homelessness, while some are killed by their partners or buyers in the prostitution industry. The absolute majority of the murderers are men.[164] To date, there are no known cases in which feminism has been the motive behind the murder of a trans person. Trans people are seemingly murdered by men because of racism, prostitution, structural economic inequalities, transphobia and homophobia.

---

[162] A. Dinno. (September 2017). 'Homicide rates of transgender individuals in the United States: 2010–2014'. *American Journal of Public Health*, Vol. 107, No. 9, pp. 1441–1447.

[163] <https://everytown.org/press/texas-moms-demand-action-everytown-respond-to-shooting-death-of-transgender-woman-in-houston/ och https://transgenderlawcenter.org/archives/14357>.

[164] Human Rights Campaign. (21 March 2019). 'Violence against the transgender community in 2017'. WWSB: 'Transgender woman admits shooting, killing transgender wife'.

Still, it is primarily feminists who are the target of the Degenderettes and other anti-terf campaigns. Had the Degenderettes invented the term MOT, Murderers of Trans People, and written "I punch MOTs," they would have focused attention on men who murder trans people and would have been able to join forces with the women's movement against male violence. Had they approached the matter from the observation that both women and trans women who are killed in prostitution are victims of the sex industry, they could have fought side by side with abolitionists. Prostitution is one of the deadliest situations a person can find herself in, yet the murders of trans women are being cynically exploited by an anti-feminist campaign in favour of legalising prostitution. The website "Stop Trans Murders" displays images of trans people who have died and then misguidedly goes on to claim the solution is legalising the buying of sex and that prostitution is necessary work.[165]

On Transgender Day of Remembrance 2020, RFSU (the Swedish Association for Sexuality Education) posted statistics about the 350 dead trans women over the past year –152 of them occurred in Brazil.[166] There too, the majority of those killed are Black and several died in prostitution. Despite this, RFSU refers to the dead as 'sex workers' and thus implicitly legitimises the cause of their death – the message is that prostitution is a legitimate form of employment for trans women. On occasion, it appears as though these statistics regarding murdered trans women are cited not out of genuine concern and desire to raise awareness, but to exploit their corpses as part of a rhetorical attack on feminists. They are, in fact, routinely pitted against statistics regarding dead women, not dead men, and not the living men who carry out the murders of nearly all people of both sexes. As well as being a tragic fact, this constitutes a missed opportunity to take action against this violence and to form a strong alliance.

The women's movement has historically welcomed male gender dissidents as allies in the fight against patriarchy and there was a time when it stood shoulder to shoulder with the LGBTQ-movement. British feminist Germaine Greer is part of this tradition. In her 1999 book. *The Whole Woman*, she writes:

---

165 <http://www.stoptransmurders.org/>.
166 <https://www.facebook.com/photo/?fbid=4121187434577937&set=pcb.4121 194371243910>.

> There has always been a confederacy between women and rebels against masculinist conditioning, be they homosexuals, transvestite or transsexual, and these are relationships that feminists should continue to foster but not at the cost of denying their own perception of female reality.[167]

This time is now long-gone and Greer's outstretched hand was met with attacks. The above quote led to her being attacked at a book signing in Wellington, New Zealand and having a bucket of glitter dumped on her. Queer Avengers, the group behind the attack, wrote in a press release that, "Transphobic feminism is so 20th century. Women's liberation must mean the right to refuse imposed gender rules, to fight for diverse gender expression,"[168] which was precisely what Greer just said. But nothing short of complete capitulation to the new theory was henceforth acceptable.

Over the past ten years, these types of attacks have grown increasingly aggressive. Not since the movement for women's suffrage have women's rights activists in the west been subjected to such massive hate campaigns. Several feminists who have spoken out about women's rights in relation to gender identity theory have been physically assaulted. In September 2017, a women's meeting titled "We Need to Talk About Gender" was held in Hyde Park in London; the location – Speakers' Corner – was decided on following the organisers receiving threats and pressure to cancel including cancellations of offers to host them from several venues.[169] At this historic meeting place where the suffragettes had met to demand the vote for women, a group of counter protestors arrived with signs that read "No Debate" and "Terfs not Welcome."[170] They violently attacked the meeting attendees and a 25-year-old man named Wolf was later sentenced for assault of a 60-year-old woman. Wolf identifies as female and had previously tweeted that he planned to attend the meeting to "fuck some terfs up" and "if you are a terf and/or dont [sic] think transwomen are

---

167 Germaine Greer. (1999/2007). *The Whole Woman*, p. 422. London: Black Swan.
168 Quoted in: Newstalk ZB. (14 March 2012). 'Germaine Greer "glitter-bombed" by Queer Avengers'. *NZ Herald*. <https://www.nzherald.co.nz/nz/germaine-greer-glitter-bombed-by-queer-avengers/YQYXQ3AP3Q2YLJHWC5UAN2G32E/>.
169 Meghan Murphy. (15 September 2017). 'Historic Speaker's Corner becomes site of anti-feminist silencing and violence'. *Feminist Current*.
170 <https://www.youtube.com/watch?time_continue=47&v=9_d3ozhSE-U>.

women, you can suck my cock you cuntface."¹⁷¹ An observer at the trial writes:

> Two dozen individuals — mostly men with masks on, some in full combat gear — accompanied Wolf to court. [...] Three of Wolf's supporters brought fighting dogs (Dobermans and Mastiffs), as well as a huge sound system blaring death metal. Half stayed outside the court, half came in. The machismo of it all was palpable. [...] By day two, Wolf's supporters had dwindled to around a dozen. All but one were men. MacLachlan's supporters were all women.¹⁷²

An odd scene indeed: a group of young, masked men gather in support of a man who has struck down a 60-year-old woman, all convinced that *they* are the women. The women's movement has gone through many ideological conflicts over the years but these have rarely been solved by assaulting one another.

Lesbian feminist Julie Bindel being attacked by a bearded man in June 2019 would, under normal circumstances, have been seen as an occurence of men's violence against women, as well as a hate crime against homosexuals. Yet when the attacker claimed that he was a woman, this analysis was entirely nullified.¹⁷³ The attacker turned out to be a rabid Twitterer, who on top of all things called himself Cathy Brennan after a famous feminist. Progressive commentators came out in support of the perpetrator and claimed that Bindel was the actual perpetrator of violence due to her views.¹⁷⁴ What we see here is a symbolic *reversal*, eerily similar to that which can occur in abusive relationships, where the perpetrator assumes the role of victim. This is generally referred to as DARVO: Deny, Attack, and Reverse Victim and Offender. Men assuming the role of women and then perpetrating violence against women while utilising the argument that they are protesting violence against women is an extremely advanced form of gaslighting which presumably has very little to do with wanting to be trans or a woman. What we are dealing with is a neo-

---

171 Maria MacLachlan. (18 April 2018). 'The ostensible trial of Tara Wolf – Part 1', peaktrans.org.
172 Jen Izaakson. (27 April 2018). 'Trans-identified male, Tara Wolf, convicted of assault after Hyde Park attack'. *Feminist Current*.
173 <https://www2.bfi.org.uk/people/cathy-brennan>.
174 <https://www.thetimes.co.uk/article/julie-bindel-the-man-in-a-skirt-called-me-a-nazi-then-attacked-8dfwk8jft?_ga=2.157655866.1864798478.1560328713-723508512.1560328712>.

patriarchal political movement whose purpose is to silence and intimidate women. By sporting a beard and behaving violently, "Brennan" sends clear signals to women that he is a dominant male, while simultaneously claiming that he is oppressed both as a woman and as a trans woman and thus deserves sympathy. But both personas in the same body are not possible: a bearded biological man who does not pass as a woman cannot be treated like, nor be oppressed like, a woman by society nor be the object of transphobia. Claiming otherwise is an advanced form of manipulation, in which both the role of the oppressor and the oppressed are occupied by "Brennan" himself, leaving the woman without a position. The underlying message is all too familiar: the woman spoke, and thus provoked the man to hit. Indeed, it is possible to analyse the violence and boycott campaigns around "terf"-accusations as patriarchy entering into DARVO-mode. While the patriarch of old would proudly state that he is the one in charge and no disobedience is tolerated, the trans-era brotherhood achieves the same by claiming victim status, and declaring that any female who disobeys is in fact a dictator.

CHAPTER 38

Sex, Race, Class, or ... An Exception to Intersectionality

If our answer to the question "Who is a woman?" becomes "anyone who defines themselves as a woman," will self-identification apply to other categories such as age, class and race? Are all categories open? This may seem a daft comparison yet it does pose a challenge to theories of intersectionality. Let us assume for a moment that this is the case. Age could be considered a spectrum – indeed, many an 80-year-old is physically more like a 60-year-old, just as there are 40-year-olds who have aged before their time due to genetic and lifestyle factors. Is it perhaps mistaken to define age solely according to our years? Were we to follow Tännsjö's proposals on how to view sex, we would also divide age into a series of different components and allow those 15-year-olds who display maturity to enter pubs but refuse entry to immature 25-year-olds. One's age could be altered on official databases without having to consult a doctor and passports would state the holder's age based on their subjective feelings. A 52-year-old Canadian man has done precisely this: he decided he was a 6-year-old girl, left his wife and child and had himself adopted by a couple.[175]

An increasing number of individuals are also claiming that they were born with the wrong skin colour. Let us imagine that this were to become a political movement: white people claiming they feel 'black inside' and

---

175 Brie Borrell. (17 January 2019). 'Trans age: The reality'. *The Pawprint*.

vice versa. They would claim they had never truly been white and that they feel more at home in 'black culture'. States would cover treatment for those who wished to change their hair and skin colour, while others would claim they were black without changing anything, since it is 'not skin colour that defines who is black', as 'black cannot be reduced to a colour'. Children who displayed 'ethnically incongruent' behaviour would be carted off to doctors for injections and surgery. Children who failed to behave according to the stereotypes presumed to match their ethnicity would be considered to be suffering to such an extent from having the wrong skin colour that the only humane option would be medical intervention to change their skin colour. White people who identify as black would be eligible to access university places and funding in those countries where quotas exist for ethnic minorities. Black people would be called 'privileged' and 'cis-coloured', since they never had to reflect on their skin colour. Battle cries such as 'Black Lives Matter' would be abolished on the grounds that some people feel excluded by such normative statements: it should rather be "transblack lives matter." Claims would be made that ethnicity was not about skin colour but an inner feeling and that white people were the most oppressed of all black people, due to their oppression not only as black people but also as 'trans-racial'. Research would frantically search for neurological differences between the races in order to identify those white people who were born with black people's brains. Anthropologists would study individuals who had crossed over to the other ethnicity *not* as part of a struggle against discrimination and apartheid, but to prove they were *really* born with the wrong skin colour. A movement of 'transblack' activists would arise, consisting of white people who, while only paying lip service to the struggle against white supremacy, spent most of their time attacking 'exclusionary' Black activists and fragmenting the anti-racist struggle.

Those white people who have attempted to change ethnicity – for example, NAACP (The National Association for the Advancement of Colored People) chapter head, American Rachel Dolezal and German model Martina Big, have been met with a resounding NO. They have been told: *if you are not born you cannot become*. Dolezal was expelled from the NAACP when it was revealed she was white and most commentators on the matter (apart from Whoopi Goldberg) felt she did not have the right to speak for black women. Dolezal herself (now Nkechi Amare Diallo) claims that she used to draw self-portraits using brown instead of beige crayons and that "race is a state of mind." Her statements seemed not to sit well with anyone. German model Martina Big (now Malaika Kubwa) appears to be accepted in Kenya, where many are happy that she wants to become Kenyan, but she has not been as successful in western anti-racist circles. In September 2020, US academic Jessica Krug was outed. She had built a career around being an Afro-Latina Bronx native whose brother had been killed by police and whose parents were drug addicts, claiming that her surname was the result of border-control officers misspelling Cruz. In reality, she was a well-to-do Jewish woman from Kansas. Following the revelation, her career collapsed overnight. She expressed her reaction in this article:

> For the better part of my adult life, every move I've made, every relationship I've formed, has been rooted in the napalm toxic soil of lies. [...] You should absolutely cancel me, and I absolutely cancel myself. [...] I have no identity outside of this. I have never developed one. I have to figure out how to be a person that I don't believe should exist.[176]

If she were to claim that she faked it till she made it, that her experience shaped her into actually becoming Afro-Latina, or that race is in the eye of the beholder (since many actually thought she was what she claimed), this would still be no help to Krug. All the experiences which resulted from passing as Black for years were invalidated since she was not Black to begin with.

It is not possible to draw exact comparisons between these individuals and trans people; both Donezal and Krug lied about their lives and invented a background they had never had. Another difference which is interesting to note is that both took on extra-radical views, as opposed to transactivists who often question the legitimacy of the women's movement. Dolezal threw herself in the struggle, teaching African American Culture and The Black Woman's Struggle, demanded racial justice and organised protests; Krug was known for hating white people, waging a war against gentrification and for denouncing Black colleagues for wanting to be white. A Tinder date of Krug later told the media that:

---

176 Jessica A. Krug. (3 September 2020). 'The truth, and the anti-black violence of my lies'. *Medium*.

"It was all F whites, F the police, F capitalism, all of that stuff."[177] They did not enter Black struggle in order to dilute it; they made it so radical it became a parody.[178] At a philosophical level, though, it is interesting to explore the ways in which sex differs from race, class and age. In her essay 'In Defence of Transracialism', philosopher Rebecca Tuvel argues that all of transgenderism's criteria can be applied to race: race as self-identification, race as lived oppression, race as social construct and a question of passing, i.e. that race is in the eye of the beholder.[179]

Tuvel's essay was widely criticised and 800 academics signed a letter in protest saying race was not comparable to sex, which led to the British feminist philosophy journal *Hypatia* removing the article. The editor, philosopher Cressida Heyes, posted an apology. She also stated race cannot be compared to sex since "beliefs about the kind of thing race is shape the possibilities for race change. In particular […] the belief that an individual's racial identity derives from her biological ancestors undermines the possibility of changing race."[180]

In other words, there is a social consensus which says that race is innate, inherited from one's parents and cannot be acquired – one cannot be born as a member of one ethnicity and die as member of another – and it is not possible within this framework to change race. Simply put, it is not possible to change race because people do not believe it is possible to change race. Converting class into a question of identity does not fly either: the aristocrat who claims he "feels like a member of the working class because he has always valued simplicity" would be met with ridicule.

What is it then about sex, and specifically the female sex, which makes it fluid while other categories are fixed? Age, class and race are, after all, considerably more fluid than sex: the former are by nature changing, and the latter are constructs devoid of meaning outside social hierarchy. It is entirely possible to imagine a society without classes. The working

---

177 <https://www.washingtonian.com/2021/01/27/the-true-story-of-jessica-krug-the-white-professor-who-posed-as-black-for-years-until-it-all-blew-up-last-fall/>.

178 <https://www.washingtonian.com/2021/01/27/the-true-story-of-jessica-krug-the-white-professor-who-posed-as-black-for-years-until-it-all-blew-up-last-fall/>.

179 Rebecca Tuvel. (Spring 2017). 'In defence of transracialism'. *Hypatia*, Vol. 32, No. 2, pp. 263–278.

180 Quoted in Tuvel 2017.

classes and capitalists have the same bodily functions and the only difference between them is their position. Cultures can have hundreds of racial categories; recall the Spanish colonial obsession with creating dozens of categories, such as *pardos, criollos, mestizos, zambos and castizos*, all depending on exactly what type of heritage one had and resulting in specific rules such as who could bring a mat to church. Individuals often have more than one ethnicity, which is not true in the case of sex. The last time anyone tried to claim that classes and races differed in their abilities was in the heavily criticised 1994 publication *The Bell Curve*, which was torn apart and never heard about again except perhaps in Ayaan Hirsi Ali's memoirs. Most of us accept the idea that race and class are social constructs, that it is possible to belong to several ethnicities and classes at once and that it is not always easy to tell where to draw the line. Despite this, there is a broad social consensus which says that race and class are real.

Sex, on the other hand, is a *reproductive function*. Even in a society with complete equality between the sexes in which all professions from CEOs to nurses comprised 50 per cent women and 50 per cent men, in which clothing and hair cuts were identical, in which we all did the dishes equally and were equally violent or nonviolent to each other, one fact would remain: women give birth to children and men do not. Although not all women give birth, all people were born of a woman. No one has yet come onto this earth in any other way: all 6 billion of us were created from embryo to human in and by a female body. Although far from all women have given birth – a fourth of all women in peasant societies never gave birth, compared to about a tenth of women today – the fact of *belonging to the childbearing class* is the source of a woman's power in a matriarchy *and* the reason for her oppression in patriarchy. No matter how many treatments and interventions a person with XY-chromosomes undergoes, he can never give birth; nor can a person with XX-chromosomes ever inseminate an ovum.

Reproduction is the most fundamental fact of life, a fact which all cultures are built on. However, gender inequality is not an automatic result of this, as there are a multitude of ways in which to organise a society based on these material preconditions, each with different outcomes. Sex is, however, the category which, more than any other, is fixed *and* which is considered fluid. For women, gender identity theory makes sex *that which we cannot flee from and that which we are not permitted to keep.*

Perhaps a connection exists here? Perhaps sex is seen as fluid precisely because it is fixed? Perhaps there is no danger to patriarchy in considering it fluid since the basic facts of oppression will stay the same? If sex-based oppression really was only a cultural construct, would it perhaps go away if we ceased naming it – is that why other systems of domination, such as racism or homophobia, still insist on *naming* their oppressed subjects, whereas patriarchy knows it doesn't have to name – women will still be women anyway?

The application of an intersectional analytical framework to sex and gender shows us that indeed, the category of sex stands out as an exception to the other categories of class, race and sexuality. Intersectionality's foremost ideological tools such as epistemic privilege, standpoint theory and cultural appropriation have been rendered inoperable when it comes to biological sex. Intersectionality, in other words, does not seem to apply to sex the same way it applies to other categories.

During the 2010s, intersectionality, an evolution of the activist notion of triple oppression (sex, race, class and how they intersect) conquered academia and social media alike. Triple oppression had been a tool of political activists in the US and Europe trying to balance the struggles of the working class with women and the Black community. It was not a user manual as much as a way to validate the experience of three groups equally. Intersectionality expanded the number of categories of oppression, and the term "check your privilege" became almost as commonplace on social media as the selfie. Donna Haraway's notion of "situated knowledges" had gained traction — the idea that your knowledge is determined by what you have witnessed, what you have experienced, and your geographical location. Thus, a man in Wall Street does not have the same worldview as a Rohingya in Myanmar. It is more likely that the man in Wall Street believes you can reach the stars if you only try hard enough and that the Rohingya believes God decides our fate. Situated knowledge tells us that, in order to understand an issue, one must have experience of it. This is also a basic tenet within Marxism: better understanding and knowledge of a situation can be gained by practical experience. A similar observation was expressed by Mao: "all genuine knowledge originates in direct experience."[181] In a sense, this insight is the basis of intersectional thinking: those with experience of racism or sexism are more likely to be able to accumulate knowledge of these phenomena than those with no experience. Theory is the compass, practice is the map. Without practice, there is no map with which to check the relevance of theories. Yet practice, according to Marxism, could never provide an analysis on its own, since it may be based on an exception – a fact which would not be understood without the help of a theory. Climbing up a mountain range, one might deduce that the whole world is made up of mountains. Those who rely solely on practice are what Mao termed vulgar "practical men" who

> ... respect experience but despise theory, and therefore cannot have a comprehensive view of an entire objective process, lack clear direction, and long-range perspective, and are complacent over occasional successes and glimpses of the truth. If such persons direct a revolution, they will lead it up a blind alley.[182]

Theory and practice are an unbeatable combination which all successful political movements have utilised. From being dismissed as partiality, practice has witnessed an upsurge and is now considered a superior source of knowledge. The "practical men" have become authorities. All this would point to women gaining ground in contemporary political debates, even having the upper hand in matters regarding the topic of sex, as women experience the oppression of patriarchy first-hand. But as we shall see, the opposite happens.

Cultural appropriation is another term which intellectuals of the underprivileged have wielded with success to refer to a dominant group's assimilation of an oppressed group's culture. James O. Young, author of 'The Ethics of Cultural Appropriation', identifies several types of appropriation: material appropriation, for instance when European museums exhibit stolen artefacts from colonised countries; stylistic appropriation, when European artists emulate the folklore of colonised

---

181 Mao Tse-tung. (1964). *On Practice: On the Relation Between Knowledge and Practice – Between Knowing and Doing*. The Maoist Documentation Project. <https://www.marxists.org/reference/archive/mao/selected-works/volume-1/mswv1_16.htm>.
182 Ibid.

countries; and subject appropriation, "when someone from one culture represents members or aspects of another culture."[183]

Cultural appropriation, CA for short, has perhaps come to be associated with online hordes mocking a white person with dreadlocks, but as Lauren Michele Jackson demonstrates in her essay collection *White Negroes: When Cornrows Were in Vogue and Other Thoughts on Cultural Appropriation*, the term raises serious questions about the transfer of power and capital.[184] An economically underprivileged group is used as a source for creating ideas and resources which then create profit for the dominant group. By way of example, the food chain Taco Bell is owned by white people, as are its European equivalents Taco Bar and Joe Peña's. The majority of cookbooks on Chinese, Indian and Mexican food marketed in Europe are written by white people. Cultural expressions of Black Americans making faces become profitable online memes for someone else. Appropriation is structural and cultural exploitation for profit.

These notions, however, are not allowed to be applied to sex. Suddenly, the entire term bank of intersectionality is no longer valid. The exact same individuals who use these terms in other circumstances, shun them when it comes to sex. When Kendall Jenner posed on the cover of *Vogue* in an afro, she was condemned for 'blackfishing' (appropriating Black people's appearance). Yet when her father Bruce Jenner changed his name to Caitlyn, got breast implants and a vagina, he was named Woman of the Year.

In the case of Kendall Jenner, many Black women pointed out the privilege of appropriation, as this one comment on the *Vogue* Instagram page: "she can wear her VOGUEtastic hair like that to 'work' with only Kardashian listed on her resume [...] Let me walk into work, an interview, meeting, conference, or HR like that with my natural hair." *Vogue* subsequently apologised for the misstep. It would appear to be a parallel case when many women pointed out that when a male Canadian schoolteacher decided to identify as female and come to class wearing massive hanging prosthetic breasts with nipples protruding, this was

---

183 James O. Young. (2000). 'The Ethics of Cultural Appropriation'. *Dalhousie Review*, Vol. 80, No. 3.
184 Lauren Michele Jackson. (2019). *White Negroes: When Cornrows Were in Vogue and Other Thoughts on Cultural Appropriation*. Boston: Beacon Press.

something a woman would not have been allowed to do. Women are constantly told it is our responsibility to dress 'down' in order to appear decent: cover nipples, make sure breasts do not move, beware of upskirts etc. Yet males wearing fetish gear to work is protected under Bill C-16 which prohibits discrimination based on gender identity, and so the school supported the teacher.[185]

Men who transition publicly have become a genre of its own, with Tiktok and Instagram accounts garnering millions of followers who applaud as grown men gradually put on dresses, shave their legs and pretend to adopt 'feminine' movements while using hashtags such as "DayThreeAsAGirl." Dulan Mulvaney is one of them, who despite being an adult male dons clothing appropriate for three-year-old girls and caricatures an extreme stereotype of femininity. One would call it cultural appropriation, but of Dylan's over seven million followers, few say anything of the sort. Most comment how pretty and graceful "she" is. Until slxthkween5.0 came along – a woman who made her own account imitating Dylan. She began posting videos of herself with a fake beard, saying exactly the same things as Dylan did, being a woman who imitates a man who imitates women. Apparently, this twist was not acceptable. Dylan hit back, thundering, "You don't get to mock my identity!" and dozens of articles were written with headlines such as "TikTok Star Dylan Mulvaney Calls Out Transphobic Troll" where some commentators, without catching the irony, claimed that what slxthkween5.0 was doing was cultural appropriation.[186] Being a woman, apparently, is for everyone – being a trans woman is protected territory.

Meredith Talusan writes in *The Guardian* that sex and race cannot be compared: Dolezal's decision to be black was a choice, while a man who decides to become a woman is merely expressing an inner truth about who he – she – is. Talusan argues this is because gender is constant:

> Doctors don't announce our race or color when we are born; they announce our gender. People who are alienated from their presumed gender and define themselves according to another gender have existed

---

185 <https://www.outkick.com/high-school-canada-trans-teacher-prosthetic-chest/>.
186 'TikTok's Dylan Mulvaney Calls Out Transphobic Troll'. *PAPER* (papermag.com). <https://www.papermag.com/dylan-mulvaney-transition-troll-2658218389.html>.

since earliest recorded history; race is a medieval European invention. Thus, Dolezal identified as black, but I *am* a woman, and other trans people *are* the gender they feel themselves to be.[187]

The concept of sex is older than the concept of race – agreed. But why should this mean that it is not possible to change race? Why is sex divided up into two: sex/gender, while age, class and race are whole concepts, where the cultural construct is inseparable from material reality? Philosopher Talia M. Bettcher and gender studies professor Susan Stryker write in an introduction to an anthology about transfeminism that an intersectional analysis demands that the oppressed subject speak for herself and define herself, to then go on to complain that

> … the *New York Times* published an op-ed piece by Elinor Burkett, 'What Makes a Woman?', in which the author, a feminist filmmaker, assumed she was entitled to answer that question in a way that prevented transgender women from being included in her definition.[188]

Oppressed subjects have a right to define themselves, unless they are women. Women should not even be allowed to discuss a definition of their own group. Bettcher and Stryker do not present a counter argument for why this is so, they simply claim that Burkett has no right to hold an opinion on the matter. The phrase "assumed she was entitled to" shows they are shocked that Burkett has the nerve to express an opinion about a group she belongs to. Instead, the authors (both born male) reference trans activist Sylvia Rivera and triumphantly insist that "the women who have tried to fight for their sex changes, or to become women, *are* the women's liberation!"[189]

The problem with intersectionality is thus not its theoretical toolbox, but that women are excluded from using it. Women are not to be granted epistemic privilege regarding their own group. They are also not to use the term male privilege, since this tool has been declared invalid by countless authoritarian gender identity theorists. For instance, Kat Callahan (born male) writes in "Cis Feminists Need to Understand 'Provisional' Male

---

187 Meredith Talusan. (12 June 2015). 'There is no comparison between transgender people and Rachel Dolezal'. *The Guardian*.
188 Talia M. Bettcher and Susan Stryker. (May 2016). 'Introduction: Trans/Feminisms'. *Transgender Studies Quarterly*, Vol. 3. <https://read.dukeupress.edu/tsq/article/3/1-2/5/91824/IntroductionTrans-Feminisms>.
189 Sylvia Rivera. (1973). Quoted in Stryker and Bettcher. Ibid. p. 9.

Privilege": "I have a lot of privilege, and most of it is not related to me being assigned male at birth." He writes that he is white and grew up in a wealthy home but that, "From a very young age, first grade or so, until high school, I had no friends."[190] Callahan writes of how he was teased and bullied as a boy, how he had a basketball thrown in his face and that teachers felt he said the wrong things so it would have been better for him to stay silent. Therefore, writes Callahan, he has "no idea what it's like to be treated as a boy."

Callahan's is a sad and unfortunately all too common tale of bullying and alienation but here it is being used to claim that it makes him less of a man. He is saying that a boy cannot have these experiences – a boy just does not get bullied, is the message, and *if he is bullied then he is not a boy*. One wonders how males can exist at all if manhood is based on throwing basketballs at other males who cease to be male the moment they get the basketball in their faces.

Despite these tenuous connections, the purpose of analyses like Callahan's is to disarm the weapon pointed at him: the term 'privileged'. By wrenching the tool out of women's hands and aiming it at them, he ensures they cannot use it against him and labels them the privileged ones. Thus, women cannot tell him to check his privilege, that he is appropriating their experience, that their knowledge is situated in a way that his isn't. These tools have been rendered ineffective and mute. The terminological apparatus of intersectionality is perfectly suited for use by women but it has been rendered harmless. The minute a man utters the words "No, *I* am the woman here," he has assumed ownership of these terms and they are turned against women.

The process is exemplified by a dispute within the British Labour Party. The party has never had a female leader: there are no rules that state the leader must be a man, yet it ends up being a man every time. To increase the number of female MPs, all-women shortlists were put in force in 1993. Since Labour's adoption of gender identity theory in 2018, anyone identifying as a woman has been eligible for inclusion on the lists: all one has to do is tick the box 'female'. Three hundred women quit the Party in protest, as the new definition meant the shortlists were

---

190 Kat Callahan. (14. July 2013). 'Cis Feminists Need To Understand "Provisional" Male Privilege.' <https://roygbiv.jezebel.com/cis-feminists-need-to-understand-provisional-male-pri-776071122>.

meaningless.[191] In 2022, Labour announced they would scrap the shortlists altogether.[192] In December 2020, Nasdaq stock exchange proposed a similar change to the makeup of the boards of all listed companies, requiring them to have at least one person who identifies as a woman and one who identifies as LGBTQ or is from a minority group. According to the proposal, it is sufficient for the woman to identify as such, "without regard to the individual's designated sex at birth."[193]

These proposals appear to be based on intersectionality, yet women's material reality is not considered important. A truly intersectional analysis would have taken it as a given that women's material reality is the basis for a *specific* oppression, just as specific as that which people from minority groups, Black people and LGBTQ people experience. Intersectionality is about exposing and understanding power structures, yet we are specifically told to ignore the power structure that is built on biological sex.

---

191 Aubrey Allegretti. (1 May 2018.). '300 women to quit Labour to protest all-women shortlist update'. *Sky News*.
192 Alexandra Rogers. (7 March 2022). 'Exclusive: Labour Drops All-Women Shortlists For Next General Election'. *HuffPost UK*. <https://www.huffingtonpost.co.uk/entry/labour-drops-use-of-all-women-shortlists-general-election-legal-advice-unlawful_uk_622226fbe4b03bc49a9a2420>.
193 <https://listingcenter.nasdaq.com/assets/RuleBook/Nasdaq/filings/SR-NASDAQ-2020-081.pdf>.

CHAPTER 39

Nature/Nurture – A Dialectical View

Let us go back to Catharine MacKinnon's words from the beginning of this book:

> My particular question was OF WHAT is sex socially constructed? The answer I gave, and still believe, is sexuality. Sexuality is itself not biological, but social, so the constructing is also the constructed, which makes sense since there is no place outside society.[194]

MacKinnon is definitely on to something here and she differs from queer theorists like Judith Butler, who seldom discuss sex-based hierarchies, in that her focus is on power and oppression.

Yet to contend that sexuality is the foundation of biological sex is akin to saying that money is the foundation of the class system – a catastrophic conflation of cause and effect. Sexual hierarchy is certainly one measure of power relations between the sexes, just as money can be a measure of class differences. However, one must go further and inquire *why* different classes have different amounts of money. The answer to this is that they have different roles in production. Similarly, we must ask why the sexes are on different rungs in the sexual hierarchy. The answer is that they have different roles in reproduction. Thus *reproduction*, and not sexuality, is the foundation of biological sex just as production is the foundation of the class system. Reproduction dictates the existence of two sexes, yet this in itself does not entail inequality: it is the *organisation* of reproduction which

---

194 Cristan Williams. (27 November 2015). 'Sex, gender, and sexuality. An interview with Catharine A. MacKinnon'. *The Conversations Project*.

determines whether inequalities exist or not, just as it is the *organisation* of production that determines whether a class system results and what divisions it comprises.

Dialectical materialism facilitates an analysis which acknowledges *both* material reality *and* socially constructed inequalities. Biological determinists, who believe that everything depends on nature and the brain, and social constructivists, who believe everything is culture and discourse, in fact share the same metaphysical worldview. As both theories are static and do not allow for movement, both actually imply that nothing can change. If everything is nature, there is no way out and if everything is culture, there is no way in. Those who claim nature determines everything are unable to answer the question: where do we go from here? And those who claim culture is king cannot answer the question: why did *we* end up *here*? For the former, life is set in stone, while for the latter it is floating at sea without a compass. Neither theory offers tools to change reality or assists us in understanding why things change. MacKinnon's assertion that "there is no place outside society" is a claustrophobic theory essentially lacking in hope. In it, women do not even exist outside patriarchy. We are created by that which we hate, sexuality is an eternal power structure with man on top and woman on the bottom and the definition of woman is she who finds herself on the bottom. According to MacKinnon, "to be a woman one does have to live women's status. Transwomen are living it, and in my experience bring a valuable perspective on it as well."[195] The second half of the statement can be true in some instances – people who transition occupy a position which affords them a unique insight into the differences between sex and gender and how women and men are treated. Yet the question remains: what is sex if we completely disregard biology? MacKinnon argues that a woman is, by definition, subordinate and that there is nothing beyond this. With such a definition, how can any change be brought about?

Dialectical materialism acknowledges the existence of the natural, a place which is independent of human society and language. Pregnancy is a material and biological fact resulting in a child being born nine months after fertilisation, regardless of how this is interpreted or understood in language and culture. It is not possible to think or talk this fact out of

---

195 Ibid.

existence – it will happen all the same. Nor is it possible for a biological man to become pregnant, regardless of how much gender roles change. We could create a world without words for the sexes, or one in which women have all the power and kill their lovers like praying mantises, or one in which men are expected to only fall in love with other men – men would still not be able to become pregnant.

In itself, this is not a controversial statement, unless one is a biological determinist. Only for biological determinists does a particular social order follow from a set of biological facts. Those who accept the premise of biological determinism – that gender roles necessarily follow from biological sex – find themselves in the position of having to deny the existence of biological sex in order to reject gender roles. This results in a position completely divorced from reality, in which our bodies become frightening and dangerous and must be ignored, as though it were our bodies that were reactionary – which of course is precisely what biological determinists believe.

A dialectical materialist, on the other hand, is capable of seeing biological sex as a reality without getting shaky. The fact that women can give birth and men cannot is so elemental that it in itself makes living conditions between the sexes fundamentally different. Regardless of the structure a society has, certain consequences exist as a result of biological sex. Women's bodies tell them when they are going to be mothers, while men become aware that they are going to be fathers when a woman informs them. No mother can doubt her motherhood, while a father can never be fully sure. Men can abandon a foetus by walking out the door, women require a doctor and abortion rights. Men can have hundreds of babies a month, women can have one baby a year. Becoming a mother involves physical pain, becoming a father does not. Being a mother alters one's body, being a father does not. Women can feed babies with their bodies, men cannot. Women bleed every month, men do not. A penis can injure a vagina, a vagina cannot injure a penis, unless it has a tight foreskin.

Yet nature alone does not create societies. Nature interacts with power structures to create what we call culture. A dialectical worldview takes into account objective facts, but unlike a metaphysical stance, it does not believe that biology is destiny. On the contrary, it is in the meeting of nature and culture that we find the most precise answers. The dialectic between nature and culture is expressed in the terms sex and gender. Yet it is not possible to claim gender is completely independent from sex, as culture is not independent from nature: the dialectic means there is a link, a communication, as both affect one another. Yvonne Hirdman notes that biology

> does not in itself lead to male supremacy. Biology does not create the male norm. Therefore, stating that something is "natural" does not mean that one must accept a series of consequences as a given, for instance that women must be tied to the home, concern themselves with small things, etc ...[196]

No societies exist in which women do not menstruate but *the way in which societies deal with menstruation* varies massively. In patrilineal societies menstruation is taboo. In matrilineal ones, celebrations are organised when girls have their first period, yet both patrilineal and matrilineal societies have developed from the same biological facts. It is possible to imagine both a society in which those who give birth rule and one in which those who inseminate do. It is also possible to imagine egalitarian societies. Yet if we are to understand why matrilineal societies seldom become matriarchies, a simple answer is that it is not necessary for a woman to lock up a man and deprive him of his freedom in order to be certain that a child is hers. She can transfer her religion and property to her children without needing to control her husband.

Patrilineal systems with private ownership of property have, on the contrary, tended to result in patriarchy and sexual oppression of women. As ecofeminist Elisabeth Hermodsson notes, "in order to be certain of fatherhood, man must control woman's sexuality [...] In order to be certain of motherhood, on the other hand, it is not necessary for man's sexuality to be controlled. Motherhood is a self-evident reality."[197] Systems for limiting women's sexuality seem to only have developed in patrilineal societies in which property is also privately owned. These systems – female genital mutilation, footbinding, clothing which conceals the female body, taboos around women leaving the house unaccompanied – have then developed into cultural features with a life of their own. It is these symbols of oppression which we today refer to as gender and gender

---

[196] Yvonne Hirdman. (2001). *Genus – om det stabilas föränderliga former*, p. 83. Stockholm: Liber.
[197] Elisabeth Hermodsson. (1999). 'Det tillåtna modersmordet'. In *Någonting annat har funnits*, p. 104. Ed. Birgitta Onsell. Stockholm: Carlsson Publishers.

roles. Sexually loaded terms like 'bastard child', virgin and promiscuous are therefore meaningless when decoupled from their roots in the organisation of reproduction, since it is woman who gives birth and thereby channels male inheritance and surname from father to son. She bears the cultural burden of sexuality precisely due to the lethal mixture of biology and patriarchy; of being the one who gives birth and thereby the one who the result of sexual intercourse stays with, while the man leaves it behind, while at the same time not having the power to decide anything about the offspring. Carrying the future but not having a say about it, such is woman's predicament under patriarchy. It is the most illogical of power relations, as it is the one who *has* who per se *doesn't have*. Yet if she didn't have, would there be a reason to oppress her? Isn't this the secret of all oppression: Africa was colonised and made poor because it had an abundance of wealth, not the opposite; the working class is exploited because it creates wealth, not because it doesn't, and animals are being chained and slaughtered because they are a source of nutrition, not because they are worthless. MacKinnon's disconnection of reproduction from sexuality and her claim that sexuality has a life of its own and creates oppression independently of other factors, renders the issue ahistorical and therefore without a solution.

A dialectical materialist approach, with terms like base and superstructure in its toolbox, is able to see how gender identity theory is emerging as the superstructure of contemporary patriarchal sexuality. Gender identity theory has become hegemonic precisely because it reflects the shifting baselines of male supremacy. The hard side: male domination of politics, sports, sexuality, public space and online debate, is perpetuated, while any possible resistance to this posed by the women's movement is disarmed by the dissolution of the category of woman. Males are perpetuated, females dissolved.

CHAPTER 40

Notes on the Word 'Woman'

Imagine that one did not know what 'woman' meant and carried out a search for the word in historical archives. Two points would soon be clear: 'woman' is a word used by men and it refers to something they do not hold in particularly high regard.

Under patriarchy, the word woman has belonged to men. From antiquity to the end of the 19th century, the word appears mainly with negative connotations: woman is a sinner, subordinate or a non-person. She first appears in the Old Testament as a support and comfort to man, called woman "for she was taken out of man," to then be punished and ordered to obey man. She is then erased from history in the long lists in which men are said to have "begat" sons on their own: Abraham begat Isaac; and Isaac begat Jacob; and Jacob begat Judas and his brethren ... The Rig Veda states her "intellect hath little weight" and that "hearts of hyenas are the hearts of women," and she is expressly forbidden from participating in ancient Greek rituals.[198] For Aristotle, woman is a "deformed" man, for Thomas Aquinas, a mistake and for Martin Luther, a creature who ought to keep seated on account of her wide hips. For Balzac, she is an appendage to and property of man, for Proudhon she is morally and intellectually inferior to the extent that she is worth 8/27 of the stronger sex, i.e. the male, as de Beauvoir has noted.[199]

---

198 Rig Veda 8:33:17 and 10:95:15; Marble slab on Thasos dated 450–425 BC.
199 <https://archive.org/stream/1949SimoneDeBeauvoirTheSecondSex/1949_simone-de-beauvoir-the-second-sex_djvu.txt see page 162>.

It is revealing, although more than a little disheartening, to search for the word woman in historical and classical texts. One very seldom finds a neutral, let alone positive, reference to her. Man after man – scientists, religious leaders, politicians – explain what a woman is and where her place ought to be. For a female reader, the weight of this several thousand years of history, long before capitalism and industrialisation, is palpably depressing in its effect.

Yet at the end of the 1700s, something happened.

Women began, in increasing numbers, reclaiming the word woman.

In 1761, Swedish author Hedvig Charlotta Nordenflycht wrote *Fruentimrets försvar* (In Defence of Women), and Mary Wollstonecraft's *A Vindication of the Rights of Woman* appeared in 1792. In the first half of the 19th century, Sojourner Truth went on a speaking tour across the United States, explaining that "As for intellect, all I can say is, if a woman have a pint, and a man a quart – why can't she have her little pint full?"[200] European authors Fredrika Bremer and Jane Austen described women's situation in novels and the first international women's congress was organised by French author Maria Deraismes in 1878. Woman after woman spoke out and what their declarations had in common was the announcement that what men had said about them for thousands of years was untrue. Men began to join the cause and Marquis de Condorcet in France and Qasim Amin in Egypt spoke out in favour of equality between the sexes.

At this point, the press started to fill up with news of women's congresses, organisations for women's suffrage, parades for women and women publicists. At the beginning of the 1900s, the word woman often appeared in relation to the suffrage movement. In the late 1900s and early 2000s, women's use of the word woman went through the roof. It is now rare to see the word used in a derogatory context outside citations of historical texts or to show a view different to that of the writer. The word woman has acquired a new meaning: it has gone from referring to an inferior being to denoting an oppressed political subject with the right to revolt. 'Woman' has become a group which does not merely exist *in itself*, but also *for itself*. (A social class which exists *in itself* has shared living conditions and a shared position but is not aware of this, while a group which exists *for itself* is aware of its own existence and living conditions

---

200 <https://www.learningforjustice.org/classroom-resources/texts/aint-i-a-woman>.

and organises politically.) The word woman became powerful, pulsating with the force of a class which is rising from several thousand years of servitude, knows its value, knows the way and knows the enemy. At the end of the 20th century, the word woman no longer belonged to patriarchy – it belonged to women.

When a tool no longer works, it is usually discarded. The word woman has, at the beginning of the 21st century, become not only an inoperable tool for patriarchy, but a dangerous one, since it has ended up in the hands of the resistance. It follows that the word must be rendered harmless.

By means of fragmenting the word, picking it apart and chopping it into pieces, reducing it to body parts, making it mean its very opposite, adding prefixes, labelling it problematic, defaming those who use it and questioning its right to exist, a linguistic war is now being waged. Its purpose is to preclude reference to, and existence of, women as political subjects. This war is not the result of a conscious conspiracy – it is an organic process which reinstates the lost power of male supremacy and it would not be possible to effect were it not interpreted as a progressive struggle. In the collective consciousness, progress, human rights and inclusion have come to be synonymous with abolishing the word woman. This has very little to do with the 'trans' issue. Trans people have ended up as pawns in the justification of a neo patriarchal backlash which is pulling the rug out from under the women's movement by eliminating its most central term.

Without the word woman, it is difficult for a women's movement to exist. Without the word woman, it is difficult to think and talk about women's situation. Without the word woman, it is impossible to understand the oppression of women.

Yet removing the word woman does not rid us of women's oppression. Women will continue to become pregnant and give birth. Women will continue to carry out the majority of all reproductive work on the planet and to own less than one per cent of its resources; we will continue to be the majority of victims of sexual offences and domestic violence; we will continue to be discriminated against in the workplace; we will continue to be sidelined and ignored in medical research; we will continue to be ridiculed and hated if we attempt to reach power; we will continue to love more and get less in return; we will continue to be drained economically, physically, sexually, emotionally.

We will just not be able to understand it or explain it. We will not know what to say. When we attempt to fight for our rights we will notice that our category has vanished. "The number you have dialled has been disconnected or is no longer in service. Please check the number."

References

4th Wave Now. (19 February 2016). 'The trans-kid honeymoon is sweet – while it lasts'.
AbbVie News Center. (20 April 2016). 'AbbVie, University of Chicago collaborate to advance cancer research'.
Al-Sibai, Noor. (6 March 2017). 'How to acknowledge your privilege at The Women's Strike'. *Bustle*.
Allegretti, Aubrey. (1 May 2018.). '300 women to quit Labour to protest all-women shortlist update'. *Sky News*.
Arcelus, Jon, Walter Pierre Bouman, Emma Haycraft and Alice Bethany Jones. (2017). 'Sport and transgender people. A systematic review of the literature relating to sport participation and competitive sport policies'. *Sports Medicine*. Vol. 47, No. 4.
Badshah, Nadeem. (7 October 2021). 'University defends "academic freedoms" after calls to sack professor'. *The Guardian*.
Baines, Camille. (21 March 2019). 'Trans woman hopes funding cut will send message to Vancouver rape crisis group'. *The Canadian Press*.
Baird, Vanessa. (1 October 2015). 'The trans revolution'. *The New Internationalist*.
Bannerman, Lucy. (20 November 2017). 'Trans teenager Lily Madigan voted in as a Labour women's officer'. *The Times*.
Barnes, Katie. (18 March 2022). 'Amid protests, Penn swimmer Lia Thomas becomes first known transgender athlete to win Division 1 national championship'. *ESPN*.
Barredo, Àlex. (25 November 2017). 'Tumblr is Tumbling'. <https://hackernoon.com/tumblr-is-tumbling-d6deb3bb831e>.
Barrett, James. (20 August 2015). Written evidence submitted by British Association of Gender Identity Specialists to the Transgender Equality Inquiry.
Bartter, Isabelle. (12 March 2019). 'Trans athletes won't be sidelined by bigotry'. *Socialist Worker*.

Batty, David. (30 July 2004.). 'Sex changes are not effective, say researchers'. *The Guardian.*

BBC News. (26 September 2018). 'Woman billboard removed after transphobia row'.

BBC. (22 May 2019). 'Twitter-ban feminist defends transgender views ahead of Holyrood meeting'.

Bermon, Stephane, David J. Handelsman and Angelica L. Hirschberg. (October 2018). 'Circulating testosterone as the hormonal basis of sex differences in athletic performance'. *Endocrine Reviews.* Vol. 39, No. 5.

Bermon, Stephane, David J. Handelsman, and Angelica L. Hirschberg. (October 2018). 'Circulating testosterone as the hormonal basis of sex differences in athletic performance'. *Endocrine Reviews.* Vol. 39. No. 5, pp. 803–829.

Bettcher, Talia M. and Susan Stryker. (May 2016). 'Introduction: Trans/Feminisms'. *Transgender Studies Quarterly.* Vol. 3. <https://read.dukeupress.edu/tsq/article/3/1-2/5/91824/IntroductionTrans-Feminisms>.

Bevan, Thomas E. (2017). *Being Transgender: What You Should Know.* Westport, Connecticut: Praeger.

Biggs, Michael. (2019). 'Britain's experiment with puberty blockers'. In Michele Moore and Heather Brunskell-Evans (eds). *Inventing Transgender Children and Young People.* Newcastle upon Tyne: Cambridge Scholars Publishing.

Biggs, Michael. (July 2019). 'The Tavistock's experiment with puberty blockers'. Oxford University.

Bilek, Jennifer. (20 February 2018). 'Who Are the Rich White Men Institutionalizing Transgender Ideology?'. *The Federalist.* <https://thefederalist.com/2018/02/20/rich-white-men-institutionalizing-transgender-ideology/>.

Bindel, Julie. (9 June 2019). 'The man in a skirt called me a Nazi – then attacked'. *TheTimes.*<https://www.thetimes.co.uk/article/julie-bindel-the-man-in-a-skirt-called-me-a-nazi-then-attacked-8dfwk8jft?_ga=2.157655866.1864798478.1560328713-723508512.1560328712>.

Bird, Jackson. (24 September 2019). 'A trans guy on adjusting to men's bathroom culture'.

BJJ World. (21 October 2018). 'Transgender MMA fighter breaks skull of her female opponent. Are we becoming too careful not to offend any group of people?'. <https://bjj-world.com/transgender-mma-fighter-fallon-fox-breaks-skull-of-her-female-opponent/>.

Borrell, Brie. (17 January 2019). 'Trans age: The reality'. *The Pawprint.*

Bowcott, Owen. (18 December 2019). 'Judge rules against researcher who lost job over transgender tweets'. *The Guardian.*

Bränström, Richard and John Pachankis. (2019). 'Reduction in mental health treatment utilization among transgender individuals after gender-affirming surgeries. A total population study'. *American Journal of Psychiatry.* <https://doi.org/10.1176/appi.ajp.2020.1778correction>.

Bränström, Richard and John Pachankis. (2020). 'Correction to Bränström and Pachankis'. *American Journal of Psychiatry*. Vol. 177, No. 8, p. 734. <https://doi.org/10.1176/appi.ajp.2020.1778correction>.
Brean, Joseph. (2 August 2018). 'Forced to share a room with transgender woman in Toronto shelter, sex abuse victim files human rights complaint'. *National Post*.
Brill, Stephanie and Rachel Pepper. (2008). *The Transgender Child: A Handbook for Families and Professionals*. Jersey City, New Jersey: Cleis Press.
Brill, Stephanie and Lisa Kenney. (2016). *The Transgender Teen: A Handbook for Parents and Professionals Supporting Transgender and Non-Binary Teens*. Jersey City: Cleis Press.
British Association for Counselling and Psychotherapy. (2017). 'Good practice across the counselling professions 001'. *Gender, Sexual, and Relationship Diversity* (GSRD).
Brynn Jones, Kelsie. (2 August 2014). 'Trans-exclusionary radical feminism. What exactly is it, and why does it hurt?' *Huffington Post*.
Bunck, M. C. and L. J. Gooren. (2004). 'Transsexuals and competitive sports'. *European Journal of Endocrinology*. Vol. 151, No. 4.
Bunim, Juliana. (17 August 2015). 'First U.S. study of transgender youth funded by NIH'. University of California.
Butler, Judith. (1991). *Gender Trouble: Feminism and the Subversion of Identity*. London: Routledge.
Byne, William, S. Tobet, L. A. Mattiace, M. S. Lasco, E. Kemether, M. A. Edgar. S. Morgello, M.S. Buchsbaum and L. B. Jones. (September 2001). 'The interstitial nuclei of the human anterior hypothalamus: an investigation of variation with sex, sexual orientation, and HIV status'. *Hormones and Behaviour*. Vol. 40, No. 2, pp. 86–92. See also <https://www.scientificamerican.com/article/massive-study-finds-no-single-genetic-cause-of-same-sex-sexual-behavior/>.
Byron, Paul and Brady Robards. (29 May 2017). 'There's something queer about Tumblr'. *The Conversation*. <http://theconversation.com/theres-something-queer-about-tumblr-73520>.
Callahan, Carey Maria Catt. (2018). 'Unheard voices of detransitioners"'. In Michele Moore and Heather Brunskell-Evans (eds). *Inventing Transgender Children and Young People*. Newcastle upon Tyne: Cambridge Scholars.
Callahan, Kat. (14. July 2013). 'Cis Feminists Need To Understand "Provisional" Male Privilege'. <https://roygbiv.jezebel.com/cis-feminists-need-to-understand-provisional-male-pri-776071122>.
Cambridge Judge Business School. 'Pre-school Activities Inventory (PSAI)' <https://www.psychometrics.cam.ac.uk/services/psychometric-tests/psai>.
Case, Laura K., David Brang, Rosalynn Landazuri, Pavitra Viswanathan and Vilayanur S. Ramachandran. (July 2017). 'Altered white matter and sensory response to bodily sensation in female-to-male transgender individuals'. *Archives of Sexual Behavior*. Vol. 46, No. 5, pp. 1223–1237.

Case, Stephanie. (9 May 2019). 'Western States Has New Rules for Transgender Athletes'. *Outside Online*.

Cashmore, Ellis. (29 June 2021). 'Will transgender athletes bring the end of women's sport as we know it?' *Fair Observer*. <https://www.fairobserver.com/culture/ellis-cashmore-transgender-athletes-womens-sport-gender-inequality-news-53621/>.

Cass, Hilary. (February 2022). 'Independent Review of Gender Identity Services for Children and Young People'. Interim report.

Centre for Reproductive Rights. (29 November 2021). 'The Disproportionate Harm of Abortion Bans: Spotlight on Dobbs vs Jackson Women's Health'. <https://reproductiverights.org/supreme-court-case-mississippi-abortion-ban-disproportionate-harm/>.

Chilton, Louis. (19 September 2020). 'Boycotting Hogwarts Legacy over JK Rowling's transgender comments won't achieve much – but it's no surprise fans are considering it'. *Independent*. <https://www.independent.co.uk/arts-entertainment/games/feature/hogwarts-legacy-jk-rowling-harry-potter-boycott-transphobia-b485188.html>.

Chisholm, Jamiyla. (11 December 2019). '170 incarcerated transgender women sue Colorado corrections for discrimination'. *Colorlines*.

ClydeFallon. (n.d). *Reddit*. Forum post. <https://www.reddit.com/r/detrans/comments/wt41ya/my_life_was_destroyed_with_15_years_old_im_17_now/>.

Cohen-Kettenis, Peggy, Henriette Delemarre-van de Waal et al. (July 2019). 'The treatment of adolescent transsexuals. Changing insights'. *The Journal of Sexual Medicine*. Vol. 5, pp. 1892–1897.

Cohen, Jodi H. and Tamar Z. Semerjian. (2008). 'The collision of trans-experience and the politics of women's ice hockey'. *International Journal of Transgenderism*. Vol. 10.

Conley-Keck, Ethan. (7 April 2019). 'Pritzker changes state's Medicaid policy to cover sex reassignment surgery' WQAD-TV.

Cortes, Laura R., Carla D. Cisternas and Nancy G. Forger. (2019). 'Does Gender Leave an Epigenetic Imprint on the Brain?'. *Frontiers in Neuroscience*. Vol. 13. <doi: 10.3389/fnins.2019.00173>.

Cristofari, S., B. Bertrand, S. Leuzzi, K. Rem, J. Rausky, M. Revol, M. Atlan and A. Stivala. (February 2019). 'Postoperative complications of male to female sex reassignment surgery. A 10-year French retrospective study'. *Annales de Chirurgie Plastique et Esthétique*. Vol. 64, No. 1, pp. 24–32. <doi: 10.1016/j.anplas.2018.08.002. E-pub. 27 September 2018>.

Daly, Mary. (1979). *Gyn/Ecology, The Metaethics of Radical Feminism*. London: The Women's Press.

de Beauvoir, Simone. (2009). *The Second Sex*. Translated by Constance Borde and Sheila Malovany-Chevallier. New York: Vintage.

De Cuypere, Griet, Gail Knudson and Jamison Green. (31 May 2013.) 'Wpath Consensus Process Regarding Transgender and Transsexual-related Diagnoses in ICD-11'. *World Professional Association for Transgender Health*.

de Vries, Annelou L. C., Jennifer K. McGuire, Thomas D. Steensma, Eva C.F. Wagenaar, Theo A. H. Doreleijers and Peggy T. Cohen-Ketteris. (October 2014). 'Young adult psychological outcome after puberty suppression and gender reassignment'. *Pediatrics*. Vol. 134, No. 4.

de Vries, Annelou L. C. (October 2020). 'Challenges in timing puberty suppression for gender-nonconforming adolescents'. *Pediatrics*. Vol. 146, No. 4. <e2020010611; DOI: 10.1542/peds.2020-010611>.

Dessens, Arianne B., Froukje M. Slijper and Stenvert L. S. Drop. (August 2005). 'Gender dysphoria and gender change in chromosomal females with congenital adrenal hyperplasia'. *Archives of Sexual Behavior*. Vol. 34, No. 4, pp. 389–397. <https://pubmed.ncbi.nlm.nih.gov/16010462/>.

Dhejne, Cecilia, Paul Lichtenstein, Marcus Boman, Anna L.V. Johansson, Niklas Långström and Mikael Landén. (22 February 2011). 'Long-term follow-up of transsexual persons undergoing sex reassignment surgery. Cohort study in Sweden'. <https://doi.org/10.1371/journal.pone.0016885 2011>.

Dinno, Alexis. (September 2017). 'Homicide rates of transgender individuals in the United States: 2010–2014'. *American Journal of Public Health*. Vol. 107, No. 9, pp. 1441–1447.

Donelly, Laura. (12 December 2019). 'Children's transgender clinic hit by 35 resignations in three years as psychologists warn of gender dysphoria overdiagnoses'. *The Telegraph*.

Drager, Harsin. (2012). 'Transforming cyber space and the trans liberation movement. A study of transmasculine youth bloggers on Tumblr.com'. Undergraduate Honors Thesis. Boulder: University of Colorado. <https://scholar.colorado.edu/concern/undergraduate_honors_theses/v979v348j>.

Dreier, Fred. (18 October 2018). 'Commentary: The complicated case of transgender cyclist Dr Rachel McKinnon'. *VeloNews*.

Drummond, Kelley D., Susan J. Bradley, Michele Peterson-Badali and Kenneth J. Zucker. (2008). 'A follow-up study of girls with gender identity disorder'. *Developmental Psychology*. Vol. 44, No. 1, pp. 34-45.

Durosomo, Damola. (n.d.). 'Chimamanda Ngozi Adichie Continues to Defend Her Comments on Trans Women During D.C. Appearance'. *OkayAfrica*.

Edenheim, Sara and Malin Rönnblom. (2016).'Representations of equality. Processes of depoliticization of the citizen-subject.' In Hilde Danielsen, Kari Jegerstedt, Ragnhild L. Muriaas and Brita Ytre-Arne (eds). *Gendered Citizenship and the Politics of Representation*. Basingstoke: Palgrave Macmillan.

Ehrensaft, Diane. (n.d.). Ph.D. 'Curriculum vitae'. <https://files.eqcf.org/wp-content/uploads/2016/09/35-Doe-MPI-UNDER-SEAL.pdf>.

Ehrensaft, Diane. (2016). *The Gender Creative Child*. New York: Workman Publishing.

Ehrensaft, Diane. (January 2009). 'One pill makes you a boy, one pill makes you a girl'. *International Journal of Applied Psychoanalytic Studies*. Vol. 6, No. 1.

Ellison, Jessie. (24 December 2012). 'For transgender youth, a home on Tumblr'. *The Daily Dot*.

Engels, Friedrich. (1982). 'The Development of Socialism from Utopia to Science'. Translated from German for *The People*, official journal of the Socialist Labor Party of America by Daniel De Leon. p. 10. <http://www.slp.org/pdf/marx/dev_soc.pdf>.

Ennis, Dawn. (7 June 2019). 'Trans powerlifter smashes records and draws backlash'. *Outsports*.

Errasti, José and Marino Pérez Álvarez. (2022). *Nadie nace en un cuerpo equivocado*. Bilbao: Deusto Publicaciones.

Ettner, Frederic M. (26 April 2018). 'Primary Care for the Transgender and Gender Non-Conforming Patient'. <https://doi.org/10.1016/j.cps.2018.03.001>.

Fairbairn, Catherine, Douglas Pyper and Baky Balogun. (February 18 2022). 'Gender Recognition Act Reform: consultation and outcome'. (Research Briefing). House of Commons Library. <https://commonslibrary.parliament.uk/research-briefings/cbp-9079/>.

FDA Adverse Advents Reporting System: Lupron (P), Lupron Depot-Ped (P). (30 June 2019). <https://fis.fda.gov/sense/app/d10be6bb-494e-4cd2-82e4-0135608ddc13/sheet/45beeb74-30ab-46be-8267-5756582633b4/state/analysis>.

Fehr, Tristan. (2020). 'Essentially a Lie: Challenging Biological Essentialist Interpretations of Transgender Neurology'. In Louie Dean Valencia-García (ed). *Far-Right Revisionism and the End of History: Alt/Histories*. London: Routledge.

Feinberg, Leslie. (1996). *Transgender Warriors: Making History from Joan of Arc to RuPaul*. Boston: Beacon Press.

Finch, Sam Dylan. (29 February 2016). '130+ examples of cis privilege in all areas of life for you to reflect on and address'. <https://everydayfeminism.com/2016/02/130-examples-cis-privilege/>.

Fine, Cordelia. (2017). *Testosterone Rex: Myths of Sex, Science and Society*. London: Icon Books.

Finlayson, Lorna, Katharine Jenkins and Rosie Worsdale. (17 October 2018). '"I'm not a transphobic, but …": A feminist case against the feminist case against trans inclusivity'. *Verso Books Blog*. <https://www.versobooks.com/blogs/4090-i-m-not-transphobic-but-a-feminist-case-against-the-feminist-case-against-trans-inclusivity>.

Fischer, Nadia. (n.d.). 'What is inclusive Language? And why should I care?' <https://www.witty.works/en/blog/post/what-is-inclusive-language>.

GenderGP. (17 January 2019). 'Treating Trans Youth with Dr Johanna Olson-Kennedy'. *The GenderGP Podcast*. <https://www.gendergp.com/gender-affirmative-johanna-olson-kennedy/>.

Georgas, K., U. Beckman, I. Bryman, A. Elander, L. Jivegård, E. Mattelin, T. Olsen Ekerhult, J. Persson, L. Sandman, G. Selvaggi, I. Stadig, U. Vikberg Adania and A. Strandell. (2018). Health Technology Assessment. 'Gender affirmation surgery for gender dysphoria – effects and risks'. *HTA report*, Västra Götalandsregionen Sahlgrenska Universitetsjukhuset.

Gershoni, Moran and Shmuel Pietrokovski. (2017). 'The landscape of sex-differential transcriptome and its consequent selection in human adults'. *BMC Biology.* Vol. 15, No. 7.

Gliske, Stephen V. (2 December 2019). 'A new theory of gender dysphoria incorporating the distress, social behavioral and body-ownership networks'. *eNeuro.* Vol. 6, No. 6. <https://doi.org/10.1523/ENEURO.0183-19.2019>.

Global Market Insights. (March 2020). 'Sex reassignment surgery market size by gender transition (Male to Female [Facial, Breast, Genitals], Female to Male [Facial, Chest, Genitals], Industry Analysis Report, Regional Outlook, Application Potential, Price Trends, Competitive market share and forecast, 2020–2026'.

Gómez-Gil, Esther, Isabel Esteva, Rocío Carrasco, M. Cruz Almaraz, Eduardo Pasaro, Manel Salamero and Antonio Guillamon. (2011). 'Birth order and ratio of brothers to sisters in Spanish transsexuals'. *Archives of Sexual Behavior.* Vol. 40, pp. 505–510. <https://doi.org/10.1007/s10508-010-9614-3>.

Greer, Germaine. (1999/2007). *The Whole Woman.* London: Black Swan.

Gregory, Andrew. (29 July 2022). 'NHS to close Tavistock gender identity clinic for children'. *The Guardian.* <https://www.theguardian.com/society/2022/jul/28/nhs-closing-down-london-gender-identity-clinic-for-children>.

Groneman, Carol. (1995). 'Nymphomania. The historical construction of female sexuality'. In Jennifer Terry and Jacqueline L. Urla. *Deviant Bodies: Critical Perspectives on Difference in Science and Popular Culture.* Bloomington: Indiana University Press.

Guillamon, Antonio, Carme Junque and Esther Gómez-Gil. (2016). 'A review of the status of brain structure research in transsexualism'. *Archives of Sexual Behavior.* Vol. 45, No. 7, pp. 1615–1648. <https://doi.org/10.1007/s10508-016-0768-5>.

Haimson, Oliver L. and Gillian R. Hayes. (2017). 'Changes in social media affect, disclosure, and sociality for a sample of transgender Americans in 2016's political climate'. Department of Informatics. Irvine: University of California Press.

Halley, April. (12 October 2019). 'Male-bodied rapists are being imprisoned with women. Why do so few people care?' *Quillette.com.*

Hargie, Owen D. W., David H. Mitchell and Ian J. A. Somerville. (22 April 2015). 'People have a knack of making you feel excluded if they catch on to your difference. Transgender experiences of exclusion in sport'. *International Review for the Sociology of Sport.* Vol. 52, No. 2.

Head, Honor. (2017). *Understanding Transgender.* London: Watts Publishing Group.

Helena. (20 March 2019). 'Tumblr: A call-out post'. *4th Wave Now.* <https://4thwavenow.com/2019/03/20/tumblr-a-call-out-post/>

Herthel, Jessica and Jazz Jennings. (2014). *Dial Books for Young Readers.* New York: Penguin Group.

Hoffman, Joanna. (19 February 2019). 'Athlete Ally: Navratilova's Statements Transphobic and Counter to our Work, Vision and Values'. *Athlete Ally.* <https://www.athleteally.org/navratilovas-statements-transphobic-counter-to-our-work-vision/>.

Hough, D. et al. (2017). 'Spatial memory is impaired by peripubertal GnRH agonist treatment and testosterone replacement in sheep'. *Psychoneuroendocrinology.* Vol. 75, pp. 173–182.

Human Rights Campaign. (21 March 2019). 'Violence against the transgender community in 2017'. WWSB: 'Transgender woman admits shooting, killing transgender wife'.

Hungerford, Elizabeth. (2016). 'Female erasure, reverse sexism, and the cisgender theory of privilege'. In Ruth Barrett (ed). *Female Erasure: What You Need to Know About Gender Politics' War on Women, the Female Sex and Human Rights.* California: Tidal Time Publishing.

IGLYO (The International Lesbian, Gay, Bisexual, Transgender, Queer & Intersex Youth & Student Organisation). (2018). 'Annual Report'. <https://www.iglyo.com/wp-content/uploads/2018/09/Board-Applications-2018.pdf>.

IGLYO, Dentons, Thomson Reuters Foundation and Nextlaw. (November 2019). 'Only adults? Good practices in legal gender recognition for youth. A report on the current state of laws and NGO advocacy in eight countries in Europe, with a focus on rights of young people'.

International Olympic Committee. (16 November 2021). 'IOC Framework on Fairness, Inclusion and Non-Discrimination on the Basis of Gender Identity and Sex Variations'.

Irwig, M. S. (September 2018). 'Cardiovascular health in transgender people'. *Reviews in Endocrine and Metabolic Disorders.* Vol. 19, No. 3, pp. 243–251. <doi:10.1007/s11154-018-9454-3>.

Izaakson, Jen. (27 April 2018). 'Trans-identified male, Tara Wolf, convicted of assault after Hyde Park attack'. *Feminist Current.*

Jackson, Lauren Michele. (2019). *White Negroes: When Cornrows Were in Vogue and Other Thoughts on Cultural Appropriation.* Boston: Beacon Press.

Jeffreys, Sheila. (2014). *Gender Hurts: A Feminist Analysis of the Politics of Transgenderism.* London: Routledge.

Jewett, Christina. (2 February 2017). 'Drug used to halt puberty in children may cause lasting health problems'. *Statnews.*

Joel, Daphna, Zohar Berman and Ido Tavor. (15 December 2015). 'Sex beyond the genitalia. The human brain mosaic'. Proceedings of the National Academy of Sciences. <http://www.pnas.org/content/112/50/15468.abstract>.

Jones, Owen. (15 December 2017). 'Anti-trans zealots, know this: history will judge you'. *The Guardian*.

Joyce, Helen. (25 July 2019). 'A Canadian human rights spectacle exposes the risks of unfettered gender self-ID'. *Quillette.com*.

Kashino, Marisa M. (27 January 2021). 'The True Story of Jess Krug, the White Professor Who Posed as Black for Years – Until It All Blew Up Last Fall'. *Washingtonian*. <https://www.washingtonian.com/2021/01/27/the-true-story-of-jessica-krug-the-white-professor-who-posed-as-black-for-years-until-it-all-blew-up-last-fall/>.

Kearns, Madeleine. (6 October 2018). 'Don't tell the parents'. *The Spectator*. <https://www.spectator.co.uk/article/don-t-tell-the-parents>.

Kennedy, Pagan. (30 March 2008). 'Q&A with Norman Spack. A doctor helps children change their gender'. *Boston Globe*.

Kenny, Dianna T. (2019). 'Gender development and the transgendering of children'. In Michele Moore and Heather Brunskell-Evans (eds). *Inventing Transgender Children and Young People*. Newcastle upon Tyne: Cambridge Scholars.

Kergil, Skylar. (2017). *Before I Had the Words*. New York: Skyhorse Publishing.

Kildevæld Simonsen, Rikke, Gert Martin Hald, Ellids Kristensen and Annamaria Giraldi. (2016). 'Long-term follow-up of individuals undergoing sex-reassignment surgery. Somatic morbidity and cause of death'. *Sexual Medicine*. Vol. 4, pp. e60–8. <https://doi.org/10.1016/j.esxm.2016.01.001>.

Killermann, Sam. (2017). 'Breaking through the binary: gender explained using continuums'. <https://www.genderbread.org/wp-content/uploads/2017/02/Breaking-through-the-Binary-by-Sam-Killermann.pdf>.

Kinkade, Tyler. (16 January 2015). 'Mount Holyoke cancels "Vagina Monologues" for not being inclusive enough'. *Huffington Post*.

Klein, David A. 'Care of a transgender adolescent'. (July 2015). *American Family Physician*. Vol. 92, No. 2.

Krug, Jessica A. (3 September 2020). 'The truth, and the anti-black violence of my lies'. *Medium*.

La Veneno. (11 November 2016). 'Las 20 mejores frases de La Veneno por las que siempre la recordaremos'. *Bekia.es*.

Lacqueur, Thomas. (1992). *Making Sex: Body and Gender from the Greeks to Freud*. Cambridge: Harvard University Press.

Landén, M., J. Wålinder, G. Hambert and B. Lundström. (1998). 'Factors predictive of regret in sex reassignment'. *Acta Psychiatrica Scandinavica*. Vol. 97, No. 4, pp. 284–289.

Lawliet, Elias. (2016). 'Criminal erasure. Interactions between transgender men and the American criminal justice system'. *Aleph, UCLA Undergraduate Research Journal for the Humanities and Social Sciences*. Vol. 13.

Lawthorn, Jared. (19 July 2019). 'Transgender man's mastectomy surgery dubbed "mutilation"'. *BBC Wales*.

Leinung, M. and C. Wu. (June 2017). 'The biologic basis of transgender identity: 2D: 4D finger length ratios implicate a role for prenatal androgen activity'. *Endocrine Practice*. Vol. 23, No. 6, pp. 669–671. <https://doi.org/10.4158/EP161528.OR>.

Littman, Lisa. (16 August 2018). 'Parent Reports of Adolescents and Young Adults Perceived to Show Signs of a Rapid Onset of Gender Dysphoria'. *Plos One*. <https://doi.org/10.1371/journal.pone.0202330>.

Lopez, German. (6 June 2016). 'How to know if your child is transgender, according to an expert'. *Vox*.

MacKinnon, Catharine A. and Durba Mitra. (2018). 'Ask a Feminist. Sexual Harassment in the Age of #MeToo'. *Signs Journal*. Vol. 4, No. 6.

MacLachlan, Maria. (18 April 2018). 'The ostensible trial of Tara Wolf – Part 1'. <www.peaktrans.org>.

Macwhirter, Iain. (17 February 2019). 'Get over it – cis women are just on the wrong side of history'. *The Herald*. <https://www.heraldscotland.com/news/17438641.iain-macwhirter-get-over-it-cis-women-are-just-on-the-wrong-side-of-history/>.

Marchiano, Lisa. (2017). 'Outbreak. On transgender teens and psychic epidemics'. *Psychological Perspectives*. Vol. 60, pp. 345–366.

Mascarelli, Amanda Leigh. (31 July 2015). 'Gender. When the body and brain disagree'. *Science News for Students*.

McCloskey, Jimmy. (17 January 2020). 'Pedophile who molested baby freed from jail after transitioning to become a woman'. *Metro UK*.

McDougle, Jonathan. (7 October 2020). 'California to house transgender inmates based on gender identity'. *CBS News*.

McGeorge, Emma. (n.d.). 'After Your SRS Surgery'. *The Pelvic Hub*. <https://www.thepelvichub.com/conditions/sr-surgery>.

McLean, Hugh. (25 October 2019). 'What Are the Positive Effects of FTM Top Surgery'. McLean Clinic Cosmetic Surgery and Medical Aesthetics Blog. <https://www.ftmtopsurgery.ca/blog/ftm-surgery/positive-effects-ftm-top-surgery/>.

McNamara, Catherine. (2010). 'Using men's changing rooms when you haven't got a penis. The constitutive potential of performing transgendered masculinities'. Central School of Speech and Drama.

Meltzer, Toby. (17 June 2016). 'Vaginoplasty procedures, complications and aftercare'. <https://transcare.ucsf.edu/guidelines/vaginoplasty>.

Meyer-Bahlburg, H. F., C. Dolezal, S. W. Baker and M. I. New. (February 2008).'Sexual orientation in women with classical or non-classical congenital adrenal hyperplasia as a function of degree of prenatal androgen excess'. *Archives of. Sexual Behavior*. Vol. 37, No. 1, pp. 85–99. <https://doi.org/10.1007/s10508-007-9265-1>.

Moi, Toril. (1999). *What Is a Woman?* Oxford: Oxford University Press.

Montañez, Amanda. (1 September 2017). 'Beyond XX and XY: The Extraordinary Complexity of Sex Determination'. *Scientific American*.

Moore, Michele. (2019). 'Rapid Onset Gender Dysphoria'. In Michele Moore and Heather Brunskell-Evans (eds). *Inventing Transgender Children and Young People*. Newcastle upon Tyne: Cambridge Scholars.

Mosbergen, Dominique. (3 September 2014). 'All-women's Mount Holyoke College changes policy to welcome transgender students'. *Huffington Post*.

Murphy, Alan. (17 September 2014). 'Exclusive: Fallon Fox' latest opponent opens up to #WhoaTV'. *whoatv.com*. <https://whoatv.com/exclusive-fallon-foxs-latest-opponent-opens-up-to-whoatv/>.

Murphy, Heather. (22 October 2019). 'Always removes female symbol from sanitary pads'. *New York Times*.

Murphy, M. J. (5 February 2020). 'Why (some) gay men won't date transmen'. *Medium.com*.

Murphy, Meghan. (15 September 2017). 'Historic Speaker's Corner becomes site of anti-feminist silencing and violence'. *Feminist Current*.

Murphy, Meghan. (7 September 2016). 'Are we women or are we menstruators'. *Feminist Current*. <https://www.feministcurrent.com/2016/09/07/are-we-women-or-are-we-menstruators/>.

Murray, Douglas. (2019). *The Madness of Crowds: Gender, Race and Identity*. London: Bloomsbury.

Najmabadi, Afsaneh. (2014). *Professing Selves: Transsexuality and Same-Sex Desire in Contemporary Iran*. Durham, NC: Duke University Press.

National Geographic. (January 2017). 'Special Issue: Gender Revolution'.

Navratilova, Martina. (17 February 2019). 'The rules on trans athletes reward cheats and punish the innocent'. *The Sunday Times*.

Navratilova, Martina. (26 June 2019). 'The trans women athletic dispute with Martina Navratilova'. BBC Documentary.

Nikkelen, Sanne and Baudewijntje Kreukels. (2018). 'Sexual experiences in transgender people. The role of desire for gender-confirming interventions, psychological wellbeing, and body satisfaction'. *Journal of Sex and Marital Therapy*. Vol. 44, No. 4.

Nimmons, David. (1 March 1994). 'Sex and the brain'. *Discover Magazine*.

Noble, Bobby. (2012). 'Trans. Panic. Some thoughts toward a theory of feminist fundamentalism'. In Anne Enke (ed). *Transfeminist Perspectives In and Beyond Transgender and Gender Studies*. Philadelphia: Temple University Press.

Nordberg, Jenny. (2015). *The Underground Girls of Kabul: In Search of a Hidden Resistance in Afghanistan*. New York: Crown Publishing Group.

O'Malley, Stella. (2019). 'Trans kids. It's time to talk'. In Michele Moore and Heather Brunskell-Evans (eds). *Inventing Transgender Children and Young People*. Newcastle upon Tyne: Cambridge Scholars.

Oliver, Brian. (30 May 2021). 'Exclusive: Rival weightlifter speaks out on transgender Hubbard's presence at Tokyo 2020'. *Inside the Games*.

Ortiz, Cristina and Valeria Vegas. (2016). ¡Digo! Ni puta, ni santa. Las memorias de La Veneno. CEDRO.

Pandey, Manish. (21 July 2022). 'Harry Potter: Quidditch renamed to Quadball over JK Rowling link'. *BBC News*.

Patrick. (2019). 'Detransition was a beautiful process'. In Michele Moore and Heather Brunskell-Evans (eds). *Inventing Transgender Children and Young People*. Newcastle upon Tyne: Cambridge Scholars Publishing. pp. 176–177.

Petrella, Dan. (26 July 2019). 'Gov. J.B. Pritzker signs law requiring one-person public bathrooms be gender-neutral'. *Chicago Tribune*.

Pfäfflin, Friedemann. (2008). 'Regrets after sex reassignment surgery', *Journal of Psychology and Human Sexuality*. Vol. 5, No. 4, pp. 69–85.

Pilgrim, David. 'Reclaiming reality and redefining realism: The challenging case of transgenderism'. *Journal of Critical Realism*. Vol. 17, No. 3, pp. 308–324.

Polderman, Tinca J. C., P. C. Baudewijntje Kreukels, Michael S. Irwig, Lauren Beach, Yee-Ming Chan, Eske M. Derks, Isabel Esteva, Jesse Ehrenfeld, Martin Den Heijer, Danielle Posthuma, Lewis Raynor, Amy Tishelman and Lea K. Davis. (January 2018). 'The biological contributions to gender identity and gender diversity. Bringing data to the table'. *Behavior Genetics*.

Pressly, Linda and Lucy Proctor. (10 March 2020). 'Ellie and Nele. From she to he – and back to she again'. *BBC News*.

Reeser, J. C. (2005.) 'Gender identity and sport: is the playing field level?'. *British Journal of Sports Medicine*. Vol. 39, No. 10.

Reginato, James. (13 June 2019). 'One "Aw, shit" wipes out a thousand "Attaboys": Why billionaire GOP donor Jennifer Pritzker is abandoning Trump after coming out as trans'. *Vanity Fair*. <https://www.vanityfair.com/news/2019/06/why-billionaire-republican-donor-jennifer-pritzker-is-abandoning-trump-after-coming-out-as-trans>.

Richard, Bernstein. (21 February 2020). 'On the left, a new clash between feminists and transgender activists'. *The Daily Signal*.

Rippon, Gina. (2019). *The Gendered Brain: The New Neuroscience that Shatters the Myth of the Female Brain*. London: Penguin Vintage.

Robles, Victor Hugo. (26 November 2016). 'Selenna, la niña trans chilena que se convirtió en un símbolo de orgullo'. *Agencia Presentes*.

Rogers, Alexandra. (7 March 2022). 'Exclusive: Labour Drops All-Women Shortlists For Next General Election'. *HuffPost UK*. <https://www.huffingtonpost.co.uk/entry/labour-drops-use-of-all-women-shortlists-general-election-legal-advice-unlawful_uk_622226fbe4b03bc49a9a2420>.

Rosenthal, Stephen. (3 April 2017). 'Care for transgender children starts with affirmation, safety'. *Healio.com*. <https://www.healio.com/endocrinology/pediatric-endocrinology/news/online/%7Ba2eedc18-0009-4682-80dd-b259bc13b45a%7D/care-fortransgender-children-starts-with-affirmation-safety>.

Rosselli, Charles E. and Scott A. Klosterman. (1 July 1998). 'Sexual differentiation of aromatase activity in the rat brain: effects of perinatal steroid exposure'. *Endocrinology.* Vol. 139, No. 7, pp. 3193–3201.

Sabet, Zarifa. (2 March 2018). 'Bacha posh. An Afghan social tradition where girls are raised as boys'. *The Newsminute.*

Sanguinetti, Emilia Philomena. (2016). *Joan of Arc: Her Trial Transcripts.* USA: Little Flower Publishing.

Sanneh, Kelefa. (26 February 2018). 'Jordan Peterson's gospel of masculinity'. *The New Yorker.*

Sargeant, Chloe. (22 January 2018). 'Until the Women's March is inclusive of all women, I can't identify with it'. *SBS News.*

Savic, Ivanka and Stefan Arver. (November 2011). 'Sex dimorphism of the brain in male-to-female transsexuals'. *Cerebral Cortex.* Vol. 21, pp. 2525–2533, <doi:10.1093/cercor/bhr032>.

Schneider, Harald J., Johanna Pickel and Gunter K. Stalla. (2006). 'Typical female 2nd-4th finger length (2D: 4D) ratios in male-to-female transsexuals – Possible implications for pre-natal androgen exposure.' *Psychoneuroendocrinology.* Number 31, pp. 265–269.

Schneider, Maiko A., Poli M. Spritzer, Bianca Machado Borba Soll, Anna M.V. Fontanari, Marina Carneiro, Fernanda Tovar-Moll, Angelo B. Costa, Dhiordan C. da Silva, Karine Schwarz, Mauricio Anes, Silza Tramontina and Maria I. R. Lobato. (14 November, 2017). 'Brain maturation, cognition and voice pattern in a gender dysphoria case under pubertal suppression'. *Frontiers in Human Neuroscience.* Vol. 11, p. 528. <https://doi.org/10.3389/fnhum.2017.00528>.

Serano, Julia. (2007). *Whipping Girl – A Transsexual Woman On Sexism and the Scapegoating of Femininity*: New York: Seal Press.

Siddique, Haroon. (10 June 2021). 'Gender-critical views are a protected belief, appeal tribunal rules'. *The Guardian.*

Siddique, Haroon. (6 July 2022). 'Maya Forstater was discriminated against over gender-critical beliefs, tribunal rules'. *The Guardian.*

Silets, Alexandra. (29 August 2013). 'Children's Gender Clinic'. *Wttw News.* <https://news.wttw.com/2013/08/29/childrens-gender-clinic>.

Simpson, Leah. (20 October 2018). 'It's definitely NOT fair: American cyclist lashes out after losing world championship to a trans woman.' *Mail Online.* <https://www.dailymail.co.uk/news/article-6296975/American-cyclist-lashes-losing-world-championship-trans-woman-wont-accept-apology.html>.

Singal, Jesse. (July/August 2018). 'When children say they're trans'. *The Atlantic.*

Singh, Simran. (1 November 2019). 'Gender identity talk cancelled at SFU campus due to "security reasons"'. *DH News.* <https://dailyhive.com/vancouver/gender-identity-meghan-murphy-sfu-cancelled>.

Slatz, Anna. (July 23 2019). 'EXCLUSIVE: 15-year-old alleged victim of Jessica Yaniv speaks out'. *PM.* <https://thepostmillennial.com/exclusive-15-year-old-alleged-victim-of-jessica-yaniv-speaks-out>.

Smith, S. E. (1 March 2019). 'Women are not the only ones who get abortions'. *Rewire News*.

Stevens, Jamie, Natalie Ramos, Shervin Shadianloo, Serena M. Chang, Myo Thwin Myint, Brandon Johnson and Alexis Chavez. (18 October 2019). 'Transgender 201: Advanced Practice in the Care of Gender-Diverse Youth'. Workshop at American Academy of Child and Adolescent Psychiatry Annual Meeting.

Stone, Natalie. (1 January 2019). 'Jazz Jennings Discusses "the Sexual Stuff" with her Doctor Ahead of Gender Confirmation Surgery'. *People*. <https://people.com/tv/jazz-jennings-talks-sexual-stuff-orgasm-libido-doctor-before-gender-confirmation-surgery>.

Strang, John F., Jason Jarin, David Call, Brett Clark, Gregory L. Wallace, Laura G. Anthony, Lauren Kenworthy and Veronica Gomez-Lobo. (2018). 'Transgender Youth Fertility Attitudes Questionnaire: Measure Development in Nonautistic and Autistic Transgender Youth and Their Parents'. *Journal of Adolescent Health*. Vol. 62, No. 2, pp. 128–135.

Summersell, Jason. (August 2018). 'Trans women are real women: a critical realist intersectional response to Pilgrim'. *Journal of Critical Realism*. Vol. 17, No. 3, pp. 329–336.

Sundar, Vaishnavi. (4 March 2020). 'I was cancelled for my tweets on transgenderism'. *Spiked Online*.

Swaab, Dick and Alicia Garcia-Falgueras. (November 2008). 'A sex difference in the hypothalamic uncinate nucleus: relationship to Gender Identity'. *Brain* 131 (Pt 12), pp. 3132–3146.

Talbot, Margaret. (11 March 2013). 'About a boy. Transgender surgery at sixteen'. *The New Yorker*.

Talusan, Meredith. (12 June 2015). 'There is no comparison between transgender people and Rachel Dolezal'. *The Guardian*.

The Football Association. (March 2016). 'A guide to including trans people in football'.

The Intercept Podcast. (29 January 2019). 'Alexandria Ocasio-Cortez on her first weeks in congress'.

The World Professional Association for Transgender Health. (n.d.). 'Standards of care for the health of transsexual, transgender, and gender nonconforming people No. 7'.

Thirani Bagri, Neha. (19 April 2017). '"Everyone treated me like a saint" – in Iran, there's only one way to survive as a transgender person'. *Quartz*.

Timpf, Katherine. (20 February 2019), 'Students drop "Vagina" from The Vagina Monologues to be more "inclusive"'. *National Review*.

TransMan's Blog. (19 August 2018). <https://mikael-nc.tumblr.com/>.

Transparency Market Research. (2018). 'Sex reassignment surgery market. Global industry analysis, size, share, growth, trends, and forecast 2018–2026'.

Travers, Ann. (2018). *The Trans Generation – How Trans Kids (and their Parents) Are Creating a Gender Revolution*. New York: New York University Press.

Truss, Elizabeth. (22 April 2020). 'Minister for Women and Equalities Liz Truss sets out priorities to Women and Equalities Select Committee'. Government Equalities Office. Speech. <https://www.gov.uk/government/speeches/minister-for-women-and-equalities-liz-truss-sets-out-priorities-to-women-and-equalities-select-committee>.

Truth, Sojourner. (n.d.). 'Ain't I A Woman?'. <https://www.learningforjustice.org/classroom-resources/texts/aint-i-a-woman>.

Tse-tung, Mao. (1964). *On Practice: On the Relation Between Knowledge and Practice – Between Knowing and Doing*. The Maoist Documentation Project. <https://www.marxists.org/reference/archive/mao/selected-works/volume-1/mswv1_16.htm>.

Tuvel, Rebecca. (Spring 2017). 'In defence of transracialism'. *Hypatia*. Vol. 32, No. 2, pp. 263–278.

UCSF Transgender Care, UCSF Health System, University of California, San Francisco. (July 2020). 'Information on Estrogen Hormone Therapy – Overview of Feminizing Hormone Therapy'. <https://transcare.ucsf.edu/article/information-estrogen-hormone-therapy>.

UPDATE: Transgender Healthcare in Oregon. (14 August 2015). TransActive Health Project.

Van Vliet, Kevin and Dick Swaab. (September 2019). 'Ik wou dat die Nashville-verklaring er niet geweest was'. *HP De Tijd*, 1.

Vergara, Eva. (23 January 2019). 'Chilean transgender school protects children from bullying'. *AP News*.

Vigo, Julian. (27 December 2018). 'Pseudo-scientific hokum and the experimentation on children's bodies'. *Forbes*.

Wallien, Madeleine S. C. and Peggy T. Cohen-Kettenis. (2008). 'Psychosexual outcome of gender dysphoric children'. *Journal of the American Academy of Child and Adolescent Psychiatry*. Vol. 47, No. 12, pp. 1413–1423.

Wei-Haas, Maya and Jackie Mansky. (18 August 2016). 'The Rise of the Modern Sportswoman'. *Smithsonian Magazine*. <https://www.smithsonianmag.com/science-nature/rise-modern-sportswoman-180960174/#Fukt0kXYIrjhYWFg.99>.

Whitman Walker Health. 'Safer Sex for Trans Bodies'. <https://assets2.hrc.org/files/assets/resources/Trans_Safer_Sex_Guide_FINAL.pdf>.

Williams, Cristan. (27 November 2015). 'Sex, gender, and sexuality. An interview with Catharine A. MacKinnon'. *The Conversations Project*.

Williams, Cristan. (28 November 2015). 'Gender Performance: An interview with Judith Butler'. <http://radfem.transadvocate.com/gender-performance-an-interview-with-judith-butler/>.

Williams, Shawna. (1 March 2018). 'Are the brains of transgender people different from those of cisgender people?'. *The Scientist*.

Winther, Sarah Marie. (16 August 2017). 'Egg-freezing is giving young trans men hope for starting a family'. *Vice Magazine*.

Wold, Agnes. (1 August 2020). 'Gender-corrective surgery promoting mental health in persons with gender dysphoria not supported by data presented in article'. *American Journal of Psychiatry*, p. 768. <https://doi.org/10.1176/appi.ajp.2020.19111170>.
Wolf, Naomi. (15 February 2013). 'Do we still need women-only spaces?' *The Guardian*.
Wolf, Naomi. (1991/2002). *The Beauty Myth: How Images of Beauty Are Used Against Women*. New York: Harper Collins.
World Health Organization. (n.d.). *ICD-11, International Classification of Diseases 11th Revision*. <https://icd.who.int/en>.
World Health Organization. *ICD-11*. 'HA61 Gender incongruence of childhood.'
World Professional Association for Transgender Health. (2018). 'Award Winners'. <https://www.wpath.org/media/cms/Documents/History/Awards/2018/Awards%20Information%20Page.pdf>.
Yadegarfard, Mohammadrasool. (20 May 2019). 'Are Iranian gay men coping with systematic suppression under islamic law? A qualitative study'. *Sexuality and Culture*.
Yang, Fu, Xiao-hai Zhu, Qing Zhang, Ning-xia Sun, Yi-xuan Ji, Jin-zhao Ma, Bang Xiao, Hai-xia Ding, Shu-han Sun and Wen Li. (2017). 'Genomic characteristics of gender dysphoria patients and identification of rare mutations in RYR3 gene'. *Scientific Report*. Vol. 7, pp. 8339.
Young, James O. (2000). 'The Ethics of Cultural Appropriation'. *Dalhousie Review*. Vol. 80, No. 3.

Index

2007 government enquiry, Swedish government, 53, 56, 59
2017 government enquiry, Swedish, 55

AbbVie, 129, 142, 164, 166
Abelson, Lars Göran, 50
Adichie, Chimamanda Ngozi, 74, 282
Åhbeck Öhman, Myra, 200
Åkerlund, Mathilda, 224, 232
Ali, Ayaan Hirsi, 296
Aliki, Silas, 244, 285
Alm, Erika, 230
Ambjörnsson, Fanny, 67
Amin, Qasim, 310
Andnor, Berit, 181
anorexia, 59, 144, 171, 177, 179, 181, 194
Anova, Swedish gender clinic, 120–124, 127, 132, 137–141, 149–150, 155, 167, 184, 186–188, 193–195
    Anova's Kid Team, 150, 184
Aquilonius, Jennie, 184
Aquinas, Thomas, 309
Arpi, Ivar, 85
Arver, Stefan, 31–32
Athlete Ally, 267
Austen, Jane, 310

bacha posh, Afghanistan, 111
Bäckman, Therese, 3
Badenoch, Isla, 114
Bah-Kuhnke, Alice, 153
Bangsuan, Vatchareeya, 243

Bannerman, Lucy, 255
Barker, Jason, 254
Barnes, Jonathan, 78
Bartter, Allan, 267
Bartter, Isabelle, 267–268
Bauhin, Caspar, 77
Baum, Joel, 183
BBC, 114, 131
Bell, Keira, 202
Bermon, Stephane, 263, 273
Berry, Halle, 22
Bettcher, Talia M., 301
Biggs, Michael, 128, 131–132
Bill C-16, Canada, 85, 237, 241, 300
Bindel, Julie, 290
biological determinism, 16–17, 23, 85, 87, 90–92, 94–95, 97, 306
biologism, 17, 46, 87, 89, 95
    challenging biological essentialist interpretations, 33
bisexuality, bisexual, 30, 39, 55, 137, 144–145, 155, 162, 164, 168, 268
Bird, Jackson, 253
Björk, Nina, 97
black American, 299
Black Lives Matter, 293
Bly, Robert, 90
Bohlin, Anna, 177
Bohlin, Rebecka, 231
Borelius, Maria, 90
Boston's Center for Transgender Medicine, 41
Brand, 231

Brändén, Henrik, 25, 39, 107
Bränström, Richard, 189–190
Bremer, Fredrika, 310
Bremer, Signe, 230
Brennan, Cathy, 290
Brents, Tammika, 266
Brill, Stephanie, 12, 40
British Association for Counselling and Psychotherapy (BACP), 18–19, 245, 288
Brunskell-Evans, Heather, 120–121, 132, 175, 191
Burkett, Elinor, 301
burrnesha, Albania, 112–114
Butler, Judith, 86, 91-92, 223, 304

Callahan, Kat, 301–302
CAMHS, Sweden's child and adolescent mental health services, 195–196
Caravella-Fader, Sarah, 265
Case, Laura, 32
Cashmere, Elle, 272
Cass, Hilary, 132, 203
Chamberland, Alexander Alvina, 229
children's transgender rights, 66, 155
  children and young people, 41, 120–121, 123, 126–127, 129, 132–134, 166, 170, 172, 175, 191
Chinn, Sarah, 69
Christenson, Åsa, 224–225
Christenson, Gerda, 225
Christian Democrat Party, 200
Cis women, 225, 233.
  cis, 29, 31–32, 34, 95, 121, 229, 232–234, 287
  cis men, 29, 31
  cis women, privileged/privilege, 225–228, 233–234, 287, 301–302
Clyde Fallon, 191
Coches, Foro, 283
Cohen, Rachel, 12
Cohen-Kettenis, Peggy, 127–128, 130–131
complex mental health needs, 144
  ADHD, 18, 144
  eating disorders, 177
congenital adrenal hyperplasia (CAH), 38–39
conservative thinkers, 85–87
Cornell University Press, 81
cultural appropriation (CA), 298–299

D'arbes, Anne, 43
Dadgostar, Nooshi, 276
Dagens Nyheter, 16, 30, 71, 85, 189–190
Dahlén, Sandra, 213
Dahlqvist, Anna, 200
Dahlström, Annika, 91
Daly, Mary, 221
Davies-Arai, Stephanie, 241
Declaration on Women's Sex-Based Rights, 237. *See also* radical feminist
definition of woman, 16–17, 19, 28, 45, 53, 71, 97, 218, 226, 262, 305
  Social constructivist approach to definition of woman, 42, 305
  definition of sex, 4, 18, 44, 47, 51, 54, 57, 61, 214, 242
  legal definition of sex, 44, 57–58, 61
Delemarre-van de Waal, Henriette, 127–128, 131
Deny, Attack, and Reverse Victim and Offender (DARVO), 290–291
Deraismes, Maria, 310
Dhejne, Cecilia, 140–141, 155, 167, 186, 258
Diagnostic and Statistical Manual of Mental Disorders (DSM-5), 130
Diallo, Nkechi Amare, 293
Dinamarca, Rossana, 276
Disorders of Sexual Development (DSD), 38, 155–156
DNA, 37, 67
Dolezal, Rachel, 293, 301
Dreier, Fred, 264–265
Dutch Protocol, for treatment of transsexualism in children, 203

Edenheim, Sara, 89, 92
Edwards, Andrea, 230–231
Ehrenberg, Johan, 106
Ehrensaft, Diane, 40, 64, 166, 182–183, 198
Einstein, Albert, 178
Ekelund, Fredrik, 19
Ekman, Kajsa Ekis, 15, 284
Electronic Medicines Compendium (EMC), 140
Employment Appeal Tribunal, 281
Encyclopaedia Britannica, 1
Endocrine Society, 130–131
Engels, Friedrich, 114–115
Ensler, Eve, 218

Index

Equality and Anti-Discrimination Ombudsman, 238–239
Equality Impact Assessments, 180
ETC, 106, 209, 231
Evans, Charlie, 177

Fabray, Lucas, 176
Fair Play for Women, 237
Fallopius, Gabriel, 77
Faludi, Susan, 91
Feinberg, Leslie, 102
female erasure/erasure of women, 225, 237
  abolishing the word woman, 216, 311
female-to-male transgender, FtM, 33, 150–151
female space, women-only space, 237, 241, 251, 258–260, 268, 274, 285
Feminine Style of Management Conference, 91
Feminist Current, 174, 210, 237, 282, 289–290
Feminist Party, 276–277
Feministiskt Initiativ (FI), 89, 95, 157
Feministiskt Perspektiv, 92, 225
Finch, Sam Dylan, 227
Fine, Cordelia, 37
Finlayson, Lorna, 257–258
first 'gender identity clinic' for young people, 128
Football Association (FA) of England, 268
Forstater, Maya, 280–281
Fox, Fallon, 266
Foxhage, Fox, 119, 122
Fraga, Paula, 237
Friedan, Betty, 89
Frisen, Louise, 123, 174, 184

Garofalo, Robert, 62, 142
gay, 11, 23, 55, 67–68, 100–102, 106, 109–110, 137, 144–148, 151, 155, 162, 168, 173, 198, 255, 267–268
Geddes, Patrick, 79
gender, 1–5, 7, 9–13, 16, 18, 20, 22–30, 32–43, 45–74, 76–78, 81–99, 101–103, 105–114, 117, 120–135, 137, 139–147, 149, 154, 156–158, 160–166, 168–174, 177–196, 198, 202–204, 207, 211–212, 214, 216–219, 222–241, 243–246, 249–253, 255, 257, 259–262, 264–272, 275–276, 278, 280–285, 288–289, 296–297, 300–302, 304–308
  as social construct, cultural construct, 11, 17, 23–24, 42–43, 46–51, 53, 55, 70, 88, 96–97, 101, 236, 295–296, 304–305
Gender and Sex Development Program, Lurie Children's Hospital, 62, 164
gender binary, 61, 178, 268
gender congruence, 58, 60, 87, 95, 182
Gender Creative Child, The, 40, 64, 183
gender dysphoria, 5, 33–34, 38–39, 59–60, 121–134, 139, 141, 144–145, 162, 164, 169–170, 174, 178, 180–181, 183, 186–187, 189, 191, 193–194, 198, 203–204, 270
gender fluidity, 16
gender identity, 2, 4–5, 9–12, 22–30, 32–37, 39–42, 46–47, 49–50, 56, 58, 60, 62–64, 70–74, 76, 83–89, 92–98, 101, 103, 107, 112, 114, 122–123, 125–126, 128, 131–132, 144–145, 154, 160, 163, 165, 169, 172–173, 187, 195–196, 198, 202–204, 207, 216, 218–219, 222–224, 230–234, 236, 239–240, 245, 250–252, 259–262, 264, 267–271, 276, 278, 280–284, 289, 297, 300–302, 308
gender identity clinic, 128, 187, 203
gender identity scale, 62, 63
gender identity theory, 2, 4–5, 9–11, 24–25, 28, 42, 47, 49–50, 70–74, 76, 83–89, 93–98, 103, 114, 216, 219, 222, 230–234, 236, 250–251, 259–261, 271, 278, 280–284, 289, 297, 302, 308
  contradictions in, 47, 74, 261
gender incongruence, 74, 147, 169–170, 190
gender non-binary, 56, 61, 68, 71, 76, 93, 165, 171, 226, 259
gender reassignment, 5, 11, 37, 43, 67–68, 72, 124, 145–146, 149, 158, 160–162, 165–166, 171, 181, 183, 188, 193, 198, 219, 229, 235, 244–245, 255, 282
  age limits, 5, 157–158. *See also* trans children, transexual children, transsexualism in children
  Sex Reassignment – Proposals for a New Law, 50
  to cure homosexuality, 67–68, 145

gender roles, 23–24, 27, 41, 51, 70, 77, 81, 83, 86–87, 89, 92, 98, 101, 103, 106, 109, 113–114, 130, 169–170, 181, 222–224, 250, 306
gender self-identification, 101, 162, 235, 237–238, 241, 249, 257
Genderbread Person, 22
Girl Project (Flicka), 181
Gisslow, Camilla, 20–21
GnRH analogues, 126, 133
   Pamorelin, 126–127
Goldberg, Whoopi, 293
Gonadotropin Releasing Hormone analogues (GnRHas), 126, 133
Goobar, Mikael Hansén, 172–173
Green Party, 158, 229
   Swedish Green Party, 229
Greer, Germaine, 285, 288–289
Gregory, Mary, 265
Groneman, Carole, 80

Haggan, 286
Hallengren, Lena, 157, 184
Hannah, Robert, 276
Haraway, Donna, 297
Harks, Matthew, 245
Harry Potter books, 281
Heape, Walter, 80
Hedberg, Timo, 174
Hedengren, Lars, 153–154
Hermodsson, Elisabeth, 307
heteronormativity, 56
Heyes, Cressida, 295
Hirdman, Yvonne, 77, 90, 307
HIV, 30, 192
Holmqvist, Sam, 108, 229
Holmström, Erik, 230
homosexuality, 30, 67–68, 110, 145, 147
Honorine, Lea, 242
hormones, 38, 161, 192, 207
   cross-sex hormones, 135–136
      hormone treatment, 3, 31, 66, 69, 122, 125, 127, 129, 135, 137–139, 144, 147, 149, 162, 164–165, 168–169, 174, 182–183, 191, 194, 203–204, 224, 230, 236, 263, 267, 269
   prescribed for children, 41, 52, 142
HSAN, 192
Hubbard, Gavin, 264
Hubbard, Laurel, 264
human rights, campaign, 156, 202, 219, 225, 287

European Convention on Human Rights, 156, 202
Human Rights Campaign Association, 219
Human Rights Tribunal, 240
UN Human Rights Declaration, 96
Hungerford, Elizabeth, 225

INAH3, subnucleus, 29–30
inclusive language, 210, 215
   preferred pronouns, 2–4, 13, 86, 173
International Federation of Bodybuilding and Fitness (IFBB), 272
International Lesbian, Gay, Bisexual, Transgender, Queer and Intersex (LGBTQI) Youth & Student Organisation (IGLYO), 162–163
International Olympic Committee (IOC), 3, 262, 264
   Rio Olympics, 262
   Tokyo Olympics, 262, 264
   Media Relations Team, 265
Internet, 47, 171, 180, 244, 247, 260, 285
   social media, 150, 173, 179–180, 283, 297
intersectionality, 292–293, 295, 297, 299, 301–303
Inventing Transgender Children and Young People, 120–121, 132, 172, 175, 191
IQ, 91, 134, 194
Iran/Iranian, 105, 109–110, 112, 272–273
Irigaray, Luce, 81
Iron John, 90
IVF, for trans people, 138–139

Jackson, Lauren Michele, 299
Jeffreys, Sheila, 96, 102
Jenkins, Katharine, 257
Jenner, Bruce, 299
Jenner, Caitlin, 249
Jenner, Kendall, 299
Jennings, Jazz, 65, 147
Joe, G.I., 63, 83
Joel, Daphna, 36–37
Johansson, Annika, 140–141
Johansson, Kristoffer, 243
Jones, Alice Bethany, 269
Jones, Kelsie Bryn, 286–287
Jones, Owen, 11

Index

Karolinska Hospital, 122, 155, 167, 188
Karolinska Institute, 31, 135, 155, 188
Keen-Minshull, Kellie-Jay, 97
Keita, Salif, 216
Kennedy, Pagan, 129, 137
Kergil, Skylar, 177
Khan, Abd Al-Ali, 105
Killermann, Sam, 22
Krug, Jessica, 294
Kubwa, Malaika, 294
    Big, Martina, 293–294
Kvindemuseet, Denmark, 211

Laboucan, Adam, 245
Labour Party, 115, 255. *See also* Left Party
    British Labour Party, 302
Lacqueur, Thomas, 76–77
Left Party, 10, 95, 157–158, 214, 276–277, 286. See also Labour Party
legal counselling for women (JURK), 239
lesbian, 30, 39, 51, 55, 108–109, 144, 147, 155, 162, 168, 173, 175–176, 185, 198, 228, 255, 266, 268, 290
    lesbian feminist, 30, 96–97, 290
LeVay, Simon, 30
Ley Trans, 101, 235, 249
LGBTQ/LGBTQI, 12, 21, 108, 110, 162–164, 166–168, 179–180, 189, 211, 243, 267, 288, 303
Liberal Democrats, Britain, 129
Liberal Party, 122, 157–158
Littman, Lisa, 144, 169
lobbying, 148
    lobbyists, 167, 196
Longstocking, Pippi, 21, 223
Lopez, German, 40, 64
López, Mario, 74
Lopez, Vanessa, 140, 198
López, Vanessa, Miss Trans Star International, 140, 198
Lurie Children's Hospital, 62, 142, 164
Luther, Martin, 309

MacKinnon, Catharine, 16, 47–49, 290, 304–305, 308
Magnusson, Lisa, 16–17
male privilege, 255, 277, 301–302
male space, 259
male to female transgender person; MtFs; MtF-TR, 31–32, 120, 151, 186.
    See also trans women, transsexual women
male/men's violence, 56, 93, 227, 239, 248–249, 257, 286, 288, 290
Manning, Chelsea, 45
Mao, Tse-tung, 298
Marchiano, Lisa, 179, 183
Mattisson, Karin, 144, 156
McKinnon, Rachel, 265–266
McLean Clinic, Canada, 150
Mead, Margaret, 223
Men's violence against women, 56, 93, 248–249, 290
Mermaids, 63, 167
metaphysical worldview, 114–115, 305
    dialectical materialism, 93, 305
    dialectical worldview, 115, 306
MeToo; #metoo movement, 48, 282
Meyer-Bahlburg, Heino, 39
Michelet, Jules, 80
Mills College, 218
Mixed Martial Arts (MMA), 266
Miyares, Alicia, 237
Moi, Toril, 16, 90, 98, 120
Montero, Irene, 101, 249
Moore, Michele, 120–121, 132, 191
Mount Holyoke, 218
Mulvaney, Dulan, 300
Munirah, 105–106
Murderers of Trans People (MOT), 288
Murphy, Erin, 218
Murphy, Meghan, 86, 210, 240, 282, 284, 289
Murray, Douglas, 85–87, 143

Najmabadi, Afsaneh, 105
National Association for the Advancement of Colored People (NAACP), 293
National College Athletic Association (NCAA), 3, 236, 265
National Geographic, 9–10
National Society for the Prevention of Cruelty to Children (NSPCC), 194
native American, 107
Navratilova, Martina, 74, 263, 266–268, 271–272
New York Times, 209, 301
NHS, Foundation Trust, 132, 137, 203
Nilsson, Helén, 244
Nilsson, Johanna, 111
Noble, Bobby, 212

Nonautistic and Autistic Transgender Youth, 136
Nord, Iwo, 230
Nordberg, Jenny, 111
Nordenflycht, Hedvig Charlotta, 310

Öberg, Katarina Görts, 141
Ocasio-Cortez, Alexandria, 226
Öhman, Myra Åhbeck, 200
Olona, Macarena, 249
Olson-Kennedy, Johanna, 143
Olsson, Ulf, 244

Pachankis, John, 189–190
Paré, Ambroise, 78
Pasquarella, Lynn, 218
Patient Information Leaflet, 126–127, 133
patriarchal view of gender, 76, 112, 211
patrilineage, 113
Paulsen, Frederik, 128
Peña, Joe, 299
Pepper, Rachel, 40
Peterson, Jordan B., 85–86
pharmaceutical industry, companies, 126, 128, 160–162, 170
   AbbVie, 129, 142, 164, 166
   Endo Pharmaceuticals, 142
   Ferring Pharmaceuticals, 128–129
   pharmaceutical companies, 126, 162, 166
Pilgrim, David, 12–13
Pirate Party, 157–158
postmodernism, 91, 93
Pre-School Activities Inventory (PSAI), 34
President, James Barrett, 245
Pritzker Group, 164–166
   Pritzker, Colonel James, 165
   Pritzker, Jennifer Natalya, 165
private ownership, 113, 307
puberty blockers, blocking puberty, for children, 5, 63, 69, 122, 125, 127–136, 138–139, 142–143, 149, 160, 183, 186, 194, 200, 202–203
Public Health Agency, 181, 185

Queer Avengers, 289
queer theory, 92–94
   Dresden Pride 2022, 285
   Pride Festival, 167
   queer activist, 13, 33, 86

QX, 189–190

Raciborski, Adam, 80
radical feminist, 86, 200, 285. *See also* Declaration on Women's Sex-Based Rights; trans-exclusive radical feminist (terf)
Ramnehill, Maria, 42, 45–46, 211, 225
Ramqvist, Karolina, 217
Real-life experience (RLE), 59
Remnets, Anna, 228
Renaissance, 78
reproduction, 1, 48, 53, 79, 93, 112–113, 213, 296, 304, 308
   reproductive rights, 210–211, 311
Rippon, Gina, 36
Rivera, Sylvia, 301
Romson, Lukas, 225
Rönnblom, Malin, 89
Rosenthal, Stephen, 142
Rowling, J. K., 281
Ruse, Austin, 85
Rydelius, Per-Anders, 150, 174
RYR3 gene, 34
Røssberg, Jan Ivar, 187

Safer, Joshua, 41
Sämfjord, Angela, 195–196
Sand, Loui, 181
Savic, Ivanka, 31–32
SCUM Manifesto, 230–231
Seals, Brandi, 286
Second Sex, The, 16–17, 274
self-identification, 5, 49, 101, 162, 238, 241, 243, 245, 249, 257, 277, 292, 295
Serano, Julia, 98, 228, 232, 251–252
Servenius, Elisa, 108
sex, 1–5, 9–10, 12–30, 32–34, 36–40, 43–44, 46–58, 60–62, 64, 66, 68–98, 102, 104–110, 112, 114, 119–136, 138–140, 142, 145–146, 148, 150–158, 161–162, 164–166, 168–170, 172, 174, 176, 178–180, 182–184, 186–188, 190–192, 194, 196–200, 204–205, 207–208, 210, 212–214, 216–217, 219–220, 222, 224–228, 230–237, 239–252, 254, 256, 258–264, 266, 268–280, 282, 284, 286, 288, 290, 292–310, 312
sex change operation, surgery, 110, 155, 157–158, 162
sexual behavior, 31–32, 34, 39

Index

sexuality, 22, 29–30, 47–49, 94, 103, 106, 113, 165, 212–213, 219, 278, 286, 297, 304–305, 307–308
Sis Sports Centre, 238
Sjöstedt, Jonas, 10, 157
Snecker, Linda, 276
Snow, John, 178
Socialist Worker, 267–268
Söder, Olle, 127, 132, 174
Söderström, Hanna, 41
Solanas, Valerie, 230
Spack, Norman P., 129, 137
split, of brain and body, 4, 38
Stahre, Ulrika, 147, 200
Starbrink, Anna, 122
Stavanger Aftenblad, 239
Stéenhof, Frida, 89
Stenhammar, Ulrika Eleonora, 27
Stewart, Jay, 10
  Gendered Intelligence, 10
Stock, Kathleen, 281
Strandhäll, Annika, 2, 11, 153–154, 181
Strömqvist, Liv, 285
Stryker, Susan, 230, 301
Suh, Krista, 220
Summersell, Jason, 13–15
Sundar, Vaishnavi, 282
Svenaeus, Fredrik, 85–87
Svenska Dagbladet, 41
Swaab, Dick, 29, 32
Swedish Agency for Health Technology Assessment and Assessment of Social Services (SBU), 179–180
Swedish Association for Sexuality Education (RFSU), 155, 157, 288
Swedish Federation for Lesbian, Gay, Bisexual, Transgender, Queer and Intersex Rights (RFSL Ungdom), 55, 137, 155, 157, 168–170, 173–174, 184, 196, 268
Swedish National Board of Health and Welfare, 5, 125, 138, 141, 147, 197
Swedish National Council for Crime Prevention, 156, 248
Swedish Prison and Probation Service, 243
Swedish Secretariat, 222–223, 232

Talusan, Meredith, 300–301
Tännsjö, Torbjörn, 85, 277
TED Talk, 22, 129
Thomas, William, 265

Thomson Reuters Foundation, 162
Thomson, Arthur, 79
Till Jerusalem, 103
trans activist, 42, 86, 98, 147, 167, 184, 225, 227, 239, 251, 255, 284–286, 294, 301
trans generation, 68
trans guidebooks, for children, 67, 69–70
trans healthcare services, 186, 189, 195, 202
trans women in prostitution/sex industry, 43, 100, 287–288
trans women, transsexual women, 13–15, 29, 31, 34, 43–46, 48–49, 71, 86, 98, 177, 209, 211, 218–220, 226–230, 232–233, 237, 251–255, 258–259, 263, 267–269, 271–272, 282, 285–288
trans, trans people, trans person, 3, 10–21, 25–26, 28–35, 39–40, 43–46, 50, 61, 67–69, 71–74, 85–87, 89, 93, 95–98, 100, 103–106, 108, 110, 119–121, 129, 132, 136–138, 144, 146, 158, 160, 163–170, 172, 175–177, 180–182, 184–186, 189–190, 196, 199–201, 207, 214, 216, 220–222, 225–226, 231, 235–236, 239–240, 242–243, 253–254, 259, 264–265, 270–271, 276–280, 282, 285–286, 288, 290, 294, 301, 311
trans children, transsexual children, transsexualism in children, 66, 127, 129–130, 200
trans man, 14, 29, 32–34, 43, 71, 108, 139, 171, 177, 198, 210, 227, 253–255, 268–269, 273–274
trans-exclusive radical feminist, terf, 244, 249, 285–286, 288–289, 291. *See also* radical feminist
Transfeminist Manifesto, 42, 47
Transfeminist Perspectives, 212
Transgender Child, The, 40, 64, 69
transphobia, 44, 97, 287, 291
transsexualism, 31, 51–52, 123, 127, 169
Transwoman Athletic Debate, The, 271
Travers, Ann, 68–69
Truth, Sojourner, 310
Tumblr, 171–173, 175–177, 179–181, 228
Tuvel, Rebecca, 295
two-sex theories, 76–77, 79, 81

University, Georgia State, 36
University, Lund, 187
University, Oxford, 128, 131
University, Tel Aviv, 36
University, Umeå, 224
University, Washington, 218
US Food and Drug Administration (FDA), 133
US National Speech and Debate Association, 3–4

Vagina Monologues, 218–219
vaginoplasty, 151, 188
Valencia-García, Louie Dean, 33
Vanbellinghen, Anna, 264
Vancouver Rape Relief and Women's Shelter, 242
Veneno, La, 100–101
Vilain, Eric, 263
Virchow, Rudolf, 80

Wagner-Assali, Jennifer, 265
Wall Street, 297
Wallin, Elisabeth Ohlson, 108
Walsh, Matt, 86
Westerhäll, Lotta Vahlne, 2–3
Westerlund, Ulrika, 55, 94–95
Western States Endurance Run (WSER), 3, 263
Whipping Girl, 98, 228, 232

White, Blaire, 198
White, Catriona, 114
White, Karen, 245
WHO, 160, 169
Williams, Cristan, 47, 49, 304
Wold, Agnes, 189–190
Wolf, Naomi, 214–215
Wollstonecraft, Mary, 310
women, 1, 3–4, 9–10, 12–20, 25–32, 34, 36, 39–40, 42–49, 52–53, 56–58, 61, 71, 74, 77–78, 81, 83–87, 89–95, 97–103, 105–110, 112–114, 120, 127, 133, 138, 155, 160, 165, 171, 174–175, 177–181, 184–185, 193, 198, 209–223, 225–234, 236–280, 282–291, 293–294, 296–303, 305–311
women's sport, 86–87, 112, 262, 264–265, 267, 270–272
sex-segregation in sports, 268
Woolf, Virginia, 89
World Anti-Doping Agency (WADA), 273
World Professional Association for Transgender Health's (WPATH), 122, 128, 130–131, 149, 164, 170
Worsdale, Rosie, 257

Yaniv, Jessica, 240
Yaniv, Jonathan, 240
YouTube, 171–172, 175–176, 180

Other books available from Spinifex Press

Being and Being Bought: Prostitution, Surrogacy and the Split Self

Kajsa Ekis Ekman

Grounded in the reality of the violence and abuse inherent in prostitution – and reeling from the death of a friend to prostitution in Spain – Kajsa Ekis Ekman exposes the many lies in the 'sex work' scenario. Trade unions aren't trade unions. Groups for prostituted women are simultaneously groups for brothel owners. And prostitution is always presented from a woman's point of view. The men who buy sex are left out.

Drawing on Marxist and feminist analyses, Ekis Ekman argues that the Self must be split from the body to make it possible to sell your body without selling yourself. The body becomes sex. Sex becomes a service. The story of the sex worker says: the Split Self is not only possible, it is the ideal.

Turning to the practice of surrogate motherhood, Kajsa Ekis Ekman identifies the same components: that the woman is neither connected to her own body nor to the child she grows in her body and gives birth to. Surrogacy becomes an extended form of prostitution. In this capitalist creation story, the parent is the one who pays. The product sold is not sex but a baby. Ekis Ekman asks: why should this not be called child trafficking?

This brilliant exposé is written with a razor-sharp intellect and disarming wit and makes us look at prostitution and surrogacy and the parallels between them in a new way.

If you've ever wondered how to respond to those who say there are no victims in prostitution or what to say when someone proposes surrogacy as a solution to childlessness - this book is a must-read.
 —Melissa Farley, Executive Director of Prostitution Research & Education, San Francisco.

ISBN 9781742198767

Vortex:
The Crisis of Patriarchy

Susan Hawthorne

In this enlightening yet devastating book, Susan Hawthorne writes with clarity and incisiveness on how patriarchy is wreaking destruction on the planet and on communities. The twin mantras of globalisation and growth expounded by the neoliberalism that has hijacked the planet are revealed in all their shabby deception.

Backed by meticulous research, the author shows how so-called advances in technology are, like a Trojan horse, used to mask sinister political agendas that sacrifice the common good for the shallow profiteering of corporations and mega-rich individuals.

The book shows a way out of the vortex: it is now up to the collective imagination and action of people everywhere to take up the challenges Susan Hawthorne shows are needed.

ISBN 9781925950168

Penile Imperialism:
The Male Sex Right and Women's Subordination

Sheila Jeffreys

In this blisteringly persuasive and piercingly intelligent book, Sheila Jeffreys argues that women live under penile imperialism, a regime in which men are assumed to have a 'sex right' of access to the bodies of women and girls.

She says that the 'sexual revolution' that began in the 1960s unleashed an explicit male sexual liberation and that even now, under current laws and cultural mores, women do not have the right to self-determination in relation to their bodies.

The power dynamics of sex, rather than being eliminated, have been eroticised, supported by state regulations and structures that have further entrenched male domination. And while men's sexual fetishisms such as BDSM and transvestism have been normalised, women now have to fight as their spaces are being erased and their voices silenced in a faux inclusivity that has 'naturalised' sexual harassment.

ISBN 9781925950700

Doublethink:
A Feminist Challenge to Transgenderism

Janice G. Raymond

In an age when falsehoods are commonly taken as truth, Janice Raymond's book illuminates the 'doublethink' of a transgender movement in which men are defined as women, women as men, he as she, dissent as heresy, science as sham, and critics as fascists. Meanwhile, trans mobs are treated as gender patriots whose main enemy is feminists and their dissent from gender orthodoxies.

Doublethink: A Feminist Challenge to Transgenderism makes us aware of the consequences of a runaway ideology and its costs – among them what is at stake when males are allowed to compete in female sports and when parents are not aware of school curricula that confuse sex with gender and that can facilitate a child's hormone treatments without parental consent.

ISBN 9781925950380

Detransition:
Beyond Before and After

Max Robinson

Many feminists are concerned about the way transgender ideology naturalizes patriarchal views of sex stereotypes, and encourages transition as a way of attempting to escape misogyny. In this brave and thoughtful book, Max Robinson goes beyond the 'before' and 'after' of the transition she underwent and takes us through the processes that led her, first, to transition in an attempt to get relief from her distress, and then to detransition as she discovered feminist thought and community.

The author makes a case for a world in which all medical interventions for the purpose of assimilation are open to criticism. This book is a far-reaching discussion of women's struggles to survive under patriarchy, which draws upon a legacy of radical and lesbian feminist ideas. Robinson's bold discussion of both transition and detransition is meant to provoke a much-needed conversation about who benefits from transgender medicine and who has to bear the hidden cost of these interventions.

ISBN 9781925950403

If you would like to know more about
Spinifex Press, write to us for a free catalogue, visit our
website or email us for further information
on how to subscribe to our monthly newsletter.

Spinifex Press
PO Box 105
Mission Beach QLD 4852
Australia

www.spinifexpress.com.au
women@spinifexpress.com.au